THE
BRAND-NAME
CALORIE COUNTER

Corinne T. Netzer

Revised Edition

A Dell Book

Published by
Dell Publishing
a division of
Bantam Doubleday Dell Publishing Group, Inc.
1540 Broadway
New York, New York 10036

ISBN: 0-440-22289-3

Printed in the United States of America

Published simultaneously in Canada

March 1998

10 9 8 7 6 5 4 3 2 1

OPM

Contents

Introduction

Eating is America's favorite pastime. If you stop and think about it, you'll probably realize that a good number of your waking hours are occupied with food. If you're not actually eating, then you're buying food, planning to buy it, preparing it, even fretting over the prices. It's almost impossible for any but the most iron-willed soul to escape the national food obsession. It is, therefore, little wonder that every month an estimated ten million Americans embark on that battle of frustration known as a *diet*.

As a perennial dieter, I can tell you that there is definite hope that you *will* lose weight if you stick to your diet. But that's the problem. Most people "fall off the wagon" after only two weeks of reducing. The sameness and boredom of crispy carrot sticks, broiled skinless chicken, and wedges of lettuce get to them, and it's all over very quickly.

The purpose of *The Brand-Name Calorie Counter* is to help you stay on your diet by relieving the tedium. For instance, you might want to substitute *Tyson*'s chicken Marsala (180 calories) for the plain broiled chicken, or have a serving of *Libby's* spaghetti and meatballs (190 calories) for lunch, or reward yourself with a slice of *Mrs. Smith's* Boston creme pie (170 calories). Dieting is not a pleasant experience, but I do believe the information contained in this book can help make it less painful by introducing variety—which is the spice not only of life but of dieting as well.

Most calorie counters list foods alphabetically. *The Brand-Name Calorie Counter* lists foods categorically. This means that all vegetables are grouped together; so are all frozen dinners, all dips, all nuts, all syrups, and so on. I can't make diet planning fun, but with this system I've made it as convenient as possible. If you're wondering what vegetable to have with your grilled fish, for example, you won't have to hopscotch from A (asparagus) to Z (zucchini)—just turn to chapter 6, "Vegetables and Vegetable Products," and the choices are there at a glance. Occasionally, you may have trouble deciding what category a food belongs in; to locate such hard-to-categorize foods quickly, just flip to the index.

This sixth edition of *The Brand-Name Calorie Counter* is completely revised because the food industry is constantly growing and improving to meet the needs of the consumer. In addition, I have again included fast-food and chain restaurants so that you may take your diet out to dinner. This section has been expanded, but if you don't find your favorites listed, it may be because the information wasn't available or because the dish varies too much from one franchise location to another.

Over the years, readers have written to tell me how they've used the book. For some, it's a planning guide for making up menus and marketing lists. Others have used it to make impossibly rigid diets more flexible and interesting by making substitutions. Still others have discovered new foods and different brands. And many people have used it as a "maintenance guide" after they've shed their unwanted pounds. Eating is very personal, and how you choose to use this book is up to you, but with it you will have the information you need to plan a varied and healthful diet—one that's interesting enough to stick with until you've achieved your goal.

The material contained in *The Brand-Name Calorie Counter* is based on information from producers, processors, and distributors of brand-name foods, and from food chains. The data contained herein are the most complete and accurate information available as this book goes to press. Please bear in mind that seasonal and regional differences can affect the nutritional values of foods. Also, the food industry often changes recipes and sizes and may discontinue products or add new ones. In the future I will revise and update this book to keep you informed.

Good luck and good dieting.

C.T.N.

Abbreviations in This Book

approx.	approximately
cont.	container
fl.	fluid
"	inch
lb.	pound
oz.	ounce
pkg.	package
pkt.	packet
tbsp.	tablespoon
tsp.	teaspoon

Chapter 1

EGGS, PANCAKES, CEREALS, AND OTHER BREAKFAST FOODS

EGGS, SUBSTITUTE, ¼ cup
See also "Vegetarian Foods, Frozen or Refrigerated"

calories

(Egg Beaters) 30
(Egg Watchers) 30
(Morningstar Farms Better'n Eggs) 20
(Morningstar Farms Scramblers) 35
(Second Nature) 40

BREAKFASTS, FREEZE-DRIED, ½ cup

calories

eggs:
   with bacon *(Mountain House)* 150
   with bacon, precooked *(Mountain House)* 120
   omelet, cheese *(Mountain House)* 180

BREAKFASTS, FROZEN, one package
See also "Breakfast Sandwiches," "French Toast, Frozen,"
"Pancakes, Frozen," and "Waffles, Frozen"

calories

egg, omelet, ham and cheese *(Weight Watchers)* 220
eggs, scrambled:
   and bacon *(Swanson Great Starts)* 290
   with Canadian bacon *(Swanson Great Starts* Low Fat/
     Cholesterol*)* 240
   with home fries *(Swanson Great Starts)* 200
   and pancake *(Swanson Great Starts* Low Fat/Cholesterol*)* . . . 220
   and sausage *(Swanson Great Starts)* 360
   and sausage, home fries *(Swanson Great Starts* Low Fat/
     Cholesterol*)* 240

Breakfasts, Frozen *(cont.)*
French toast:
    cinnamon swirl *(Swanson Great Starts)* 440
    with sausage *(Swanson Great Starts)* 410
    sticks, with syrup *(Swanson Kids Breakfast Blast)* 320
pancakes:
    (Swanson Kids Breakfast Blast Mini) 320
    with bacon *(Swanson Great Starts)* 400
    with sausage *(Swanson Great Starts)* 490
    silver dollar, eggs and *(Swanson Great Starts)* 250
    silver dollar, and sausage *(Swanson Great Starts)* 340
waffles *(Swanson Kids Breakfast Blast)* 330

BREAKFAST SANDWICHES, one serving
See also "Breakfasts, Frozen" and "Sandwiches, Frozen or Refrigerated"

---

                                           calories

bacon *(Schwan's Bright Starts* Singles) 440
burrito:
    (Schwan's Bright Starts) 280
    black bean *(Amy's)* 230
    egg, scrambled *(Swanson Great Starts* Original) 200
    egg, scrambled, with bacon *(Swanson Great Starts)* 250
    ham and cheese *(Swanson Great Starts)* 210
    hot and spicy *(Swanson Great Starts)* 220
    sausage *(Swanson Great Starts)* 240
egg:
    with cheese *(Swanson Great Starts)* 350
    muffin *(Weight Watchers)* 210
    muffin, with bacon and cheese *(Swanson Great Starts)* 290
    muffin, with Canadian bacon and cheese *(Hormel Quick*
       Meal) 260
    muffin, with ham *(Schwan's)* 230
    muffin, with sausage and cheese *(Hormel Quick Meal)* 390
    omelet *(Weight Watchers* Classic) 220
sausage biscuit:
    (Hormel Quick Meal) 350
    (Schwan's Twin Pack) 340
    (Weight Watchers) 230
    with cheese *(Hormel Quick Meal)* 410
    with egg *(Hormel Quick Meal)* 390

with gravy *(Schwan's)*, 4.4-oz. piece 250
vegetarian *(Morningstar Farms)*:
   bagel, with scrambler, patty, and cheese 320
   muffin, with scrambler and patty 240
   muffin, with scrambler, patty, and cheese 280
western *(Schwan's Bright Starts* Singles) 410

FRENCH TOAST, FROZEN
See also "Breakfasts, Frozen"

	calories
apple cinnamon stick *(Schwan's)*, 5 pieces	450
plain or cinnamon swirl *(Aunt Jemima)*, 2 pieces	240

PANCAKES, FROZEN, three pieces, except as noted
See also "Breakfasts, Frozen" and "Pancakes & Waffles, Mixes"

	calories
(Aunt Jemima Lowfat)	130
(Aunt Jemima Original)	200
(Downyflake)	270
(Hungry Jack Microwave Original)	270
blueberry *(Aunt Jemima)*	210
blueberry *(Hungry Jack* Microwave)	230

buttermilk:
   (Aunt Jemima) 180
   (Hungry Jack Microwave) 280
   (Schwan's) 260
   mini *(Hungry Jack* Microwave), 11 pieces 260

PANCAKES & WAFFLES, MIXES
See also "Pancakes, Frozen" and "Waffles, Frozen"

	calories
(Aunt Jemima Original), 1/3 cup	150
(Aunt Jemima Original Complete), 1/3 cup	190
(Betty Crocker Complete or Buttermilk Complete), 1/3 cup	200
(Bisquick Shake 'N Pour), 1/2 cup	210
(Gladiola), 1/2 cup	240
(Hungry Jack Original), 1/3 cup	150
(Hungry Jack Premeasured), 1/2 pkt.	200

Pancakes & Waffles, Mixes *(cont.)*

(Hungry Jack Extra Lights), ⅓ cup	160
(Hungry Jack Hungry Lights Complete), ⅓ cup	150
(Martha White FlapStax), ½ cup	240
blueberry *(Bisquick Shake 'N Pour)*, ½ cup	220
buckwheat *(Arrowhead Mills)*, ⅓ cup	140
buckwheat *(Aunt Jemima)*, ¼ cup	120
buttermilk:	
(Arrowhead Mills), ¼ cup	120
(Aunt Jemima Complete), ⅓ cup	190
(Aunt Jemima Complete Reduced Calorie), ⅓ cup	140
(Bisquick Shake 'N Pour), ½ cup	200
(Hungry Jack/Hungry Jack Complete), ⅓ cup	160
(Robin Hood), ⅓ cup	180
corn, blue *(Arrowhead Mills)*, ⅓ cup	150
gluten-free or kamut *(Arrowhead Mills)*, ¼ cup	130
multigrain or whole grain *(Arrowhead Mills)*, ¼ cup	120
oat bran or wild rice *(Arrowhead Mills)*, ⅓ cup	140
whole wheat *(Aunt Jemima)*, ¼ cup	130

WAFFLES, FROZEN, two pieces, except as noted
See also "Breakfasts, Frozen" and "Pancakes & Waffles, Mixes"

---

	calories
(Aunt Jemima Original)	200
(Belgian Chef), 1 piece	170
(Downyflake Homestyle)	170
(Downyflake Homestyle Low Fat)	140
(Eggo Homestyle)	220
(Eggo Minis Homestyle), 3 sets	240
(Eggo Nutri · Grain)	190
(Eggo Special K)	140
(Schwan's), 4 pieces	400
apple cinnamon *(Downyflake)*	190
apple cinnamon *(Eggo)*	220
blueberry:	
(Aunt Jemima)	190
(Downyflake)	190
(Eggo)	220
(Eggo Minis), 3 sets	240

buttermilk:
 (Aunt Jemima) 170
 (Downyflake) 170
 (Eggo) 220
cinnamon *(Aunt Jemima)* 180
cinnamon toast *(Eggo)*, 3 sets 280
low fat *(Aunt Jemima)* 160
multibran *(Eggo Nutri · Grain)* 80
nut and honey *(Eggo)* 240
oat bran *(Eggo Common Sense)* 200
oat bran, with fruit and nut *(Eggo Common Sense)* 220
oatmeal or whole-grain *(Aunt Jemima)* 170
raisin and bran *(Eggo Nutri · Grain)* 210
strawberry *(Eggo)* 220

TOASTER MUFFINS & PASTRIES, one piece, except as noted
See also "Muffins" and "Granola & Snack Bars"

---

               calories

apple, blueberry, cherry, strawberry, or raspberry *(Toaster
 Strudel)* 180
apple cinnamon *(Pop-Tarts)* 210
apple cinnamon *(Thomas' Toast-R-Cakes)* 100
banana nut *(Thomas' Toast-R-Cakes)* 110
blueberry:
 (Pop-Tarts) 210
 (Thomas' Toast-R-Cakes) 100
 (Toaster Strudel) 180
 frosted *(Pop-Tarts)* 200
 frosted *(Toastettes)* 190
brown sugar cinnamon:
 (Pop-Tarts) 220
 frosted *(Pop-Tarts)* 210
 frosted *(Toastettes)* 190
cherry:
 (Pop-Tarts) 200
 (Toaster Strudel) 180
 frosted *(Pop-Tarts)* 200
 frosted *(Toastettes)* 190
chocolate:
 (Pop-Tarts Minis), 1 pkt. 170
 fudge, frosted *(Pop-Tarts)* 200

Toaster Muffins & Pastries, chocolate *(cont.)*

graham *(Pop-Tarts)* 210
chocolate vanilla creme, frosted *(Pop-Tarts)* 200
cinnamon *(Toaster Strudel)* 190
corn *(Thomas' Toast-R-Cakes)* 110
cream cheese, all varieties *(Toaster Strudel)* 190
fudge, frosted *(Toastettes)* 190
grape, frosted *(Pop-Tarts)* 200
grape, frosted *(Pop-Tarts Minis)*, 1 pkt. 170
raisin bran *(Thomas' Toast-R-Cakes)* 90
raspberry *(Toaster Strudel)* 180
raspberry, frosted *(Pop-Tarts)* 210
S'mores *(Pop-Tarts)* 200
strawberry:
    (Pop-Tarts) 200
    (Pop-Tarts Minis), 1 pkt. 170
    (Thomas' Toast-R-Cakes) 110
    (Toaster Strudel) 180
    (Toastettes) 190
    frosted *(Pop-Tarts)* 200
    frosted *(Toastettes)* 190

CEREALS, READY-TO-EAT
*See also "Cereals, Cooking Type" and "Cereal & Grain
Products"*

---

                                                        calories
amaranth flakes *(Arrowhead Mills)*, 1 cup 130
bran *(see also "oat bran," below)*:
    (Kellogg's All-Bran), ½ cup 80
    (Kellogg's All-Bran Extra Fiber), ½ cup 50
    (Kellogg's Bran Buds), ⅓ cup 70
    (Kellogg's Frosted Bran), ¾ cup 100
    (Kellogg's Fruitful Bran), 1¼ cups 170
    (Nabisco 100% Bran), ⅓ cup 80
    (Post Bran'nola), ½ cup 200
    flakes *(Arrowhead Mills)*, 1 cup 100
    flakes *(Kellogg's Complete)*, ¾ cup 100
    flakes *(New Morning Multi-Bran)*, 1 cup 110
    flakes *(Post)*, ⅔ cup 90
    raisin *(Kellogg's)*, 1 cup 170
    raisin *(Malt-O-Meal)*, 1 cup 180

raisin *(New Morning Multi-Bran)*, 1 cup 90
raisin *(Post)*, 1 cup 190
raisin *(Post Bran'nola)*, ¹⁄₂ cup 200
with raisins *(Total Raisin Bran)*, 1 cup 180
with raisins and nuts *(Raisin Nut Bran)*, ³⁄₄ cup 210

corn:
   (Arrowhead Mills Maple Corns), 1 cup 190
   (Barbara's Frosted Funnies), 1 cup 110
   (Barbara's Puffins), ³⁄₄ cup 90
   (Cap 'N Crunch), ³⁄₄ cup 110
   (Cocoa Comets), ³⁄₄ cup 120
   (Colossal Crunch/Berry Colossal Crunch), ³⁄₄ cup 120
   (Corn Burst), 1 cup 110
   (Kellogg's Corn Pops), 1 cup 110
   (Nut & Honey Crunch), 1¹⁄₄ cups 220
   (Perky's Nutty Rice), ³⁄₄ cup 220
   (Post Toasties), 1 cup 100
   almond raisin *(New Morning Crunchy)*, ³⁄₄ cup 110
   bran *(Quaker Crunchy)*, ³⁄₄ cup 90
   with cranberries *(Cap'N Crunch)*, ³⁄₄ cup 100
   chocolate flavor *(Cocoa Puffs)*, 1 cup 120
   chocolate flavor *(Coco-Roos)*, ³⁄₄ cup 120
   flakes *(Arrowhead Mills)*, 1 cup 100
   flakes *(Barbara's)*, 1 cup 110
   flakes *(Country Corn Flakes)*, 1 cup 120
   flakes *(Kellogg's Corn Flakes)*, 1 cup 110
   flakes *(Kellogg's Frosted Flakes)*, ³⁄₄ cup 120
   flakes *(Malt-O-Meal Frosted)*, ³⁄₄ cup 110
   flakes *(New Morning)*, 1 cup 120
   flakes *(Total Corn Flakes)*, 1¹⁄₃ cups 110
   flakes, frosted *(Quaker By the Bag)*, ³⁄₄ cup 120
   flakes, honey frosted *(New Morning)*, ²⁄₃ cup 120
   honey roasted pecan *(Kellogg's Temptations)*, 1 cup 120
   with marshmallow bits *(Count Chocula/Franken Berry)*,
     1 cup 120
   peanut butter *(Cap'N Crunch)*, ³⁄₄ cup 110
   puffed *(Arrowhead Mills)*, 1 cup 80
   puffed, honey *(Health Valley)*, 1 cup 80
   puffs *(Body Buddies)*, 1 cup 120
   Quakes *(Quaker By the Bag)*, ³⁄₄ cup 120

corn and oat:
   cinnamon *(Kellogg's Mini Buns)*, ³⁄₄ cup 120

Cereals, Ready-to-Eat, corn and oat *(cont.)*
vanilla almond *(Kellogg's Temptations)*, ³/₄ cup 120
corn and rice *(Kellogg's Crispix)*, 1 cup 110
corn and rice *(Kellogg's Double Dip Crunch)*, ³/₄ cup 110
granola:
    (C. W. Post Hearty), ²/₃ cup 280
    (Heartland), ¹/₂ cup 300
    (Heartland Lowfat), ¹/₂ cup 210
    (Kellogg's Lowfat), ¹/₂ cup 210
    (New Morning Oatiola), ³/₄ cup 200
    almond *(Sun Country)*, ¹/₂ cup 270
    with blueberries and milk *(Mountain House)*, ¹/₃ cup 120
    carob cashew *(Roman Meal)*, ¹/₂ cup 190
    figs and filberts *(Roman Meal)*, ¹/₂ cup 190
    honey nut *(Roman Meal)*, ¹/₂ cup 210
    low fat, with fruit *(Nature Valley)*, ²/₃ cup 210
    raisin *(Heartland)*, ¹/₂ cup 290
    raisin *(Kellogg's* Low Fat), ²/₃ cup 210
    raisin and date *(Sun Country)*, ¹/₂ cup 260
    raisin nut *(Roman Meal)*, ¹/₂ cup 210
kamut:
    (New Morning Kamutios), 1 cup 120
    flakes *(Arrowhead Mills)*, 1 cup 120
    puffed *(Arrowhead Mills)*, 1 cup 50
millet, puffed *(Arrowhead Mills)*, 1 cup 90
mixed/multi grain:
    (Apple Jacks), 1 cup 110
    (Arrowhead Mills Crispy Puffs), 1 cup 80
    (Barbara's Shredded Spoonfuls), ³/₄ cup 120
    (Barbara's High 5), ³/₄ cup 100
    (Basic 4), 1 cup 210
    (Berry Berry Kix), ³/₄ cup 120
    (Cinnamon Toast Crunch), ³/₄ cup 130
    (Fiber One), ¹/₂ cup 60
    (Froot Loops), 1 cup 120
    (Fruiteo's), 1 cup 120
    (Golden Grahams), ³/₄ cup 120
    (Grape-Nuts), ¹/₂ cup 200
    (Grape-Nuts Flakes), ³/₄ cup 100
    (Just Right Crunchy Nuggets), 1 cup 200
    (Kaboom), 1¹/₄ cups 120
    (Kellogg's Mueslix Crispy), ²/₃ cup 200

(Kellogg's Mueslix Golden Crunch), ¾ cup 210
(Kix), 1⅓ cups 120
(Multi·Grain Cheerios), 1 cup 110
(Product 19), 1 cup 110
(Quaker 100% Natural), ½ cup 220
(Quaker 100% Natural Low Fat), ½ cup 210
(Quaker 100% Natural with Raisins), ½ cup 230
(Quaker Life), ¾ cup 120
(S'mores Grahams), ¾ cup 120
(Team Flakes), 1¼ cups 220
(Tootie Fruities), 1 cup 110
(Total Whole Grain), ¾ cup 110
(Trix), 1 cup 120
all varieties *(Granola O's)*, ¾ cup 120
all varieties *(Health Valley Honey Clusters & Flakes)*, ¾ cup . 130
brown sugar cinnamon *(Pop-Tarts Crunch)*, ¾ cup 120
cocoa *(Startoons)*, 1 cup 110
dates, raisins, and walnuts *(Fruit & Fibre)*, 1 cup 210
flakes *(Arrowhead Mills)*, 1 cup 140
flakes *(Healthy Choice)*, 1 cup 100
fruit-nut *(Just Right)*, 1 cup 210
granola, *see "granola," above*
honey *(Startoons)*, 1 cup 110
peaches, raisins, and almonds *(Fruit & Fibre)*, 1 cup 210
pecan *(Great Grains)*, ⅔ cup 220
raisins, dates, and pecans *(Great Grains)*, ⅔ cup 210
raisins, oats, and almonds *(Healthy Choice)*, 1 cup 200
squares *(Healthy Choice)*, 1¼ cups 190
strawberry *(Pop-Tarts Crunch)*, ¾ cup 120
oat:
(Alpha-Bits), 1 cup 130
(Apple Cinnamon Cheerios), ¾ cup 120
(Arrowhead Mills Nature O's), 1 cup 130
(Barbara's Breakfast O's), 1 cup 120
(Cheerios), 1 cup 110
(Frosted Cheerios), 1 cup 120
(Honey Bunches of Oats), ¾ cup 120
(Honey Nut Cheerios), 1 cup 120
(Kellogg's Nut & Honey Crunch O's), ¾ cup 120
(New Morning Oatios Original), 1 cup 120
(Quaker Cinnamon Squares), 1 cup 230
(Quaker Oat Squares), 1 cup 220

Cereals, Ready-to-Eat, oat *(cont.)*

(Toasty O's/Honey & Nut *Toasty O's)*, 1 cup 110
(Toasty O's Frosted), 1 cup 120
almonds *(General Mills* Oatmeal Crisp Almond), 1 cup 220
almonds *(Honey Bunches of Oats)*, ¾ cup 130
apple cinnamon *(General Mills* Oatmeal Crisp), 1 cup 210
apple cinnamon *(New Morning Oatios)*, 1 cup 90
apple cinnamon *(Toasty O's)*, ¾ cup 120
blueberry *(New Morning Oatiola)*, 1 cup 200
cinnamon *(Quaker Life)*, 1 cup 120
cinnamon raisin *(Nature Valley* 100% Natural Oat
   Cinnamon & Raisin), ¾ cup 240
cocoa *(New Morning Oatios)*, 1 cup 170
fruit and nut *(Nature Valley* 100% Natural Oat Fruit & Nut),
   ⅔ cup 250
and honey *(Nature Valley* 100% Natural Oat Toasted Oats
   & Honey), ¾ cup 250
honey almond *(New Morning Oatios)*, 1 cup 100
honey graham *(Quaker Oh!s)*, ¾ cup 110
honey nut *(Quaker By the Bag)*, 1 cup 110
marshmallow *(Alpha-Bits)*, 1 cup 120
marshmallow *(Lucky Charms)*, 1 cup 120
marshmallow *(Mateys)*, 1 cup 120
with raisins *(General Mills* Oatmeal Raisin Crisp), 1 cup . . . 210
oat bran:
(Common Sense), ¾ cup 110
(Cracklin' Oat Bran), ¾ cup 230
(New Morning Ultimate Oat Bran), 1 cup 110
(Quaker), 1¼ cups 210
flakes *(Arrowhead Mills)*, 1 cup 110
oatmeal, toasted, plain or honey nut *(Quaker)*, 1 cup 190
rice:
(Apple Cinnamon Rice Krispies), ¾ cup 110
(Cocoa Krispies), ¾ cup 120
(Frosted Krispies), ¾ cup 110
(Fruity Marshmallow Krispies), ¾ cup 110
(Perky's Nutty Rice), ¾ cup 210
(Rice Krispies), 1¼ cups 110
(Rice Krispies Treats), ¾ cup 120
(Special K), 1 cup 110
crispy *(Malt-O-Meal)*, 1 cup 110
puffed *(Arrowhead Mills)*, 1 cup 90

puffed *(Malt-O-Meal)*, 1 cup 60
puffed *(Quaker)*, 1 cup 50
puffed *(Quaker By the Bag Popeye)*, 1 cup 50
rice, brown, crisp:
   (Barbara's), 1 cup 120
   (Health Valley), 1 cup 110
   (New Morning), 1 cup 110
   frosted *(New Morning)*, 1 cup 210
rice and corn, almond raisin *(Nutri · Grain)*, 1¼ cups 200
rice and rye *(Kellogg's Apple Raisin Crisp)*, 1 cup 180
spelt flakes *(Arrowhead Mills)*, 1 cup 100
wheat:
   (Clusters), 1 cup 210
   (Golden Puffs), ¾ cup 120
   (Honey Frosted Wheaties), ¾ cup 120
   (Kellogg's Apple Cinnamon/Blueberry Squares), ¾ cup 180
   (Kellogg's Frosted Mini-Wheats), 1 cup 190
   (Kellogg's Raisin Squares), ¾ cup 180
   (Kellogg's Smacks), ¾ cup 110
   (Kellogg's Strawberry Squares), ¾ cup 180
   (Nabisco Frosted Wheat Bites), 1 cup 190
   (Nutri · Grain Golden), ¾ cup 100
   (Wheaties), 1 cup 110
   blueberry or strawberry *(Nabisco Wheat Bites)*, ¾ cup 170
   honey grahams *(New Morning)*, 2 pieces 120
   puffed *(Arrowhead Mills)*, 1 cup 90
   puffed *(Malt-O-Meal)*, 1 cup 50
   puffed *(Quaker)*, 1 cup 50
   puffed *(Quaker By the Bag Popeye)*, 1¼ cups 50
   raisin *(Nutri · Grain Golden)*, 1¼ cups 180
   with raisins *(Crispy Wheats 'n Raisins)*, 1 cup 190
   raspberry *(Nabisco Wheat Bites)*, ¾ cup 160
wheat, shredded:
   (Barbara's), 2 pieces 140
   (Nabisco), 2 pieces 160
   (Nabisco Shredded Wheat 'n Bran), 1¼ cups 200
   (Nabisco Spoon Size), 1 cup 170
   (Quaker), 3 pieces 220
wheat and barley *(Perky's Nutty Wheat & Barley)*, ¾ cup 220
wheat bran, see "bran"

CEREALS, COOKING TYPE, one packet, except as noted
*See also "Cereals, Ready-to-Eat" and "Cereal & Grain
Products"*

---

calories

barley:
  (Arrowhead Mills Bits O Barley), ⅓ cup 140
  banana nut *(Fantastic Cup)*, 1.6 oz. 170
mixed/multi grain:
  (Mother's), ½ cup 130
  (Pritikin) 160
  (Quaker), ½ cup 130
  (Roman Meal) 130
  (Roman Meal Instant) 100
  3-grain, maple raisin *(Fantastic* Cup), 1.8 oz. 180
  3-grain, strawberry banana *(Fantastic* Cup), 1.7 oz. 180
  4-grain, with flax *(Arrowhead Mills)*, ¼ cup 150
  7-grain *(Arrowhead Mills)*, ⅓ cup 140
  7-grain *(Arrowhead Mills* Wheat Free), ¼ cup 120
  apple cinnamon *(Roman Meal)* 120
  apple cinnamon *(Roman Meal* Instant) 110
  raisin date-nut *(Roman Meal)* 140
  raisin date-nut *(Roman Meal* Instant) 120
oat bran:
  (Mother's), ½ cup 150
  (Quaker), ½ cup 150
  mango *(Fantastic* Cup), 1.8 oz. 180
oat flakes, raisin and spice *(H–O* Instant) 150
oatmeal, instant:
  (Arrowhead Mills) 110
  (H–O), ½ cup 150
  (Maypo), ⅓ cup 150
  (Quaker) 100
  (Quaker Microwave) 110
  (Roman Meal Premium) 220
  apple cinnamon *(Fantastic* Cup), 1.7 oz. 170
  apple spice or cinnamon double raisin *(Quaker* Microwave) . 170
  with apples and cinnamon *(Quaker)* 130
  bananas and cream *(Quaker)* 140
  blueberries and cream *(Quaker)* 130
  brown sugar cinnamon or honey bran *(Quaker* Microwave) . . . 150

chocolate chip cookie, cookies 'n cream, or oatmeal raisin
   cookie *(Quaker Kids' Choice)* 160
cinnamon raisin almond *(Arrowhead Mills)* 130
cinnamon spice *(Quaker)* 170
cinnamon toast *(Quaker)* 130
cranberry orange *(Fantastic* Cup), 1.7 oz. 180
maple *(Maypo),* ½ cup 190
maple, apple, spice *(Arrowhead Mills)* 130
maple brown sugar *(Quaker)* 160
peaches and cream *(Quaker)* 130
raisin, date, walnut *(Quaker)* 140
raisin spice *(Quaker)* 160
raspberry, strawberries'n stuff, or strawberry-banana
   (Quaker Kids' Choice) 150
strawberries and cream *(Quaker)* 130
oats *(H–O* Quick), ½ cup 150
oats *(H–O* Quick Oats'n Fiber) 110
oats, rolled:
   (H–O Instant) 110
   (H–O Sweet & Mellow Instant) 150
   (Mother's), ½ cup 150
  ✳*(Quaker* Quick/Old Fashioned), ½ cup 150
   almond raisin *(H–O* Explo Instant) 160
   apple and cinnamon *(H–O* Instant) 130
   apple maple spice *(H–O* Explo Instant) 170
   apricot honey *(H–O* Explo Instant) 170
   banana creme *(H–O* Explo Instant) 170
   maple and brown sugar *(H–O* Instant) 160
oats, toasted *(H–O* Old Fashioned), ⅓ cup 160
rice:
   (Arrowhead Mills Rice & Shine), ¼ cup 150
   all varieties, except almond *(Lundberg* Hot 'n Creamy),
    ⅓ cup 190
   almond, sweet *(Lundberg* Hot 'n Creamy), ⅓ cup 200
   cinnamon raisin *(Lundberg* Hot 'n Creamy), ⅓ cup 190
rye, cream of *(Roman Meal)* 110
rye, cream of *(Roman Meal* Instant) 100
wheat:
   (Arrowhead Mills Bear Mush), ¼ cup 160
   (H–O Farina), 3 tbsp. 120
   (Malt-O-Meal Quick), 3 tbsp. 120
   (Mother's), ½ cup 130

Cereals, Cooking Type, wheat *(cont.)*

   (Wheat Hearts), ¼ cup 130
   (Wheatena), ⅓ cup 150
   all varieties *(Malt-O-Meal)*, 3 tbsp. 120
   n'berries *(Fantastic* Cup), 1.7 oz. 170
   cracked *(Arrowhead Mills)*, ¼ cup 170
   and oat, peachberry *(Fantastic* Cup), 1.8 oz. 190
   whole *(Quaker)*, ½ cup 130

CEREAL & GRAIN PRODUCTS, dry
See also "Cereals, Ready-to-Eat," "Cereals, Cooking Type,"
"Flour," and "Grain Dishes, Mixes"

---

                                           calories

amaranth seed *(Arrowhead Mills)*, ¼ cup 170
barley:
   flakes *(Arrowhead Mills)*, ⅓ cup 110
   pearled *(Arrowhead Mills)*, ¼ cup 170
   pearled *(Goya)*, ¼ cup 100
   pearled *(Quaker Scotch* Quick), ⅓ cup 170
   pearled, medium *(Quaker Scotch)*, ¼ cup 170
buckwheat groats, brown *(Arrowhead Mills)*, ¼ cup 140
bulgur, *see "wheat," below*
corn grits *(see also "hominy")*:
   (Albers Quick Hominy), ¼ cup 140
   (Cee-Leci/Dixie Lily/Jim Dandy), ¼ cup 170
   (Goya), ¼ cup 180
   instant *(Quaker* Original), 1-oz. pkt. 100
   instant, with bacon bits, butter flavor, cheddar, zesty
      cheddar, or sausage bits *(Quaker)*, 1-oz. pkt. 100
   instant, with ham bits *(Quaker)*, 1-oz. pkt. 90
   instant, with sausage bits *(Quaker)*, 1-oz. pkt. 100
   iron-fortified *(Jim Dandy)*, ¼ cup 140
   quick *(Cee-Leci/Dixie Lily/Jim Dandy)*, ¼ cup 160
   white *(Arrowhead Mills)*, ¼ cup 140
   white *(Quaker* Hominy), ¼ cup 140
   white *(Quaker* Quick Hominy), ¼ cup 130
   yellow *(Arrowhead Mills)*, ¼ cup 130
   yellow *(Dixie Lily/Martha White)*, ¼ cup 150
   yellow *(Quaker* Quick Hominy), ¼ cup 120
cornmeal, 3 tbsp., except as noted:
   blue or hi-lysine *(Arrowhead Mills)*, ¼ cup 130

blue and red *(Frieda's)*, ½ cup 214
coarse *(Goya)* 110
degerminated *(Jim Dandy)* 120
fine *(Goya)* 100
self-rising *(Dixie Lily/Martha White/Pekerson's)* 110
self-rising, buttermilk *(Dixie Lily Mix)* 140
self-rising, degerminated *(Jim Dandy)* 110
self-rising, stone-ground *(Cabin Home/Pine Mountain)* 110
self-rising, white *(Cee-Leci/Dixie Lily/Hay Market/Mother's Best/Omega)* 140
self-rising, white, regular or buttermilk *(Aunt Jemima Mix)* . .80
self-rising, white, regular or degerminated *(Aunt Jemima)* . .90
self-rising, white, plain or honey *(Martha White)* 140
self-rising, yellow, buttermilk *(Martha White Mix)* 150
white *(Arrowhead Mills)*, ¼ cup 120
white *(Dixie Lily/Hay Market/Martha White/Pekerson's)* 120
white *(Goya)*, 2½ tbsp. 100
white or yellow *(Albers)* 110
whole ground *(Cabin Home/Martha White/Pine Mountain)* . . . 110
yellow *(Arrowhead Mills)*, ¼ cup 120
yellow *(Aunt Jemima Mix)* 80
yellow *(Goya)*, 2½ tbsp. 110
yellow *(Martha White)* 120
couscous:
  (Arrowhead Mills), ¼ cup 170
  (Fantastic Foods), ¼ cup 210
  whole wheat *(Fantastic Foods)*, ¼ cup 210
flax seed *(Arrowhead Mills)*, 3 tbsp. 140
hominy, ½ cup:
  golden *(Allens/Uncle William)* 120
  golden *(Goya)* 120
  golden *(Sun-Vista)* 70
  golden *(Van Camp's)* 80
  Mexican *(Allens/Uncle William)* 120
  white *(Allens/Uncle William)* 100
  white *(Goya)* 100
  white *(Sun-Vista)* 65
  white *(Van Camp's)* 80
masa harina *(Quaker Enriched)*, ¼ cup 110
masa harina *(Quaker Preparada Para Tortillas)*, ⅓ cup 160
millet, hulled *(Arrowhead Mills)*, ¼ cup 150

Cereal & Grain Products *(cont.)*

oat:

    bran, dry *(Arrowhead Mills)*, ⅓ cup 150

    groats *(Arrowhead Mills)*, ¼ cup 160

    flakes, rolled *(Arrowhead Mills)*, ⅓ cup 130

    steel-cut *(Arrowhead Mills)*, ¼ cup 170

quinoa:

    (Eden), ¼ cup 170

    black and white *(Frieda's)*, 2 oz. dry or ½ cup cooked 218

    seeds *(Arrowhead Mills)*, ¼ cup 140

rye, whole-grain *(Arrowhead Mills)*, ¼ cup 160

rye flakes, rolled *(Arrowhead Mills)*, ⅓ cup 110

spelt flakes *(Arrowhead Mills)*, 1 cup 100

teff seed *(Arrowhead Mills)*, 2 oz. 200

wheat:

    bran *(Arrowhead Mills)*, ¼ cup 30

    bran *(Shiloh Farms)*, ¼ cup 30

    bran, toasted *(Kretschmer)*, ¼ cup 30

    bran, unprocessed *(Quaker)*, ⅓ cup 30

    bulgur, dry *(Arrowhead Mills)*, ¼ cup 150

    flakes *(Arrowhead Mills)*, ⅓ cup 110

    germ *(Kretschmer)*, 2 tbsp. 50

    germ, honey crunch *(Kretschmer)*, 1⅔ tbsp. 50

    germ, raw *(Arrowhead Mills)*, 3 tbsp. 50

    nuts *(Sonoma)*, 2 tbsp. 60

    whole-grain, hard red or winter *(Arrowhead Mills)*, ¼ cup . . 160

Chapter 2

BREADSTUFFS, CRACKERS, AND FLOUR PRODUCTS

BREAD, one slice, except as noted
See also "Bread, Pita or Pocket," "Bread Dough, Ready-to-Bake," "Bread Mix," and "Sweet Breads, Mixes"

	calories
(Arnold Bran'nola Country)	.90
(Arnold/Brownberry Bran'nola Original)	.90
apple honey wheat *(Brownberry)*	.60
apple walnut *(Pepperidge Farm)*	.80
bran:	
honey *(Pepperidge Farm)*	.90
light *(August Bros./Brownberry Bakery* Country), 2 slices	.80
whole *(Brownberry)*	.60
brown, canned *(S&W),* ½″ slice, 1.6 oz.	.90
brown, canned, plain or raisin *(B&M),* ½″ slice	130
buttermilk *(Arnold)*	100
cinnamon *(Brownberry)*	.80
cinnamon *(Pepperidge Farm)*	.80
cranberry *(Arnold)*	.70
date nut *(Thomas'),* 1 oz.	.80
French:	
(Arnold Francisco), 1 oz.	.70
(Pepperidge Farm), ⅛ loaf	130
(Pepperidge Farm Sliced), ⅛ loaf	120
twin *(Brownberry Francisco Intl.)*	.80
golden, light *(Brownberry Bakery),* 2 slices	.80
golden swirl *(Pepperidge Farm* Vermont Maple)	.90
Italian:	
(Arnold Francisco), 2 slices	110
(Arnold Savoni's)	.60
(Wonder, 20 oz.)	.80
brown and serve *(Pepperidge Farm),* ⅛ loaf	130
light *(Arnold/Brownberry Bakery),* 2 slices	.80

Bread, Italian *(cont.)*
    light *(Wonder, 1 lb.)* 40
    stick *(Arnold Francisco, 10 oz.)*, 1 oz. 70
    stick, sliced *(Arnold Francisco, 1 lb.)* 70
    thick *(Brownberry Francisco Intl.)*, 2 slices 110
kamut, sprout *(Shiloh Farms Egyptian)* 90
mixed/multi grain:
    (Brownberry Hearth) 90
    (Merita Autumn) 80
    (Roman Meal Round Top/Sun Grain) 70
    5, sprouted *(Shiloh Farms/Shiloh Farms No Salt)* 90
    7 or 12 *(Roman Meal)* 70
    7, hearty *(Pepperidge Farm)* 100
    7, light *(Pepperidge Farm)*, 3 slices 140
    7, light *(Roman Meal)*, 2 slices 80
    7, sprouted *(Breads for Life/Shiloh Farms/Shiloh Farms No
      Salt)* 90
    7, white *(Arnold/Brownberry Bran'nola)* 90
    9 *(Pepperidge Farm)* 90
    12 *(Arnold Bran'nola)* 90
    12 *(Brownberry)*, 2 slices 110
    crunchy *(Pepperidge Farm)* 90
    nutty *(Arnold Bran'nola/Brownberry Bran'nola)* 90
    with oat bran *(Roman Meal)* 70
    sprouted *(Shiloh Farms Sandwich)* 80
    whole *(Pepperidge Farm 100%)* 90
nut *(Brownberry Natural Health)* 70
oat:
    (Brownberry Bran'nola) .90
    (Roman Meal) 70
    crunchy, hearty *(Pepperidge Farm)* 100
oat bran, honey or honey nut *(Roman Meal)* 70
oat bran, light *(Roman Meal)*, 2 slices 80
oatmeal:
    (Brownberry Natural) 70
    (Pepperidge Farm) 80
    light *(Arnold/Brownberry Bakery)*, 2 slices 80
    light *(Pepperidge Farm)*, 3 slices 140
    soft *(Brownberry)* 70
    soft or thin *(Pepperidge Farm)* 60
orange raisin *(Brownberry)* .70
poppy seed, hazelnut *(Roman Meal)* 110

potato:
(Arnold Country) 100
country *(Wonder,* 20 oz.) 80
hearty *(Pepperidge Farm* Russet) 90
pumpernickel:
(Arnold/Arnold August Bros., 1 lb./*Arnold Levy's)* 80
(Arnold August Bros., 24 oz.) 90
dark *(Pepperidge Farm)* 80
party *(Pepperidge Farm),* 8 slices 110
rye *(Brownberry)* 70
raisin:
(Arnold Sunmaid) 70
cinnamon *(Arnold/Brownberry)* 70
cinnamon *(Pepperidge Farm)* 80
walnut *(Brownberry)* .80
whole wheat *(Shiloh Farms),* 2 slices 140
rye:
(Arnold Deli) 80
(Brownberry Hearth) .90
Dijon *(Arnold* Real Jewish) 80
Dijon, thin *(Pepperidge Farm),* 2 slices 100
dill *(Arnold)* 80
dill *(Brownberry)* 70
hearty or soft *(Beefsteak)* 70
onion *(Arnold August Bros.)* 80
onion *(Pepperidge Farm)* 80
onion, with seeds *(Arnold August Bros.)* 90
party *(Pepperidge Farm),* 8 slices 110
seeded *(Arnold August Bros.,* 1 lb.) 80
seeded *(Arnold/Brownberry* Natural/*Levy's* Real Jewish) 70
seeded or unseeded *(Arnold August Bros.,* 24 oz.) 90
seeded or unseeded *(Pepperidge Farm)* 80
soft *(Arnold* Country) 70
soft, light *(Arnold/Brownberry Bakery),* 2 slices 80
soft, seeded or unseeded *(Arnold Bakery)* 80
thin *(Arnold Levy's Melba),* 2 slices 90
unseeded *(Arnold* Real Jewish, 1 lb./2 lb.) 70
unseeded *(Arnold August Bros.,* 1 lb.) 80
unseeded *(Arnold Levy's* Real Jewish/*Brownberry* Natural) . . .70
unseeded, thin *(Arnold August Bros.),* 2 slices 90
unseeded, thin *(Brownberry),* 2 slices 100
rye and pump *(Arnold August Bros.)* 90

Bread (cont.)
sourdough:

    (Arnold August Bros.) 110
    (Arnold Francisco) 90
    brown and serve (Arnold Francisco), 1 oz. 70
    light (Arnold), 2 slices 80
    light (Pepperidge Farm), 3 slices 130
    thick (Brownberry Francisco Intl.) 90
    whole-grain (Roman Meal) .70
spelt (Shiloh Farms) 100
stick, sliced (Arnold August Bros.), 2 slices 110
stick, sliced (Brownberry Francisco) 100
toast, Texas (Arnold August Bros.) 150
Vienna, light (Pepperidge Farm), 3 slices 130
Vienna, thick (Pepperidge Farm) 70
wheat:
    (Arnold Brick Oven) 80
    (Arnold Brick Oven, 8 oz./1 lb.), 2 slices 110
    (Arnold/Brownberry Country/Brownberry Hearth) 90
    (Arnold Sunny Valley), 2 slices 100
    (Brownberry Natural) 80
    (Home Pride Butter Top) .70
    (Pepperidge Farm/Pepperidge Farm Natural) 90
    (Pepperidge Farm Family) 70
    (Roman Meal Natural) 90
    (Shiloh Farms Homestyle), ½" slice, 2 oz. 160
    (Wonder/Wonder Family) .70
    cracked, thin (Pepperidge Farm) 70
    dark or hearty (Arnold/Brownberry Bran'nola) 90
    light (Pepperidge Farm), 3 slices 130
    light (Roman Meal), 2 slices 80
    light, golden (Arnold), 2 slices 80
    light, hearty (Roman Meal Light), 2 slices 80
    sesame, hearty (Pepperidge Farm) 100
    soft (Brownberry) 80
    soft (Brownberry, 16 oz.), 2 slices 110
    very thin (Pepperidge Farm), 3 slices 110
wheat or white (Home Pride, 20 oz.) 70
wheat, whole:
    (Arnold Stoneground, 1 lb. 4 oz.) 60
    (Arnold Stoneground, 2 lb.), 2 slices 100
    (Merita 100%) 70

(Roman Meal) 60
(Shiloh Farms/Shiloh Farms No Salt), 2 slices 140
(Wonder, 24 oz.) 80
light (Roman Meal), 2 slices 80
soft or thin (Pepperidge Farm) 60
wheatberry, honey:
  (Arnold) 70
  (Arnold Bran'nola) .90
  (Roman Meal) 70
  hearty (Pepperidge Farm) 100
  light (Roman Meal), 2 slices 80
white:
  (Arnold Brick Oven) 80
  (Arnold Brick Oven, 8 oz.), 2 slices 120
  (Arnold Brick Oven, 1 lb.), 2 slices 130
  (Arnold Country) 100
  (Arnold Sunny Valley), 2 slices 100
  (Brownberry Country) 90
  (Brownberry Natural), 2 slices 120
  (Home Pride Butter Top) 70
  — (Wonder, 12 oz.), 2 slices 100
  — (Wonder, 1 lb.) .60
  (Wonder, 22 oz.), 2 slices 120
  hearty (Pepperidge Farm/Pepperidge Farm Country) 90
  light (Arnold/Brownberry Bakery), 2 slices 80
  light (Roman Meal), 2 slices 80
  sandwich (Pepperidge Farm), 2 slices 130
  sandwich (Roman Meal), 2 slices 110
  soft (Arnold Country/Brownberry) 80
  soft (Brownberry, 16 oz.), 2 slices 110
  thin (Pepperidge Farm/Pepperidge Farm Large Family) 80
  toasting (Pepperidge Farm) 90
  very thin (Pepperidge Farm), 3 slices 110

BREAD, PITA OR POCKET
See also "Bread" and "Shells & Wrappers"

                             calories

(Arnold), 2-oz. piece 140
(Arnold), 3-oz. piece 210
(Cedar's), ½ piece, 1.5 oz. 122
(Cedar's Mountain Bread), 2-oz. piece 180

Bread, Pita or Pocket *(cont.)*

(Pepperidge Farm), 1 piece 150
(Pepperidge Farm Mini), 1-oz. piece 70
(Thomas' Sahara), 2-oz. piece 150
(Thomas' Sahara), 3-oz. piece 220
(Thomas' Sahara Mini), 1-oz. piece 70
6-grain *(Cedar's)*, ½ piece, 1.5 oz. 94
6-grain *(Cedar's* Mountain Bread), 2-oz. piece 200
garlic *(Arnold)*, 1 piece 160
oat bran *(Thomas' Sahara)*, 1 piece 130
onion *(Arnold)*, 1 piece 150
onion *(Thomas' Sahara)*, 1 piece 140
salsa *(Thomas' Sahara)*, 1 piece 170
sourdough *(Thomas' Sahara)*, 1 piece 150
wheat:
    (Arnold), 2-oz. piece 140
    (Arnold), 3-oz. piece 200
    (Cedar's Mountain Bread), 2-oz. piece 180
    (Thomas' Sahara), 2-oz. piece 130
    (Thomas' Sahara Mini), 1-oz. piece 60
    whole *(Cedar's)*, ½ piece, 1.5 oz. 129
wheat or white *(Arnold 4")*, 1-oz. piece 70
wheat or white *(Cedar's* Mountainette), 1.1-oz. piece 135

BREAD, FROZEN, ⅙ loaf or package, except as noted
See also "Bread Dough, Ready-to-Bake"

	calories
cheddar, two *(Pepperidge Farm)*	210
corn bread *(Marie Callender's)*, 1.9-oz. piece	150
five cheese and garlic *(Schwan's)*	320
garlic or garlic Parmesan *(Pepperidge Farm)*	160
garlic mozzarella *(Pepperidge Farm)*	200
garlic sourdough *(Pepperidge Farm)*	180
Monterey Jack/jalapeño cheese *(Pepperidge Farm)*	200

BREAD DOUGH, READY-TO-BAKE*
*See also "Bread," "Bread, Frozen," "Bread Mix," "Sweet
Breads, Mixes," and "Breadsticks & Snacks"*

---

                                                                    calories

frozen, white or honey wheat *(Schwan's)*, ⅛ loaf 130
refrigerated:
   breadsticks *(Pepperidge Farm Brown and Serve)*, 1 piece . 150
   breadsticks *(Pillsbury)*, 1 piece 110
   breadsticks, sesame, thin *(Pepperidge Farm)*, 7 sticks 60
   corn bread twists *(Pillsbury)*, 1 piece 140
   French *(Pillsbury)*, ⅕ loaf 150

BREAD MIX, dry, except as noted
*See also "Bread," "Bread Dough, Ready-to-Bake," and "Sweet
Breads, Mixes"*

---

                                                                    calories

beer *(Buckeye)*, ¹/₁₄ pkg. 130
beer, whole wheat *(Buckeye)*, ¹/₁₄ pkg. 120
cheddar cheese *(Dromedary)*, ⅑ pkg. 140
corn bread:
   (Arrowhead Mills), ¼ cup 120
   (Ballard), ¹/₁₈ pkg. 110
   (Ballard), ¹/₁₈ bread* 130
   (Buckeye), ¹/₁₆ pkg. 130
   (Dromedary), ¹/₁₀ pkg. 140
   buttermilk *(Martha White)*, ⅕ bread* 150
   buttermilk *(Martha White Cotton Pickin')*, ⅕ pkg. 130
   buttermilk or yellow *(Martha White)*, ⅕ pkg. 130
   chili fiesta *(Martha White)*, ⅙ bread* 190
   golden honey *(Martha White)*, ⅙ bread* 170
   golden honey, Mexican or chili fiesta *(Martha White)*,
      ⅙ pkg. 110
   Mexican *(Gladiola)*, ⅙ pkg. 110
   Mexican *(Gladiola)*, ⅙ bread* 130
   Mexican *(Martha White)*, ⅙ bread* 140
   white *(Martha White Light Crust)*, ⅙ pkg. 110
   white or yellow *(Gladiola)*, ⅙ pkg. 110

---

* *Prepared according to package directions*

Bread Mix, corn bread *(cont.)*
 white or yellow *(Gladiola/Martha White* Light Crust), ⅙
  bread* 140
 yellow *(Martha White),* ⅕ bread* 140
 yellow *(Martha White* Light Crust), ⅙ pkg. 120
herb, Italian *(Dromedary),* ⅑ pkg. 140
kamut *(Arrowhead Mills),* ⅓ cup 140
multi-grain *(Arrowhead Mills),* ⅓ cup 160
oatmeal, honey *(Dromedary),* ⅑ pkg. 150
rye *(Arrowhead Mills),* ⅓ cup 160
sourdough *(Buckeye),* 1/14 pkg. 130
sourdough *(Dromedary),* ⅑ pkg. 140
spelt *(Arrowhead Mills),* ⅓ cup 150
wheat:
 cracked *(Pillsbury* Bread Machine), 1/12 loaf* 130
 stone-ground *(Dromedary),* ⅑ pkg. 140
 whole *(Arrowhead Mills),* ⅓ cup 150
white:
 (Arrowhead Mills), ⅓ cup 150
 country *(Dromedary),* ⅑ pkg. 140
 crusty *(Pillsbury* Bread Machine), 1/12 loaf 130

SWEET BREADS, MIXES, dry, except as noted
*See also "Bread," "Bread Dough, Ready-to-Bake," "Bread
Mix," "Muffins, Mixes," "Rolls, Frozen or Refrigerated," and
"Rolls, Mixes"*

---

                                                        calories
(Buckeye), 1/16 pkg. 110
apple cinnamon *(Dromedary),* ⅑ pkg. 140
apple cinnamon or blueberry *(Pillsbury),* 1/12 pkg. 140
apple cinnamon or blueberry *(Pillsbury),* 1/12 loaf* 180
banana or pumpkin *(Pillsbury),* 1/12 pkg. 130
banana or pumpkin *(Pillsbury),* 1/12 loaf* 170
carrot *(Pillsbury),* 1/16 pkg. 110
carrot *(Pillsbury),* 1/16 loaf* 140
cinnamon swirl *(Pillsbury),* 1/12 pkg. 180
cinnamon swirl *(Pillsbury),* 1/12 loaf* 220
cranberry *(Pillsbury),* 1/12 pkg. 140
cranberry *(Pillsbury),* 1/12 loaf* 160

* Prepared according to package directions

date *(Pillsbury)*, 1/12 pkg. 150
date *(Pillsbury)*, 1/12 loaf* 180
date nut *(Dromedary)*, 1/12 pkg. 180
gingerbread *(Dromedary)*, 1/6 pkg. 260
gingerbread *(Pillsbury)*, 1/8 loaf* 220
lemon poppyseed *(Pillsbury)*, 1/12 pkg. 160
lemon poppyseed *(Pillsbury)*, 1/12 loaf* 180
nut *(Pillsbury)*, 1/12 pkg. 150
nut *(Pillsbury)*, 1/12 loaf* 170
pumpkin *(Pillsbury)*, 1/12 pkg. 130
pumpkin *(Pillsbury)*, 1/12 loaf* 170

BAGELS, one piece
See also "Bagels, Frozen"

---

calories

plain:
   (Awrey's), 2.6 oz. 200
   (Awrey's), 4 oz. 280
   (Thomas') 150
blueberry *(Awrey's)* 280
cinnamon raisin *(Awry's)*, 2.6 oz. 200
cinnamon raisin *(Awrey's)*, 4 oz. 270
cinnamon raisin or egg *(Thomas')* 160
mini *(Awrey's)* 100
onion or multi-grain *(Thomas')* 150

BAGELS, FROZEN, one piece, except as noted
See also "Bagels"

---

calories

plain:
   (Lender's) 160
   (Lender's Bagelettes), 2 pieces 140
   (Lender's Big'N Crusty) 220
blueberry or cinnamon raisin *(Lender's)* 200
cinnamon raisin *(Lender's Big'N Crusty)* 240
cinnamon raisin *(Sara Lee)* 220
egg *(Lender's)* 160
egg *(Lender's Big'N Crusty)* 230

---

* Prepared according to package directions

Bagels, Frozen *(cont.)*
garlic *(Lender's)* 150
oat bran *(Lender's)* 190
onion *(Lender's)* 160
onion *(Lender's Big'N Crusty)* 220
poppy or sesame *(Lender's)* 150
pumpernickel or rye *(Lender's)* 150
soft *(Lender's Original)* 210

BISCUITS
See also "Rolls"

---

calories

packaged:
    (Arnold Old Fashioned), 2 pieces 130
    (Awrey's Country), 1 piece 140
    (Awrey's Round), 1 oz. 70
    (Awrey's Round), 2 oz. 150
    (Awrey's Round), 3 oz. 230
frozen, cinnamon raisin, iced *(Schwan's)*, 1 piece 300
frozen, garlic and cheese *(Pepperidge Farm)*, 1 piece 170
mix:
    (Arrowhead Mills), 1/4 cup 120
    (Bisquick), 1/3 cup 170
    (Gold Medal Biscuit Mix), 1/3 cup 170
    (Gold Medal Biscuit Mix), 2 biscuits* 180
    buttermilk *(Gladiola Biscuit Mix)*, 1/3 cup 160
    buttermilk *(Martha White Bismix)*, 1/2 cup 150
    buttermilk *(Martha White Bismix)*, 1/2 cup* 160
    lower fat *(Bisquick Reduced Fat)*, 1/3 cup 150
refrigerated, 1 piece, except as noted:
    (Big Country Butter Tastin') 100
    (Grands! Butter Tastin') 200
    (Grands! Butter Tastin' Reduced Fat/Grands! Homestyle) . . . 190
    (Ovenready), 3 pieces 150
    baking powder or buttermilk *(1869 Brand)* 100
    buttermilk *(Big Country)* 100
    buttermilk *(Grands! Reduced Fat)* 190
    buttermilk *(Ovenready)*, 3 pieces 150
    buttermilk or cinnamon raisin *(Grands!)* 200

---

* *Prepared according to package directions*

flaky *(Grands!)* 190
fluffy, extra *(Grands!)* 200
rich, extra *(Grands!)* 220
Southern style *(Big Country)* 100
Southern style *(Grands!)* 200

MUFFINS, one piece, except as noted
*See also "Muffins, Frozen or Refrigerated," "Muffins, Mixes,"
and "Toaster Muffins & Pastries"*

---

 calories

(Arnold Bran'nola) 130
(Arnold Extra Crisp) 120
almond poppy seed *(Aunt Fanny's)*, 2 pieces 310
apple:
   (Awrey's), 1.5 oz. 130
   (Awrey's), 2.5 oz. 250
   bran *(Aunt Fanny's)*, 2 pieces 290
banana nut:
   (Aunt Fanny's), 2 pieces 320
   (Awrey's Grande) 400
   (Tastykake), ½ piece, 2 oz. 120
   (Tastykake Family) 220
   mini *(Awrey's)*, 2 pieces 200
   mini *(Hostess)*, 3 pieces 160
blueberry:
   (Aunt Fanny's), 2 pieces 290
   (Awrey's), 1.5 oz. 130
   (Awrey's), 2.5 oz. 210
   (Awrey's Grande) 340
   (Entenmann's) 160
   (Entenmann's Fat Free) 120
   (Tastykake), ½ piece, 2 oz. 230
   (Tastykake Family) 170
   (Tastykake Low Fat), ½ piece, 2 oz. 150
   loaf *(Hostess)*, 3.8 oz. 440
   mini *(Awrey's)*, 2 pieces 180
   mini *(Hostess)*, 3 pieces 150
   top *(Awrey's)*, 2.5 oz. 210
carrot raisin *(Awrey's* Grande) 360
cheese streusel *(Awrey's* Grande) 380
chocolate chocolate chip *(Awrey's* Grande) 460

Muffins *(cont.)*

cinnamon apple or chocolate chip, mini *(Hostess)*, 3 pieces . . . 160
corn:
   (Awrey's), 1.5 oz. 130
   (Awrey's), 2.5 oz. 220
   (Tastykake), ½ piece, 2 oz. 220
   (Tastykake Golden Family) 190
cranberry nut *(Awrey's)* 120
cranberry orange *(Tastykake Low Fat)*, ½ piece, 2 oz. 160
English:
   (Awrey's) 140
   (Pepperidge Farm) 130
   (Roman Meal) 135
   (Tastykake) 130
   (Thomas') 120
   (Wonder) 120
   7-grain or sourdough *(Pepperidge Farm)* 130
   blueberry, cranberry, or raisin *(Thomas')* 140
   cinnamon raisin *(Pepperidge Farm)* 140
   cinnamon raisin *(Tastykake)* 110
   honey wheat *(Thomas')* 110
   oat bran or sourdough *(Thomas')* 120
   sandwich size *(Thomas' 4 Pack/Twin)* 190
   sourdough *(Tastykake)* 130
   sourdough, sandwich size *(Thomas' Em's)* 200
   wheat, sandwich size *(Thomas' Em's)* 180
lemon poppy seed:
   (Awrey's) 170
   (Awrey's Grande) 390
   mini *(Awrey's)*, 2 pieces 90
oat bran *(Hostess)*, 2 pieces 320
onion, sandwich size *(Thomas' Em's)* 180
raisin *(Arnold)* 150
raisin bran:
   (Awrey's), 1.5 oz. 110
   (Awrey's), 2.5 oz. 190
   (Awrey's Grande) 350
   (Tastykake Low Fat), ½ piece, 2 oz. 170
   top *(Awrey's)* 190
raspberry, loaf *(Hostess)*, 3.8 oz. 440
sourdough *(Arnold)* 120

MUFFINS, FROZEN OR REFRIGERATED, one piece
See also "Muffins" and "Muffins, Mixes"

calories

apple oatmeal *(Pepperidge Farm Wholesome Choice)*	160
banana *(Weight Watchers Fat Free)*	170
blueberry *(Pepperidge Farm Wholesome Choice)*	140
blueberry *(Weight Watchers Fat Free)*	160
bran, harvest honey *(Weight Watchers Fat Free)*	160
bran, with raisins *(Pepperidge Farm Wholesome Choice)*	150
chocolate chocolate chip *(Weight Watchers)*	190
corn *(Pepperidge Farm Wholesome Choice)*	150
corn *(Sara Lee)*	260
English *(Thomas')*	120
English, honey wheat *(Thomas')*	110

MUFFINS, MIXES, one piece*, except as noted
See also "Muffins," "Muffins, Frozen or Refrigerated," and "Sweet Breads, Mixes"

calories

apple cinnamon:

(Betty Crocker), ¼ cup mix	110
(Betty Crocker)	140
(Martha White), ¼ cup mix	170
(Martha White)	180
(Pillsbury), ⅓ cup mix	170
(Pillsbury)	180
(Robin Hood), ⅙ pkg. mix	130
(Robin Hood)	170
low fat *(Martha White Low Fat)*	160
low-fat recipe *(Betty Crocker Fat Free)*	120
low-fat recipe *(Sweet Rewards Fat Free)*	120
no-cholesterol recipe *(Betty Crocker)*	130
non fat *(Betty Crocker Fat Free)*, ¼ cup mix	120
non fat *(Betty Crocker Fat Free)*	120
non fat *(Sweet Rewards Fat Free)*, ¼ cup mix	120
non fat *(Sweet Rewards Fat Free)*	120

banana nut:

(Betty Crocker), 3 tbsp. mix	130

* Prepared according to package directions

Muffins, Mixes, banana nut *(cont.)*
  (Betty Crocker) 150
  (Gold Medal/Robin Hood), 1/6 pkg. mix 130
  (Gold Medal/Robin Hood) 170
  (Martha White), 1/3 cup mix 180
  (Martha White) 200
  no-cholesterol recipe *(Betty Crocker)* 130
blackberry *(Martha White),* 1/4 cup mix 170
blackberry *(Martha White)* 180
blueberry:
  (Betty Crocker), 1/4 cup mix 120
  (Betty Crocker) 140
  (Betty Crocker Fat Free), 3 tbsp. mix or 1 muffin 120
  (Duncan Hines), 1/12 pkg. mix 150
  (Duncan Hines) 160
  (Duncan Hines Bakery Style), 1/12 pkg. mix 170
  (Duncan Hines Bakery Style) 190
  (Martha White), 1/4 cup mix 170
  (Martha White) 180
  (Martha White Low Fat/*Pillsbury* Low Fat) 160
  (Pillsbury), 1/3 cup mix 170
  (Pillsbury) 180
  (Robin Hood), 1/6 pkg. mix 120
  (Robin Hood) 160
  (SnackWell's) 120
  (Sweet Rewards Fat Free) 120
  double *(Martha White),* 1/4 cup mix 160
  double *(Martha White)* 180
  low-fat recipe *(Betty Crocker* Fat Free) 120
  no-cholesterol recipe *(Betty Crocker)* 130
  no-cholesterol recipe *(Duncan Hines* Bakery Style) 180
  wild *(Betty Crocker),* 1/4 cup mix 140
  wild *(Betty Crocker)* 170
  wild *(Sweet Rewards* Fat Free), 1/4 cup mix or 1 muffin 120
  wild, no-cholesterol recipe *(Betty Crocker)* 150
bran:
  (Martha White), 1/3 cup mix 160
  (Martha White) 190
  multi *(Buckeye),* 1/12 pkg. mix 110
  oat *(Arrowhead Mills),* 1/3 cup mix 160
  oat *(Martha White),* 1/3 cup mix 170
  oat *(Martha White)* 200

wheat *(Arrowhead Mills)*, ⅓ cup mix 150
caramel nut *(Gold Medal/Robin Hood)*, ⅙ pkg. mix. 130
caramel nut *(Gold Medal/Robin Hood)* 170
chocolate chip:
   (Duncan Hines), 1/12 pkg. mix 180
   (Duncan Hines) 190
   chocolate *(Martha White)*, ¼ cup mix 150
   chocolate *(Martha White)* 200
   chocolate *(Pillsbury)*, ⅓ cup mix 180
   chocolate *(Pillsbury)* 190
cinnamon:
   streusel *(Betty Crocker)*, ¼ cup mix 160
   streusel *(Betty Crocker)* 170
   swirl *(Duncan Hines)*, 1/12 pkg. mix 190
   swirl *(Duncan Hines)* 200
corn:
   (Flako), ⅓ cup mix 160
   (Gladiola), ¼ cup mix 140
   (Gladiola) 200
   (Gold Medal), ⅙ pkg. mix 110
   (Gold Medal) 160
   (Martha White), ⅓ cup mix 160
   (Martha White) 180
honey pecan *(Martha White)*, ⅓ cup mix 160
honey pecan *(Martha White)* 180
lemon poppy seed:
   (Betty Crocker), ¼ cup mix 150
   (Betty Crocker) 190
   (Martha White), ⅓ cup mix 160
   (Martha White) 240
   no-cholesterol/low-fat recipe *(Betty Crocker)* . . . 150
oatmeal raisin *(Martha White)*, ¼ cup mix 150
oatmeal raisin *(Martha White)* 200
raspberry:
   (Martha White), ¼ cup mix 170
   (Martha White) 180
   swirl *(Duncan Hines)*, 1/12 pkg. mix 150
   swirl *(Duncan Hines)* 160
strawberry:
   (Martha White), ¼ cup mix 170
   (Martha White) 180
   (Pillsbury), ⅓ cup mix 170

Muffins, Mixes, strawberry *(cont.)*

    (Pillsbury) 180
    low fat *(Martha White* Low Fat*)* 160

ROLLS, one piece, except as noted
See also "Biscuits," "Rolls, Frozen or Refrigerated," "Rolls, Mixes," and "Snack Cakes & Pastries"

---

                                                 calories

(Arnold Francisco 3"*)* 90
(Arnold Bran'nola Buns*)* 130
assorted *(Brownberry* Hearth*)* 120
brown and serve:
    (Pepperidge Farm Hearth*)*, 3 rolls 150
    (Roman Meal), 2 rolls 140
    (Wonder 12 oz.*)* 70
    club *(Pepperidge Farm)* 120
    French *(Pepperidge Farm,* 3/pkg.*)* 240
    French *(Pepperidge Farm,* 2/pkg.*)*, ½ roll 180
    sourdough *(Arnold Francisco)* 80
crescent, butter *(Pepperidge Farm* Heat & Serve*)* 110
croissant:
    butter *(Awrey's)*, 1.5-oz. roll 140
    butter *(Awrey's)*, 2-oz. roll 190
    butter *(Awrey's Tip-to-Tip)* 290
    butter *(Pepperidge Farm* Petite*)* 130
    dill and onion or pesto Parmesan *(Awrey's)* 210
    margarine *(Awrey's Tip-to-Tip)* 140
    margarine, sandwich *(Awrey's)*, 1.8-oz. roll 180
    margarine, sandwich *(Awrey's)*, 2.5-oz. roll 250
    margarine, sandwich, wheat *(Awrey's)* 250
dill and onion or garlic and pepper *(Awrey's* Deli Rounds*)* 150
dinner:
    (Arnold 12 Pack/24 Pack*)* 110
    (Arnold August Bros.*)* .90
    (Arnold Bran'nola) 70
    (Brownberry Francisco Intl.*)* 120
    (Pepperidge Farm Country Style*)*, 3 rolls 150
    (Roman Meal), 2 rolls 150
    all varieties *(Awrey's)*, 2 rolls, 1.6 oz. 110
    finger, Parker House, poppy seed, or sesame seed
        (Pepperidge Farm), 3 rolls 150

    potato *(Pepperidge Farm* Deli Classic) 80
    potato or sesame seed *(Arnold)*, 2 rolls 110
    wheat *(Arnold August Bros.)* 100
    white *(Arnold August Bros.)* 90
egg, twist *(Arnold Levy* Old Country) 170
French:
    (Arnold 6″) 160
    (Brownberry Francisco Intl. 6″) 170
    7-grain *(Pepperidge Farm,* 9/pkg.) 80
    mini *(Arnold Francisco)* 110
    regular or sourdough *(Pepperidge Farm)* 100
golden twist *(Pepperidge Farm* Heat & Serve) 110
hamburger:
    (Arnold 8 Pack) 130
    (Arnold 12 Pack) 120
    (Arnold August Bros.) 140
    (Pepperidge Farm) 130
    (Roman Meal) 120
    (Wonder 4″) 130
    wheat *(Arnold August Bros.)* 130
hoagie, *see also "sub," below:*
    (Awrey's) 230
    (Pepperidge Farm Deli Classic/*Pepperidge Farm* Multi-
      Grain) 200
    (Wonder Deli) 190
hot dog/frankfurter:
    (Arnold 11 oz.) 100
    (Arnold 12 oz./12 Pack) 110
    (Arnold Bran'nola/*Arnold* New England/*Brownberry)* 110
    (Pepperidge Farm) 140
    (Roman Meal) 110
    (Wonder Foot Long Coneys) 190
    Dijon *(Pepperidge Farm)* 140
    potato *(Arnold)* 120
    wheat *(Brownberry)* 110
Italian *(Arnold Savoni* 8″) 280
kaiser:
    (Arnold August Bros.) 160
    (Arnold Francisco 6″/*Arnold Levy* Old Country) 170
    (Awrey's) 190
    (Brownberry Hearth) 150
    (Brownberry Francisco) 170

Rolls *(cont.)*

onion *(Arnold* Deli) 170
onion *(Arnold August Bros./Arnold Levy* Old Country) 160
party *(Pepperidge Farm* 20), 5 rolls 170
potato, plain or with sesame *(Arnold)* 150
sandwich roll/bun:
   (Pepperidge Farm Hearty) 230
   (Roman Meal) 185
   multigrain or onion *(Pepperidge Farm)* 150
   potato *(Brownberry)* 150
   potato *(Pepperidge Farm)* 160
   sesame, soft *(Arnold)* 140
   sesame seed *(Pepperidge Farm)*. 140
   soft *(Arnold* 8 Pack) 140
   soft *(Arnold* 12 Pack) 130
   sourdough *(Pepperidge Farm)* 170
   wheat *(Brownberry)* 130
   white *(Brownberry)* 140
sesame *(Arnold August Bros.)* 170
sesame *(Arnold* Sandwich) 140
sourdough *(Arnold Francisco)* 90
steak *(Arnold* Premium/*Arnold August Bros./Arnold Francisco)* . 170
sub, *see also "hoagie," above:*
   (Arnold August Bros.) 170
   (Arnold Levy Old Country) 140
   super loaf *(Arnold Francisco)*, 1 oz. 70
tea *(Wonder)* 80

ROLLS, FROZEN OR REFRIGERATED, one piece, except as
noted
See also "Rolls"

---

                          calories

(Rich's Homestyle), 2 rolls 150
crescent *(Pillsbury* Reduced Fat) 100
crescent, plain or cheese *(Pillsbury)* 110
croissant *(Sara Lee* Original) 170
croissant, petite *(Sara Lee)*, 2 rolls 230
dinner, wheat or white *(Pillsbury)* 110

ROLLS, MIXES,
See also "Rolls"

calories

(Dromedary), ¹/₁₆ pkg. 100
(Pillsbury), ¹/₄ cup 110
(Pillsbury), ¹/₁₅ pkg.* 130

BREADSTICKS & SNACKS
See also "Bread Dough, Ready-to-Bake"

calories

bagel chips, 1 oz.:
   cheese, three *(Pepperidge Farm)* 140
   onion and garlic *(Pepperidge Farm)* 110
   onion multigrain *(Pepperidge Farm)* 120
bread crisps, cinnamon raisin *(Pepperidge Farm)*, 1 oz. 130
bread crisps, garlic butter *(Pepperidge Farm)*, 1 oz. 140
breadstick dough, *see "Bread Dough, Ready-to-Bake," page 00*
breadsticks:
   (Stella D'Oro Sodium Free), 1 stick 45
   all varieties *(Stella D'Oro Fat Free Original Deli)*, 5 sticks 60
   all varieties *(Stella D'Oro Fat Free Original Grissini)*, 3
     sticks 60
   all varieties *(Stella D'Oro Fat Free Traditional)*, 2 sticks 70
   butter or dill and onion *(Awrey's)*, 2 sticks 130
   cheddar, thin *(Pepperidge Farm)*, 7 sticks 70
   with cheese *(Handi-Snacks)*, 1 stick 130
   cheese, three *(Pepperidge Farm)*, 9 sticks 140
   garlic *(Stella D'Oro)*, 1 stick 40
   garlic and pepper or Italian spice *(Awrey's)*, 2 sticks 140
   onion, thin *(Pepperidge Farm)*, 7 sticks 70
   pretzel *(Pepperidge Farm)*, 9 sticks 130
   pumpernickel *(Pepperidge Farm)*, 9 sticks 150
   regular, onion or wheat *(Stella D'Oro)*, 1 stick 40
   sesame *(Pepperidge Farm)*, 9 sticks 160
   sesame *(Stella D'Oro)*, 1 stick 50

* *Prepared according to package directions*

CROUTONS, two tablespoons or ¼ ounce, except as noted
See also "Stuffing & Stuffing Mixes" and "Crumbs & Meal"

---

	calories
Caesar or cheddar *(Brownberry)*	.30
Caesar, cheese and garlic, ranch, or seasoned *(Pepperidge Farm)*	.35
Caesar or spicy Italian *(Pepperidge Farm* Fat Free), 6 pieces, .3 oz.	.30
cheddar and Romano *(Pepperidge Farm)*	.30
cheese and garlic, onion and garlic, ranch, or seasoned:	
(Arnold Crispy)	.30
(Brownberry)	.30
cracked pepper and Parmesan or zesty Italian *(Pepperidge Farm)*	.35
garlic *(Old London* Restaurant Style)	.30
herb, fine *(Arnold* Crispy)	.30
Italian *(Arnold* Crispy)	.30
Italian *(Old London* Restaurant Style)	.30
olive oil and garlic or onion and garlic *(Pepperidge Farm)*	.30
sourdough *(Old London* Restaurant Style)	.30
sourdough, cheese *(Pepperidge Farm)*	.30
toasted *(Brownberry)*	.30

STUFFING & STUFFING MIXES
See also "Croutons" and "Crumbs & Meal"

---

	calories
stuffing:	
(Arnold Unspiced), 2 cups	250
apple and raisin *(Pepperidge Farm)*, ½ cup	140
Cajun rice *(Good Harvest)*, ½ cup	130
chicken, classic *(Pepperidge Farm)*, ½ cup	130
corn bread *(Arnold/Brownberry)*, 2 cups	250
corn bread *(Pepperidge Farm)*, ¾ cup	170
corn bread, honey pecan *(Pepperidge Farm)*, ½ cup	140
country style or cube *(Pepperidge Farm)*, ¾ cup	140
cube, bread, unseasoned *(Brownberry)*, 2 cups	240
garden and herb, country *(Pepperidge Farm)*, ½ cup	150
herb seasoned *(Brownberry)*, 1 cup	200
herb seasoned *(Pepperidge Farm)*, ¾ cup	170
herb seasoned or sage and onion *(Arnold)*, 2 cups	240

sage and onion *(Brownberry 7 oz./14 oz.)*, 2 cups 240
sage and onion *(Pepperidge Farm)*, ½ cup 150
Santa Fe *(Good Harvest)*, ½ cup 110
seasoned *(Arnold)*, 2 cups 250
sourdough, San Francisco *(Good Harvest)*, ½ cup 110
vegetable, harvest, and almond *(Pepperidge Farm)*, ½ cup . 140
wild rice and mushroom *(Pepperidge Farm)*, ⅔ cup 170
wild rice trio *(Good Harvest)*, ½ cup 140
stuffing mix, ⅙ box dry, except as noted:
  (Kellogg's Croutettes), 1 cup 120
  for beef, pork, or turkey *(Stove Top)* 110
  chicken flavor *(Stove Top/Stove Top Lower Sodium)* 110
  chicken flavor *(Stove Top Microwave)* 130
  chicken flavor, with rice *(Rice-A-Roni)*, 1 cup* 170
  corn bread or savory herb *(Stove Top)* 110
  corn bread, homestyle *(Stove Top Microwave)* 120
  corn bread, with rice *(Rice-A-Roni)*, 1 cup* 170
  herb *(Stove Top Flexible Serve)*, 1 oz. 120
  herb and butter *(Rice-A-Roni)*, 1 cup* 170
  long grain and wild rice or mushroom and onion *(Stove
    Top)* 110
  San Francisco style *(Stove Top)* 110
  with wild rice *(Rice-A-Roni)*, 1 cup* 170

CRUMBS & MEAL
See also "Croutons" and "Stuffing & Stuffing Mixes"

                                          calories

bread crumbs, ¼ cup or 1 oz., except as noted:
  (Contadina), ⅓ cup 100
  (Devonsheer/Old London) 100
  garlic and herb, lemon herb, or Parmesan *(Progresso)* . . . 100
  Italian *(Devonsheer)* 100
  Italian or plain *(Progresso)* 110
  seasoned *(Old London)* 100
  tomato basil *(Progresso)* 120
corn flake crumbs *(Kellogg's)*, 2 tbsp. 40
cracker crumbs and meal:
  crumbs *(Ritz)*, ⅓ cup 140
  crumbs, saltine *(Premium Fat Free)*, ¼ cup 100

* Prepared according to package directions

Crumbs & Meal *(cont.)*
  matzo meal *(Manischewitz)*, ¼ cup 130
  matzo meal *(Streit's)*, ¼ cup 110

SHELLS & WRAPPERS
See also "Bread, Pita or Pocket" and "Pastry & Pie Crusts"

---

	calories

crepe *(Frieda's)*, 1 piece 45
egg roll wrapper:
  (Frieda's), 2 pieces, 1.7 oz. 132
  (Nasoya), 1.5 oz. 117
pizza crust, ¼ crust:
  (Pillsbury) 180
  (Totino's) 180
  mix *(Martha White)*, ¼ crust* 170
  mix *(Robin Hood)*, ¼ crust* 160
  mix, deep pan *(Martha White)*, ⅕ crust* 150
taco shell:
  (Gebhardt), 3 shells 155
  (Lawry's), 2 shells 120
  (Lawry's Super Size), 2 shells 180
  (Old El Paso Super), 2 shells 200
  (Pancho Villa), 3 shells 180
  (Rosarita), 3 shells 155
  golden or white corn *(Old El Paso)*, 3 shells 170
  mini *(Old El Paso)*, 7 shells 170
  tostada *(Lawry's)*, 2 shells 110
  tostada *(Old El Paso)*, 3 shells 170
  tostada *(Rosarita)*, 2 shells 125
  white corn *(Chi-Chi's)*, 2 shells 170
tortilla:
  corn *(Tyson)*, 3 pieces 140
  corn, white *(Goya)*, 2 pieces 120
  flour *(Cedar's Boston)*, 1.1-oz. piece 100
  flour *(Cedar's Boston)*, 2.6-oz. piece 200
  flour *(Goya)*, 1 piece 110
  flour *(Mesa 6")*, 1 piece 80
  flour *(Old El Paso)*, 1 piece 140
  flour *(Tyson)*, 1.4-oz. piece 120

* Prepared according to package directions

flour *(Tyson),* 1.9-oz. piece 170
flour, heat pressed *(Tyson),* 2 pieces 180
flour, refrigerated *(Old El Paso),* 1 piece 130
flour, refrigerated *(Old El Paso* Low Fat), 1 piece 110
flour, small *(Goya),* 1 piece 80
mix, flour *(Burris Light Crust),* ⅓ cup 160
soft taco *(Old El Paso),* 2 pieces 170
soft taco, refrigerated *(Old El Paso),* 1 piece 110
wonton:
    (Frieda's), 1 piece 13
    (Nasoya), 5 pieces 90

FLOUR, ¼ cup, except as noted
*See also "Cereal & Grain Products" and "Baking Powder,
Soda, & Starch"*

---

                                                          calories

all-purpose, *see "wheat," below*
amaranth, kamut, or millet *(Arrowhead Mills)* 110
barley *(Arrowhead Mills)* 75
buckwheat *(Arrowhead Mills)* 100
chickpea *(Arrowhead Mills),* 2 oz. 200
garbanzo *(Arrowhead Mills)* 90
oat *(Arrowhead Mills),* ⅓ cup 120
rice:
    (Goya), 3 tbsp. 120
    brown *(Arrowhead Mills)* 120
    white *(Arrowhead Mills)* 160
rye *(Arrowhead Mills)* 100
rye, medium *(Pillsbury)* 100
rye-wheat *(Pillsbury* Bohemian Style) 100
semolina, mix *(Arrowhead Mills),* ½ cup 240
soy *(Arrowhead Mills),* ½ cup 200
spelt *(Arrowhead Mills)* 100
teff *(Arrowhead Mills),* 2 oz. 200
wheat:
    (All Trump) 100
    (Gladiola HD) 120
    (La Pina) 100
    (Wondra) 100
    all-purpose, white *(Gold Medal)* 100
    all-purpose, white *(Goya)* 100

Flour, wheat *(cont.)*

all-purpose, white *(Red Band)*	100
all-purpose, white *(Robin Hood)*	100
all-purpose, white bleached *(Burris Light Crust/Dixie Lily/Gladiola/Light Crust/Omega/Martha White/Mother's Best)*	110
all-purpose, white bleached *(Pillsbury)*	110
all-purpose, white unbleached *(Arrowhead Mills)*, 1/3 cup	160
all-purpose, white unbleached *(Gold Medal)*	100
all-purpose, white unbleached *(Pillsbury)*	100
all-purpose, white unbleached *(Robin Hood)*	100
all-purpose, white unbleached, whole-grain *(Arrowhead Mills)*	110
bread, wheat blend *(Gold Medal)*	110
bread, white *(Gold Medal)*	100
bread, white *(Pillsbury)*	110
cake, white *(Betty Crocker Softasilk)*	100
cake, white *(Martha White)*	100
cake, white *(Swan's Down)*	100
gluten *(Arrowhead Mills)*, 3 tbsp.	35
gluten *(General Mills* Supreme Hygluten)	100
pastry, soft, white unbleached *(Arrowhead Mills)*	100
pastry, soft, whole-grain *(Arrowhead Mills)*, 1/3 cup	100
presifted, white *(Pillsbury* Shake & Blend)	110
self-rising, white *(Gold Medal)*	100
self-rising, white *(Red Band)*	100
self-rising, white *(Robin Hood)*	100
self-rising, white bleached *(Dixie Lily/Gladiola/Hollyhock/Omega/Martha White/Mother's Best)*	110
self-rising, white bleached or unbleached *(Pillsbury)*	100
whole-grain, stone-ground *(Arrowhead Mills)*,	130
whole wheat *(Gold Medal)*	90
whole wheat *(Martha White)*	120
whole wheat *(Pillsbury)*	120

YEAST, BAKER'S

	calories
all varieties *(Fleischmann's)*, 1/4 tsp.	0

BAKING POWDER, SODA, & STARCH
See also "Flour"

	calories
arrowroot *(Durkee)*, ¼ tsp.	0
baking powder *(Calumet)*, ¼ tsp.	0
baking powder *(Davis)*, 1 tsp.	8
baking soda *(Tone's)*, 1 tsp.	0
cornstarch *(Argo/Kingsford)*, 1 tbsp.	30
cream of tartar *(Tone's)*, 1 tsp.	2
tapioca, dry *(Minute)*, 1½ tsp.	20

CRACKERS
See also "Rice & Grain Cakes," "Chips, Crisps, & Similar Snacks," and "Corn Chips, Puffs, & Similar Snacks"

	calories
bacon flavor *(Nabisco)*, 15 pieces, 1.1 oz.	160
(Barbara's Rite Lite), 5 pieces, .5 oz.	55
butter/butter flavor:	
(Goya Tropical), 4 pieces	140
(Hi-Ho), 9 pieces, 1.1 oz.	160
(Keebler Club Partners), 4 pieces, .5 oz.	70
(Ritz), 5 pieces, .6 oz.	80
(Ritz Low Sodium), 5 pieces, .6 oz.	80
(Ritz Air Crisps), 24 pieces	140
(Toasted Complements Buttercrisp), 9 pieces, 1 oz.	140
(Town House), 5 pieces, .6 oz.	80
mini *(Ritz Bits)*, 48 pieces, 1.1 oz.	160
thins *(Pepperidge Farm)*, 4 pieces, .5 oz.	70
cheese:	
(Appeteasers Original), 1 oz.	130
(Barbara's Bites Original/Hot & Spicy), 26 pieces, 1.1 oz.	120
(Krispy Mild Cheddar), 5 pieces, .5 oz.	60
(Nips), 29 pieces, 1.1 oz.	150
(Nips Air Crisps), 32 pieces	130
(SnackWell's), 38 pieces, 1.1 oz.	130
(Tid-Bit), 32 pieces, 1.1 oz.	150
chili *(Munch 'ems)*, 28 pieces, 1.1 oz.	130
garlic herb *(Appeteasers)*, 1 oz.	130
Parmesan *(Goldfish)*, 60 pieces, 1.1 oz.	140
salsa *(SnackWell's)*, 32 pieces	120

Crackers, cheese *(cont.)*

Swiss *(Nabisco Swiss)*, 15 pieces, 1 oz. 140
zesty *(SnackWell's)*, 32 pieces, 1.1 oz. 120

cheese, cheddar:

(Better Cheddars/Better Cheddars Low Sodium)*, 22 pieces,
   1.1 oz. 150
(Better Cheddars Reduced Fat)*, 24 pieces, 1.1 oz. 140
(Cheez-It/Cheez-It Low Sodium)*, 27 pieces, 1.1 oz. 160
(Cheez-It Reduced Fat)*, 30 pieces, 1.1 oz. 130
(Combos), 1 oz. 140
(Combos), 1.7-oz. bag 250
(Frito-Lays'), 1 pkg. 220
(Goldfish), 55 pieces, 1.1 oz. 140
(Goldfish Reduced Sodium)*, 60 pieces, 1.1 oz. 150
(Munch 'ems), 30 pieces, 1.1 oz. 130
(Snorkels), 56 pieces, 1.1 oz. 140
double *(Appeteasers)*, 1 oz. 130
hot and spicy *(Cheez-It)*, 26 pieces, 1.1 oz. 160
white *(Cheez-It)*, 26 pieces, 1.1 oz. 160
white *(Wheatables)*, 27 pieces, 1.1 oz. 130

cheese sandwich:

(Handi-Snacks Cheez'n Crackers)*, 1.1-oz. piece 130
(Little Debbie), 1.4 oz. 200
(Ritz), 1.4-oz. pkg. 210
(Ritz Bits), 14 pieces, 1.1 oz. 160
bacon, jalapeño cheddar, or wheat *(Frito-Lay's)*, 1 pkg. 200
cheddar, golden toast *(Frito-Lay's)*, 1 pkg. 230
cream cheese and chive, golden toast *(Frito-Lay's)*, 1 pkg. . 240
peanut butter, *see "peanut butter," below*

(Chicken in a Biskit), 14 pieces, 1.1 oz. 160

cracked pepper, *see "water or soda," below*

croissant *(Carr's)*, 3 pieces, .5 oz. 70

flatbread:

(Lavosh Hawaii Classic)*, 8 pieces, 1 oz. 120
(New York), .4-oz. piece 45
(New York Everything)*, .4-oz. piece 45
(New York Fat Free)*, .4-oz. piece 40
10-grain *(California Crisps)*, 2 pieces, .5 oz. 59
10-grain *(Lavosh Hawaii)*, 8 pieces, 1 oz. 110
all varieties *(J. J. Flats)*, .5-oz. piece 50
Cajun *(New York)*, .4-oz. piece 45
caraway rye or peppercorn *(Lavosh Hawaii)*, 8 pieces, 1 oz. . 115

cracked pepper, garlic, roasted, honey cinnamon,
   pumpernickel, or garden vegetable *(New York Fat Free)*,
   .4-oz. piece 40
  garlic *(California Crisps)*, 2 pieces, .5 oz. 65
  onion *(New York)*, .4-oz. piece 40
  onion or poppy *(California Crisps)*, 2 pieces, .5 oz. 66
  onion, slightly *(Lavosh Hawaii)*, 8 pieces, 1 oz. 120
  poppy, pumpernickel sesame, or sesame *(New York)*,
   .4-oz. piece 50
  pumpernickel onion *(New York)*, .4-oz. piece 40
  rosemary garlic *(Lavosh Hawaii)*, 8 pieces, 1 oz. 125
golden *(SnackWell's* Classic), 6 pieces, .5 oz. 60
(Goldfish Original), 55 pieces, 1.1 oz. 140
(Goya Snack), 11 pieces 140
(Goya Tropical), 4 pieces 140
graham, *see "Cookies," page 313*
(Munch 'ems), 30 pieces, 1.1 oz. 130
matzo, 1 oz.:
  (Manischewitz Everything!) 110
  (Manischewitz Unsalted) 110
  garlic *(Manischewitz* Savory) 100
  rye *(Manischewitz)* 110
melba rounds/snacks, 5 pieces, .5 oz.:
  plain *(Devonsheer)* 50
  bacon, cheese, garlic, Mexicali corn, onion, rye, white,
   sesame, or whole-grain *(Old London)* 60
  garlic or sesame *(Devonsheer)* 60
  honey bran, savory herb, onion, 12-grain, or vegetable
   (Devonsheer) 50
melba toast, 3 pieces, .5 oz.:
  plain or wheat *(Devonsheer/Devonsheer* No Salt) 50
  onion, rye, wheat, or white *(Old London)* 50
  rye, 12-grain, or vegetable *(Devonsheer)* 50
  sesame *(Devonsheer/Devonsheer* No Salt) 50
  sesame *(Old London/Old London* No Salt) 50
  whole-grain *(Old London)* 45
  whole-grain *(Old London* No Salt) 50
milk *(Royal Lunch)*, .4-oz. piece 50
multi-grain:
  (Hi-Ho), 9 pieces, 1.1 oz. 160
  (Wheat Thins), 17 pieces, 1.1 oz. 130
  5-grain *(Harvest Crisps)*, 13 pieces, 1.1 oz. 130

Crackers *(cont.)*
oat *(Harvest Crisps)*, 13 pieces, 1.1 oz. 140
oat *(Oat Thins)*, 18 pieces, 1.1 oz. 140
onion:
    (Toasted Complements), 9 pieces, 1 oz. 140
    French *(SnackWell's)*, 32 pieces, 1.1 oz. 120
    French *(Wheatables)*, 27 pieces, 1.1 oz. 130
pappadum *(Patak's)*, 3 pieces 80
peanut butter *(Handi-Snacks)*, 1.1-oz. piece 180
peanut butter *(Handi-Snacks* Grahamstick), 1.1-oz. piece 170
peanut butter sandwich:
    (Ritz), 13 pieces, 1.1 oz. 150
    cheese *(Frito-Lay's)*, 1 pkg. 200
    cheese *(Little Debbie)*, 1.4 oz. 200
    cheese *(Nabs)*, 6 pieces, 1.4 oz. 190
    cheese *(Planters)*, 1.4-oz. pkg. 190
    toast *(Little Debbie)*, 1.4 oz. 190
    toast *(Frito-Lay's)*, 1 pkg. 190
    toast *(Nabs)*, 6 pieces, 1.4 oz. 190
    toast *(Planters)*, 1.4-oz. pkg. 190
    toast *(Sunshine)*, 1.2-oz. pkg. 180
pizza:
    (Goldfish), 55 pieces, 1.1 oz. 140
    all varieties *(Health Valley)*, 6 pieces 50
    bites *(Barbara's)*, 26 pieces, 1.1 oz. 120
potato, au gratin, barbecue, or sour cream and chives
    (No Fries), 1.1 oz. 110
(Pretzel Air Crisps), 22 pieces 110
ranch *(Munch 'ems)*, 33 pieces, 1.1 oz. 130
ranch *(SnackWell's)*, 32 pieces 120
rice:
    brown *(Eden)*, 5 pieces, 1.1 oz. 120
    and seaweed *(Eden* Nori Maki), 15 pieces, 1.1 oz. 110
    rice bran *(Health Valley)*, 6 pieces, 1 oz. 110
salsa *(Munch 'ems)*, 28 pieces, 1.1 oz. 130
saltine, 5 pieces, .5 oz., except as noted:
    (Dux), 2 pieces 40
    (Krispy/Krispy Fat Free/*Krispy* Unsalted Top) 60
    (Premium/Premium Low Sodium/*Premium* Unsalted Top) . . .60
    (Premium Fat Free) 50
    (Zesta) 60
    cracked pepper *(Krispy)* 60

saltine, mini *(Premium Bits)*, 34 pieces, 1.1 oz. 150
sesame:
   (Breton), 10 pieces, 1.5 oz. 220
   (Pepperidge Farm), 3 pieces, .5 oz. 70
   (Toasted Complements), 10 pieces, 1 oz. 140
sesame cheese *(Twigs)*, 15 pieces, 1.1 oz. 150
(Sociables), 7 pieces, .5 oz. .80
soup and oyster, .5 oz.:
   (Krispy) 60
   (Oysterettes) 60
   (Premium) 60
sour cream and onion *(Munch 'ems)*, 33 pieces, 1.1 oz. 130
(Uneeda), 2 pieces, .5 oz. 60
vegetable *(Garden Crisps)*, 15 pieces, 1.1 oz. 130
vegetable *(Vegetable Thins)*, 14 pieces, 1.1 oz. 160
water or soda:
   (Breton/Breton 50% Less Salt), 10 pieces, 1.5 oz. 210
   (Breton Light), 10 pieces, 1.5 oz. 200
   (Cabaret), 10 pieces, 1.7 oz. 230
   (Carr's Table Water), 5 pieces, .6 oz. 70
   (Crown Pilot), .6-oz. piece 70
   (Dux), 2 pieces 40
   (Hi-Ho), 9 pieces, 1.1 oz. 160
   (Pepperidge Farm Original), 5 pieces, .5 oz. 60
   (Vivant), 10 pieces, 1.5 oz. 210
   cracked pepper *(Carr's Table Water)*, 5 pieces, .6 oz. 70
   cracked pepper *(Hi-Ho)*, 9 pieces, 1.1 oz. 160
   cracked pepper *(Pepperidge Farm)*, 5 pieces, .5 oz. 60
   cracked pepper *(SnackWell's)*, 7 pieces, .5 oz. 60
   poppy sesame *(Carr's)*, 4 pieces, .5 oz. 80
   sesame *(Breton)*, 10 pieces, .5 oz. 220
   sesame *(Carr's Table Water)*, 5 pieces, .6 oz. 70
wheat:
   (SnackWell's Fat Free), 5 pieces, .5 oz. 60
   (Stoned Wheat Thins/Stoned Wheat Thins Lower Sodium),
      2 pieces 60
   (Toasted Complements), 9 pieces, 1 oz. 140
   (Triscuit), 7 pieces, 1.1 oz. 140
   (Triscuit Low Sodium), 7 pieces, 1.1 oz. 150
   (Triscuit Reduced Fat), 8 pieces, 1.1 oz. 130
   (Waverly), 5 pieces, .5 oz. 70
   (Wheat Thins/Wheat Thins Low Salt), 16 pieces, 1 oz. 140

Crackers, wheat *(cont.)*
    (Wheat Thins Reduced Fat), 18 pieces, 1 oz. 120
    (Wheat Thins Air Crisps), 24 pieces 130
    (Wheatables), 29 pieces, 1.1 oz. 150
    (Wheatsworth), 5 pieces, .6 oz. 80
    all varieties *(Barbara's* Wheatines), .5-oz. square 60
    cracked *(Pepperidge Farm),* 2 pieces, .5 oz. 70
    hearty *(Pepperidge Farm),* 3 pieces, .5 oz. 80
    herb, garden *(Triscuit),* 6 pieces, 1 oz. 130
    ranch *(Wheatables),* 29 pieces, 1.1 oz. 150
    and rye *(Triscuit* Deli), 7 pieces, 1.1 oz. 140
wheat, whole:
    (Carr's), 2 pieces, .6 oz. 80
    (Health Valley No Salt), 5 pieces 50
    (Hi-Ho), 9 pieces, 1.1 oz. 150
    (Krispy), 5 pieces, .5 oz. 60
    all varieties *(Health Valley),* 5 pieces 50
    and bran *(Triscuit),* 7 pieces, 1.1 oz. 140
(Zwieback), .3-oz. piece 35

RICE & GRAIN CAKES, one cake, except as noted
See also "Crackers" and "Granola & Snack Bars"

---

                                        calories
popcorn bar, caramel or chocolate *(Pop Secret),* 1 bar 70
popcorn cakes:
    all varieties *(Orville Redenbacher* Mini), 1.1 oz. 100
    butter *(Orville Redenbacher),* 3 cakes 115
    butter *(Quaker* Mini), 6 cakes 50
    caramel *(Orville Redenbacher),* 2 cakes 80
    cheddar, white *(Lundberg* Mini), 5 cakes 70
    cheddar, white *(Orville Redenbacher),* 3 cakes 110
rice cakes:
    plain *(Quaker* Salted/Salt Free) 35
    all varieties *(Lundberg/Lundberg* Unsalted) 60
    all varieties *(Pritikin/Pritikin* Unsalted) 35
    all varieties, bars *(Health Valley* Crisp Fat Free) 110
    all varieties, except cheddar *(Quaker* Mini), 5 cakes 50
    all varieties, except cheddar popped corn, caramel popped
      corn, and banana nut *(Mother's)* 35
    apple cinnamon *(Crispy Cakes)* 35
    apple cinnamon *(Quaker)* 50

apple crisp *(Pritikin* Mini), 5 cakes 50
banana nut or caramel popped corn *(Mother's)* 50
blueberry, strawberry, or chocolate crunch *(Quaker)* 50
brown *(Lundberg* Mini), 5 cakes 60
brown, toasted *(Crispy Cakes)* 30
butter popped corn *(Quaker)* 35
caramel corn, cinnamon crunch, or banana nut *(Quaker)* 50
caramel nut *(Pritikin* Mini), 5 cakes 50
cheddar *(Crispy Cakes)* 35
cheddar, white, or Monterey Jack *(Quaker)* 40
cheddar, white *(Quaker* Mini), 6 cakes 50
cheddar popped corn *(Mother's)* 40
cheese, nacho *(Lundberg* Mini), 5 cakes 60
dill, creamy *(Lundberg* Mini), 5 cakes 60
pizza or ranch *(Crispy Cakes)* 30
vegetable, garden *(Crispy Cakes)* 35

Chapter 3

CREAM, MILK, MILK BEVERAGES, AND YOGURT

> **MILK**
> *See also "Cream," "Flavored Milk Beverages," and "Nondairy 'Milk' Beverages"*

	calories
condensed, sweetened, canned, 2 tbsp.:	
(Borden)	130
(Carnation)	130
(Eagle/Magnolia Brand/Meadow Gold/Star)	130
(Goya)	130
low-fat (Borden)	120
low-fat (Eagle)	120
skim (Borden Fat Free)	110
skim (Eagle Fat Free)	110
dairy pack and packaged, 8 fl. oz.:	
(Lactaid Calcium Fortified/Nonfat)	90
(Lactaid 100)	100
1% (America's Choice)	100
1% (Crowley)	110
1% (Lactaid)	110
1% (The Organic Cow of Vermont)	110
1% (Parmalat)	110
2% (America's Choice)	130
2% (Crowley)	130
2% (Lactaid 100)	130
2% (Parmalat)	130
buttermilk (Friendship Lowfat)	120
skim (The Organic Cow of Vermont)	90
skim (Parmalat)	90
skim (Weight Watchers)	90
whole (America's Choice)	150
whole (The Organic Cow of Vermont)	160
whole (Parmalat)	160

dry, nonfat, instant *(Carnation)*, 1/3 cup 80
evaporated, canned, 2 tbsp.:
    (Carnation) 40
    (Pet) 40
    low-fat or skim *(Carnation)* 25
    skim *(Pet)* 20
goat, dairy pack *(Meyenberg)*, 1 cup 140

CREAM
See also "Milk," "Sour Cream," and "Creamers, Nondairy"

                                          calories

half and half, 2 tbsp.:
    (America's Choice) 40
    (Land O'Lakes Fat Free) 20
    (Land O'Lakes Gourmet) 40
heavy, dairy pack *(America's Choice)*, 1 tbsp. 50
heavy, dairy pack *(Crowley)*, 1 tbsp. 50
light, canned *(Nestlé Crema)*, 1 tbsp. 30
light, dairy pack *(Crowley)*, 1 tbsp. 30

SOUR CREAM, two tablespoons
See also "Cream"

                                          calories

(Breakstone's) 60
(Friendship) 60
(Heluva Good) 60
(Knudsen Hampshire) 60
(Land O'Lakes) 60
(Sealtest) 60
half and half *(Breakstone's)* .45
light:
    (Friendship) 35
    (Heluva Good) 40
    (Knudsen Light) 40
    (Land O'Lakes Light) 35
    (Sealtest Light) 40
nondairy, plain or flavored *(Sour Supreme)* 50
nonfat:
    (Breakstone's/Sealtest Free) 35
    (Friendship) 20

Sour Cream, nonfat *(cont.)*

(Heluva Good). 20
(Land O'Lakes No Fat) 30
(Naturally Yours) 20

CREAMERS, NONDAIRY, one tablespoon, except as noted
See also "Cream"

calories

(Coffee-mate) 20
(Coffee-mate Fat Free) 10
(Coffee-mate Lite) 10
(Rich's Coffee Rich) 25
(Rich's Coffee Rich Light) 15
(Rich's Farm Rich) 20
(Rich's Farm Rich Fat Free) 10
(Rich's Farm Rich Light) 10
flavored, all flavors, liquid (Coffee-mate) 40
flavored, all flavors, powdered (Coffee-mate), 1⅓ tbsp. 60
powdered (Coffee-mate/Coffee-mate Lite), 1 tsp. 10
powdered (Cremora/Cremora Fat Free/Lite), 1 tsp. 10

FLAVORED MILK BEVERAGES
See also "Milk," and "Cocoa & Flavored Mixes, Dry"

calories

banana flavor, low-fat, dairy pack (Nestlé Quik), 1 cup 200
bananaberry shake, dairy pack (Nestlé Killer), 14 oz. 450
Butterfinger, dairy pack (Nestlé Quik), 1 cup 200
chocolate drink (Yoo-Hoo), 9 fl. oz. 150
chocolate drink (Yoo-Hoo), 11-fl.-oz. can 180
• chocolate flavor:
    (Sego) Lite), 10 oz. 150
    almond or creamy milk (Sweet Success), 10 oz. 200
    almond, creamy milk, or fudge (Sweet Success), 12 oz. . . . 220
    creamy milk (Nestlé Instant Breakfast),
        10 oz. 220
    fudge, mocha, or raspberry truffle (Sweet Success), 10 oz. . 200
    regular or Dutch (Sego Lite), 10 oz. 150
    regular or malt (Sego), 10 oz. 240
chocolate milk, dairy pack, 8 fl. oz.:
    (Crowley's) 220

(Nestlé Quik) 230
  fat-free *(Hershey's)* 130
  low-fat *(Hershey's)* 190
  low-fat *(Lactaid 1%)* 180
  low-fat *(Nestlé Quik)* 190
  low-fat *(Nestlé Quik Aseptic)* 200
chocolate milk, lowfat, packaged *(Parmalat)*, 8 fl. oz. 180
chocolate shake, dairy pack *(Nestlé Killer)*, 14 oz. 470
chocolate shake, dairy pack *(Nestlé Quik)*, 9 oz. 300
eggnog, dairy pack, ½ cup:
  (Borden) 160
  (Borden Light) 150
  (Crowley) 190
  (Crowley Light) 120
  (Crowley Nonfat) 130
mocha drink, dairy pack *(Nestlé Mocha Cooler)*, 1 cup 170
mocha drink, cafe, canned *(Carnation Instant Breakfast)*,
  10 fl. oz. 220
root beer shake, dairy pack *(Nestlé Killer)*, 14 oz. 460
strawberry flavor, canned, 10 fl. oz.:
  (Sego) 240
  (Sego Lite) 150
  creme *(Carnation Instant Breakfast)* 220
strawberry milk, dairy pack:
  (Nestlé Quik), 1 cup 230
  low-fat *(Nestlé Quik)*, 1 cup 200
  low-fat *(Nestlé Quik)*, 8-oz. container 210
  banana *(Nestlé Quik)*, 1 cup 200
strawberry shake, dairy pack *(Nestlé Killer)*, 14 oz. 420
strawberry shake, dairy pack *(Nestlé Quik)*, 9 oz. 270
vanilla flavor, canned, 10 fl. oz.:
  (Sego) 240
  (Sego Lite) 150
  creme *(Sweet Success)* 200
  French *(Sego Lite)* 150
vanilla shake, dairy pack *(Nestlé Killer)*, 14 oz. 430
vanilla shake, dairy pack *(Nestlé Quik)*, 9 oz. 280

YOGURT
See also "Frozen Yogurt" and "Frozen Yogurt Bars & Cup"

calories

plain:
    (Breyers), 8 oz. 130
    (Dannon Lowfat), 8 oz. 140
    (Dannon Lowfat), 1 cup 150
    (Dannon Nonfat), 8 oz. 110
    (Dannon Nonfat), 1 cup 120
    (Friendship), 1 cup 150
    (Ultimate 90), 8 oz. 90
    (Weight Watchers Nonfat), 1 cup 90
    (Yoplait), 6 oz. 100
    (Yoplait Extra Creamy Nonfat), 8 oz. 130
all flavors:
    (Colombo Light), 8 oz. 100
    (Dannon Light), 8 oz. 100
    (Dannon Sprinkl'ins Magic Crystals), 4.1 oz. 110
    (Yoplait Custard Style), 4 oz. 130
    (Yoplait Custard Style), 6 oz. 190
    (Weight Watchers Nonfat), 1 cup 90
    (Yoplait Light), 6 oz. 90
    except banana creme strawberry *(Dannon Double Delights)*,
        8 oz. 170
    except cherry cheesecake *(Yoplait* Crunch 'n Yogurt Light),
        7 oz. 140
    except coconut cream pie *(Yoplait)*, 6 oz. 180
    except vanilla chocolate crunch *(Dannon Light 'n Crunchy)*,
        8 oz. 140
all fruit flavors:
    (Dannon Chunky Fruit), 6 oz. 110
    (Dannon Fruit on Bottom), 8 oz. 240
    (Dannon Fruit on Bottom Minipack), 4.4 oz. 130
    (Dannon Minipack), 4.4 oz. 120
    (Dannon Sprinkl'ins Rainbow Sprinkles), 4.1 oz. 130
    (Light 'N Lively Free 50 Cal), 4.4 oz. 50
    (Yoplait), 4 oz. 120
    (Yoplait Fruit-on-the-Bottom Fat Free), 6 oz. 160
    (Yoplait Trix), 4 oz. 110
    (Yoplait Trix), 6 oz. 160
    except banana/strawberry *(Colombo* Fat Free), 8 oz. 200

banana *(Tropifruita)*, 6 oz. 150
banana creme strawberry *(Dannon Double Delights)*, 6 oz. 160
banana-strawberry *(Colombo Fat Free)*, 8 oz. 220
berry, mixed:
    (Breyers), 8 oz. 250
    (Knudsen Free), 6 oz. 170
    (Light n' Lively Free), 6 oz. 170
blueberry:
    (Breyers), 8 oz. 250
    (Dannon Danimals), 4.4 oz. 130
    (Knudsen Cal 70), 6 oz. 70
    (Light n' Lively Multi), 4.4 oz. 140
    (Light n' Lively Free), 6 oz. 190
    (Light n' Lively Free 70 Cal), 6 oz. 70
    and creme *(Ultimate 90)*, 8 oz. 90
cappuccino *(Ultimate 90)*, 8 oz. 90
cappuccino, all flavors *(Colombo Fat Free)*, 8 oz. 170
cherry, black:
    (Breyers), 8 oz. 260
    (Knudsen Cal 70), 6 oz. 70
    (Light n' Lively Free 70 Cal), 6 oz. 70
cherry cheesecake *(Yoplait Crunch 'n Yogurt Light)*, 7 oz. 130
cherry jubilee *(Ultimate 90)*, 8 oz. 90
coconut cream pie *(Yoplait)*, 6 oz. 200
coffee:
    (Breyers), 8 oz. 220
    (Dannon Natural Flavored), 8 oz. 210
    (Dannon Natural Flavored), 1 cup 230
cranberry raspberry *(Dannon Natural Flavored)*, 8 oz. 210
cranberry raspberry *(Ultimate 90)*, 8 oz. 90
guava *(Tropifruita)*, 6 oz. 150
lemon:
    (Dannon Natural Flavored), 8 oz. 210
    (Dannon Natural Flavored), 1 cup 230
    (Knudsen Cal 70), 6 oz. 70
    (Knudsen Free), 6 oz. 160
    (Light n' Lively Free), 6 oz. 170
    (Light n' Lively Free 70 Cal), 6 oz. 70
    creamy *(Breyers)*, 8 oz. 220
lemon chiffon:
    (Ultimate 90), 8 oz. 90
    with blueberry *(Dannon Light'n Crunchy)*, 8 oz. 140

Yogurt *(cont.)*

lemon ice or grape lemonade *(Dannon Danimals)*, 4.4 oz. 120
mango *(Tropifruita)*, 6 oz. 150
orange-banana *(Dannon Danimals)*, 4.4 oz. 130
papaya-pineapple *(Tropifruita)*, 6 oz. 150
peach:
   (Breyers), 8 oz. 250
   (Knudsen Cal 70), 6 oz. 70
   (Knudsen Free), 6 oz. 170
   (Light n' Lively Multi), 4.4 oz. 140
   (Light n' Lively Free), 6 oz. 170
   (Light n' Lively Free 70 Cal), 6 oz. 70
   (Ultimate 90), 8 oz. 90
piña colada *(Tropifruita)*, 6 oz. 150
pineapple:
   (Breyers), 8 oz. 250
   (Knudsen Cal 70), 6 oz. 70
   (Light n' Lively Multi), 4.4 oz. 140
raspberry:
   (Dannon Danimals), 4.4 oz. 120
   (Light n' Lively Multi), 4.4 oz. 130
   creme *(Ultimate 90)*, 8 oz. .90
raspberry or strawberry:
   (Breyers), 8 oz. 250
   (Knudsen Cal 70), 6 oz. 70
   (Knudsen Free), 6 oz. 160
   (Light n' Lively Free), 6 oz. 180
   (Light n' Lively Free 70 Cal), 6 oz. 70
strawberry:
   (Dannon Danimals), 4.4 oz. 130
   (Light n' Lively Multi), 4.4 oz. 140
   (Tropifruita), 6 oz. 150
   (Ultimate 90), 8 oz. 90
   (Yoplait), 4 oz. 140
   (Yoplait), 6 oz. 180
   fruit basket *(Knudsen Cal 70)*, 6 oz. 70
   fruit cup *(Light n' Lively Free)*, 6 oz. 170
   fruit cup *(Light n' Lively* Multi), 4.4 oz. 140
   fruit cup *(Light n' Lively Free* 70 Cal), 6 oz. 70
   wild *(Light n' Lively* Kidpack), 4.4 oz. 140
strawberry-banana:
   (Breyers), 8 oz. 250

(Knudsen 70), 6 oz. 70
(Light n' Lively Multi), 4.4 oz. 140
(Light n' Lively Free 70 Cal), 6 oz. 70
(Tropifruita), 6 oz. 150
(Ultimate 90), 8 oz. 90
(Yoplait), 4 oz. 140
(Yoplait), 6 oz. 180
strawberry-kiwi *(Tropifruita)*, 6 oz. 150
tropical punch *(Dannon Danimals)*, 4.4 oz. 130
vanilla:
   (Breyers), 8 oz. 220
   (Dannon Natural Flavored), 8 oz. 210
   (Dannon Natural Flavored), 1 cup 230
   (Dannon Danimals), 4.4 oz. 120
   (Knudsen Cal 70), 6 oz. 70
   (Knudsen Free), 6 oz. 170
   (Light n' Lively Free), 6 oz. 160
   (Ultimate 90), 8 oz. 90
   (Yoplait Extra Creamy Non-Fat), 8 oz. 210
   chocolate crunch *(Dannon Light 'n Crunchy)*, 8 oz. 130

Chapter 4

CHEESE AND CHEESE PRODUCTS

CHEESE*, one ounce, except as noted
*See also "Cheese, Substitute or Imitation," "Cheese Food,"
"Cheese Product," and "Cheese Spreads"*

	calories
American, processed:	
(Boar's Head Loaf)	100
(Borden), ⅔-oz. slice	70
(Borden), ¾-oz. slice	80
(Borden Loaf)	110
(Harvest Moon), ⅔-oz. slice	70
(Kraft Deluxe Loaf)	100
(Kraft Deluxe Slice), ⅔-oz. slice	70
(Kraft Deluxe Slice), ¾-oz. slice	80
(Kraft Deluxe Slice), 1-oz. slice	110
(Old English Loaf)	100
(Old English Slice), 1-oz. slice	110
(Schwan's), ⅔-oz. slice	70
(Weight Watchers Reduced Sodium), ¾-oz. slice	30
sharp *(Borden)*	110
(Bel Paese):	
medallions, ¾ oz.	65
with basil and sun-dried tomatoes	101
flavored varieties	110
blue *(Kraft)*	100
blue, crumbled *(Sargento),* ¼ cup, 1 oz.	100
brick *(Kraft)*	110

* Note: Unless otherwise noted, data listed for a cheese apply to all the forms in which
it may be packaged—slices, loaves, wedges, and the like. Be careful not to confuse
"real" cheese with a "cheese spread" or a "cheese food" that bears the same or a
similar name. Generally, it isn't hard to differentiate between cheese and cheese
spreads, but cheese foods sometimes pose a problem (especially when packaged in
slices). Check the label if you're confused about a product; if it is a cheese food, the
label will say so.

butterkase, plain or smoked *(Boar's Head)* 100
cheddar:
    (Alpine Lace Reduced Fat) 80
    (Boar's Head Double Gloucester) 110
    (Cracker Barrel) 110
    (Cracker Barrel 1/3 Less Fat) 80
    (Dorman) 110
    (Dorman Reduced Fat) 80
    (Heluva Good Low Sodium) 110
    (Land O'Lakes) 110
    (Land O'Lakes Cheddarella) 100
    mild *(Heluva* Good Reduced Fat) 80
    mild *(Kraft* 1/3 Less Fat) 80
    mild, light, snack *(MooTown Snackers)*, .8-oz. piece 60
    mild or sharp *(MooTown Snackers)*, .8-oz. piece 100
    mild or sharp *(Weight Watchers)* 80
    mild, sharp, or extra sharp *(Heluva* Good) 110
    nacho, with peppers *(Kraft)* 110
    sharp *(Boar's Head* Slicing) 110
    sharp *(Kraft* Less Fat) 80
    sharp *(Sargento* Sliced) 110
    sharp *(Weight Watchers* Fat Free), 3/4-oz. slice 30
cheddar, shredded:
    (Kraft), 1/4 cup 120
    fat free *(Kraft Healthy Favorites)*, 1/4 cup 45
    fine *(Kraft)*, 1/4 cup .90
    mild *(Heluva* Good), 1/4 cup 110
    mild *(Kraft* 1/3 Less Fat), 1/4 cup 90
    mild *(Sargento Preferred Light)*, 1/4 cup 70
    mild or sharp *(Sargento)*, 1/4 cup 110
    sharp *(Cracker Barrel* 1/3 Less Fat), 1/4 cup 80
    sharp, New York State *(Heluva* Good) 110
Colby:
    (Alpine Lace Reduced Fat) 80
    (Dorman Sandwich), 1.1-oz. slice 130
    (Kraft) 110
    (Kraft 1/3 Less Fat) .80
    (Sargento Sliced) 110
    mild *(Heluva* Good Longhorn) 117
Colby Jack:
    (Heluva Good) 110
    shredded *(Heluva* Good), 1/4 cup 110

Cheese, Colby Jack *(cont.)*
  shredded *(Sargento)*, 1/4 cup 110
  snack *(MooTown Snackers)*, .8 oz. 90
Colby Monterey Jack *(Kraft)* 110
Colby Monterey Jack, shredded *(Kraft)*, 1/4 cup 120
cottage cheese, *see "Cottage Cheese," page 67*
cream cheese:
  (Boar's Head) 100
  (Philadelphia Brand) 100
  (Western Creamy), 2 tbsp., 1.1 oz. 70
  (Western Creamy Light), 2 tbsp., 1.1 oz. 50
  with chive or pimiento *(Philadelphia Brand)* 90
  fat free *(Philadelphia Brand)* 25
cream cheese, soft, 2 tbsp.:
  plain *(Friendship)* 100
  plain *(Philadelphia Brand)* 100
  plain, fat free *(Philadelphia Brand)* 30
  plain, light *(Philadelphia Brand)* 70
  plain, reduced fat *(Friendship)* 50
  with chives and onion or herb and garlic *(Philadelphia
    Brand)* 110
  with olive and pimiento *(Philadelphia Brand)* 100
  with pineapple or strawberries *(Philadelphia Brand)* 100
  with smoked salmon *(Philadelphia Brand)* 100
cream cheese, whipped, 3 tbsp.:
  plain *(Breakstone's Temp-Tee)* 110
  plain *(Philadelphia Brand)* 110
  with smoked salmon *(Philadelphia Brand)* 100
curd, extra sharp *(Heluva* Good) 110
Edam *(Boar's Head)* .90
Edam *(Dorman* Sliced) 90
farmer:
  (Friendship) 50
  (Kraft) 100
  (Western Creamy), 2.3 oz. 100
  dry *(Western Creamy* Fat Free), 2 oz. 50
feta:
  (Alpine Lace Reduced Fat) 60
  (Classika Portions) 100
  (Krinos Imported) .90
fontina *(Classica)* 110
Gorgonzola *(Galbani* Dolcelatte) 93

Gouda:
    (Boar's Head) 110
    (Dorman Sliced) 100
    (Kraft) 110
Havarti:
    (Boar's Head) 110
    (Dorman Sliced) 100
    (Kraft Casino) 120
hoop cheese *(Friendship)* 20
hot pepper *(Alpine Lace)* 80
Italian *(Classica Italiana)* 110
Italian blend, shredded *(Heluva Good)*, ¼ cup 90
Italian style:
    grated *(Kraft* ⅓ Less Fat), 2 tsp. 25
    grated *(Weight Watchers* Fat Free Topping), 1 tbsp. 20
    shredded *(Sargento Recipe Blend)*, ¼ cup 90
Jarlsberg *(Sargento)*, 1.2-oz. slice 120
(Laughing Cow Babybel 7 oz.) 100
(Laughing Cow Babybel Mini), ¾-oz. piece 70
(Laughing Cow Original Wedge) 70
Limburger *(Kraft Mohawk Valley)* 90
mascarpone *(Classica* Domestic) 120
mascarpone *(Galbani* Imported) 140
Mexican, 4, shredded *(Sargento Recipe Blend)*, ¼ cup 110
Monterey Jack:
    (Boar's Head) 100
    (Dorman) 100
    (Dorman), 1.2-oz. slice 130
    (Dorman Reduced Fat) 80
    (Dorman Reduced Fat), 1.5-oz. slice 120
    (Kraft) 110
    (Kraft ⅓ Less Fat) 80
    (Land O'Lakes) 110
    (Sargento Sliced) 100
    regular or jalapeño *(Heluva* Good) 100
    shredded *(Dorman)*, ⅓ cup, 1 oz. 80
    shredded *(Kraft)*, ¼ cup 110
    shredded *(Sargento)*, ¼ cup 100
    jalapeño *(Boar's Head)* 100
    jalapeño *(Kraft)* 110
    peppers *(Kraft* ⅓ Less Fat) 80

Cheese *(cont.)*
mozzarella:
    (Boar's Head) 90
    (Polly-O Fat Free) 35
    (Polly-O Fior Di Latte) 80
    (Polly-O Lite) 60
    whole milk *(Heluva* Good) 80
    whole milk *(Polly-O)* 80
    part skim *(Alpine Lace* Reduced Fat) 70
    part skim *(Dorman)* 80
    part skim *(Kraft)* 80
    part skim *(Polly-O)*, ¼ cup 90
    part skim, regular or string *(Heluva* Good) 70
    sliced *(Sargento)*, 1.6-oz. slice 130
    sliced *(Sargento Preferred Light)*, 1.6 oz. 90
mozzarella, shredded, ¼ cup:
    (Heluva Good) 80
    (Sargento) 80
    (Sargento Preferred Light) 70
    whole milk *(Kraft)* 90
    whole milk *(Polly-O)* 90
    part skim *(Kraft)* 90
    part skim *(Kraft* ⅓ Less Fat) 80
    part skim *(Polly-O)* 80
    part skim, fine *(Kraft)* 70
    fat free *(Kraft Healthy Favorites)* 50
    fat free *(Polly-O)* 45
    light *(Polly-O* Lite) 60
Muenster:
    (Alpine Lace Reduced Sodium) 100
    (Boar's Head) 100
    (Boar's Head Low Sodium) 100
    (Dorman), 1-oz. slice 100
    (Dorman), 1.5-oz. slice 160
    (Dorman Reduced Fat), 1.5 oz. 120
    (Dorman Reduced Sodium), 1.5 oz. 160
    (Heluva Good) 100
    (Kraft) 110
    (Sargento Sliced) 100
Neufchâtel *(Philadelphia Brand)* 70
Parmesan, grated:
    (Classica), 1 tbsp. 20

(Kraft), 2 tsp. 20
(Kraft Italian Blend), 2 tsp. 25
(Polly-O), 2 tsp. 25
(Sargento), 1 tbsp. .25
Parmesan, shredded:
   (Classica), 1 tbsp. 20
   (Kraft), 2 tsp. 20
   (Sargento), ¼ cup 110
Parmesan-Romano, grated *(Sargento)*, 1 tbsp. 25
Parmesan-Romano, shredded *(Sargento)*, ¼ cup 110
pimiento, processed *(Kraft* Deluxe) 100
pizza, shredded, ¼ cup:
   (Heluva Good) 90
   (Sargento) 90
   (Sargento Pizza Double Cheese) 90
   cheddar, mild, and mozzarella *(Kraft)* 90
   four cheese *(Kraft)* 90
   mozzarella and cheddar *(Kraft)* 100
   mozzarella and smoked provolone *(Kraft)* 90
provolone:
   (Alpine Lace Reduced Fat) 70
   (Boar's Head) 100
   (Dorman) 100
   (Dorman Reduced Fat), 1.5 oz. 120
   (Sargento Sliced) 100
   smoke flavor *(Kraft)* 100
ricotta, ¼ cup:
   (Breakstone's) 110
   (Polly-O Light) .70
   (Sargento Light) 60
   (Sargento Old Fashioned) 90
   whole milk *(Polly-O)* 110
   part skim *(Polly-O)* 90
   part skim *(Sargento)* 80
   fat free *(Polly-O)* 50
Romano, grated:
   (Kraft), 2 tsp. .25
   dry *(Classica* Pecorino), 1 tbsp. 20
   fresh *(Classica* Pecorino), 1 tbsp. 20
Romano, shredded *(Classica* Pecorino), 1 tbsp. 20
Romano-Parmesan, grated *(Polly-O)*, 2 tsp. 25

Cheese *(cont.)*
string:
 (Polly-O) 80
 (Polly-O Light Mozzarella) 60
 snack *(Handi-Snacks/Kraft),* 1 piece 80
 snack *(MooTown Snackers),* .8 oz. 70
 snack *(Polly-O),* ³/₄ oz. 60
 snack, light *(MooTown Snackers),* .8 oz. 60
Swiss:
 (Alpine Lace Reduced Fat) 90
 (Boar's Head Domestic) 100
 (Boar's Head Gold Label Imported/No Salt) 110
 (Borden) 100
 (Dorman), 1.2-oz. slice 130
 (Dorman Low Sodium), 1.2-oz. slice 130
 (Dorman Reduced Fat), 1.2-oz. slice 100
 (Dorman Sandwich) 100
 (Dorman Very Low Sodium) 110
 (Kraft) 110
 (Sargento Sliced), ³/₄-oz. slice 80
 (Sargento Preferred Light Sliced) 80
 (Sargento Wafer Thin Sliced), 2 slices 110
 (Weight Watchers Fat Free), ³/₄-oz. slice 30
 baby *(Boar's Head)* 110
 baby *(Cracker Barrel)* 110
 processed *(Kraft* Deluxe), ³/₄-oz. slice 70
 processed *(Kraft* Deluxe), 1-oz. slice 90
 shredded *(Kraft),* ¹/₄ cup 110
 shredded *(Sargento),* ¹/₄ cup 110
taco, shredded, ¹/₄ cup:
 (Heluva Good) .110
 (Sargento) 110
 (Sargento Preferred Light) 70
 cheddar and Monterey Jack *(Kraft)* 100
 nacho and taco *(Sargento)* 110
(Tal-Fino Taleggio) .110

CHEESE, SUBSTITUTE OR IMITATION
See also "Cheese," "Cheese Food," "Cheese Product," and "Vegetarian Foods, Frozen or Refrigerated"

	calories
(Sandwich-Mate), .7-oz. slice	60
all varieties:	
(AlmondRella), 1 oz.	60
(Smart Beat), ²/₃ oz.	25
(TofuRella), 1 oz.	80
(VeganRella), 1 oz.	60
(Weight Watchers Fat Free Slices)*, ³/₄-oz. slice	30
(Zero-FatRella), 1 oz.	40
American flavor:	
(Borden), 1 slice	60
(Cheeztwo/Sandwich-Mate), 1 slice	60
(Golden Image), ³/₄ oz.	70
(Lunchwagon), ²/₃ oz.	60
(Lunchwagon), ³/₄ oz.	70
(Smart Beat Fat Free)*, ²/₃ oz.	25
shredded *(Harvest Moon)*, ¹/₄ cup	120
Swiss *(Borden)*, 1 slice	60
cheddar flavor:	
(Borden/Bordern Taco Mate)*, 1 oz.	100
fortified *(Borden)*, 1 oz.	100
shredded *(Harvest Moon)*, ¹/₄ cup	120
shredded *(Sargento)*, ¹/₄ cup	90
"cream cheese," all varieties *(Tofutti Better than Cream Cheese)*, 1 oz.	80
Jamaican Jack style *(HempRella)*, 1 oz.	70
Monterey Jack *(Borden)*, 1 oz.	90
mozzarella, shredded:	
(Borden), 1 oz.	90
(Harvest Moon), ¹/₄ cup	110
(Sargento), ¹/₄ cup	80
Swiss *(Borden)*, 1 slice	60

CHEESE FOOD
See also "Cheese," "Cheese, Substitute or Imitation," "Cheese Product," and "Cheese Spreads"

---

                                                              calories

American:
  (Borden), .7-oz. slice 70
  (Heluva Good), 1 oz. 70
  (Kraft Singles), ⅔-oz. slice 60
  (Kraft Singles), ¾-oz. slice 70
  (Kraft Singles), 1.2-oz. slice 110
  grated *(Kraft)*, 1 tbsp. .25
cheddar:
  sharp *(Kaukauna* Premium Blend), 1 oz. 100
  sharp *(Kaukauna Lite 50)*, 1 oz. 70
  sharp or extra sharp *(Cracker Barrel)*, 2 tbsp. 100
  sharp or extra sharp *(Kaukauna)*, 1 oz. 90
with garlic *(Kraft)*, 1 oz. 90
with jalapeños:
  (Kraft), 1 oz. 90
  (Kraft Mexican Singles), ¾-oz. slice 70
  shredded, hot or mild *(Velveeta* Mexican), ¼ cup 130
Monterey *(Kraft* Singles), ¾-oz. slice 70
with pimiento *(Kraft* Singles), ⅔-oz. slice 60
with pimiento *(Kraft* Singles), ¾-oz. slice 70
port wine:
  (Kaukauna), 1 oz. 90
  (Kaukauna Premium Blend), 1 oz. 100
  (Kaukauna Lite), 1 oz. 70
  (Wispride Cup), 2 tbsp. 100
  (Wispride Light Cup), 2 tbsp. 80
sharp *(Kraft* Singles), ¾-oz. slice 70
shredded *(Velveeta)*, ¼ cup 130
smoke flavor *(Kaukauna* Smokey), 1 oz. 90
smoke flavor *(Kaukauna Lite 50* Smokey), 1 oz. 70
Swiss:
  (Borden), 1 slice 70
  (Kraft Singles), ¾-oz. slice 70
  almond *(Kaukauna)*, 1 oz. 90
  almond *(Kaukauna Lite 50)*, 1 oz. 70

CHEESE PRODUCT, processed
*See also "Cheese," "Cheese, Substitute or Imitation," and
"Cheese Food"*

	calories
(Cheeze Whiz Light), 2 tbsp.	.80
(Kraft Free Singles), ⅔-oz. slice	.30
(Kraft Free Singles), ¾-oz. slice	.30
(Velveeta Light), 1 oz.	.60
all varieties *(Borden* Fat Free), 1 slice	.25
all varieties *(Lite-Line),* .7-oz. slice	.30

American flavor:

(Alpine Lace), 1 oz.	.80
(Alpine Lace Nonfat), ¾-oz. slice	.30
(Alpine Lace Nonfat), 1 oz.	.45
(Borden Fat Free), ¾-oz. slice	.45
(Borden Light), ¾-oz. slice	.45
(Borden Lowfat), 1 slice	.30
(Harvest Moon), ⅔ oz.	.50
(Kraft Deluxe 25% Less Fat), ¾-oz. slice	.70
(Kraft Singles Less Fat), ¾-oz. slice	.50
(Light N' Lively 50% Less Fat), ¾-oz. slice	.50
(Light N' Lively White 50% Less Fat), ¾-oz. slice	.50

cheddar flavor:

(Alpine Lace Nonfat), 1 oz.	.45
all varieties *(Spreadery),* 2 tbsp.	.80
sharp *(Kraft* Singles ⅓ Less Fat), ¾-oz. slice	.50
sharp *(Kraft Free* Singles), ¾-oz. slice	.30

mozzarella *(Alpine Lace* Nonfat), 1 oz.	.45

Neufchâtel, 2 tbsp.:

garlic herb *(Spreadery)*	.80
ranch *(Spreadery)*	.80
vegetable *(Spreadery)*	.70
pimiento *(Spreadery),* 2 tbsp.	100

Swiss flavor:

(Kraft Singles Less Fat), ¾-oz. slice	.50
(Kraft Free Singles), ¾-oz. slice	.30

CHEESE SPREADS, two tablespoons, except as noted
*See also "Cheese," "Cheese Food," "Cheese Product," and
"Dips"*

	calories
(Cheez Whiz)	90
(Squeeze-A-Snak)	90
(Velveeta), 1 oz.	80
(Velveeta Italiana), 1 oz.	80
all varieties *(Heluva Good)*	90
American:	
(Borden), 1 oz.	80
(Easy Cheese)	100
(Harvest Moon), ²/₃ oz.	60
(Harvest Moon), ³/₄ oz.	60
(The Big!), 1 slice	80
with bacon *(Kraft)*	90
blue cheese *(Kraft Roka)*	80
cheddar, regular, bacon, or sharp *(Easy Cheese)*	100
with jalapeños:	
(Cheez Whiz)	90
(Kraft), 1 oz.	80
hot or mild *(Velveeta Mexican)*, 1 oz.	80
Limburger *(Mohawk Valley)*	80
nacho *(Easy Cheese)*	100
nacho *(The Big!)*, 1 slice	80
Neufchâtel, garden vegetable, garlic and herb,	
or ranch *(Kaukauna)*, 1 oz.	80
nut log, sharp *(Wispride)*	100
olive and pimiento *(Kraft)*	70
pimiento:	
(Kraft)	80
(Price's)	80
(Price's Light)	60
pineapple *(Kraft)*	70
salsa, hot *(Cheez Whiz)*	90
salsa, mild *(Cheez Whiz)*	90
sharp *(Old English)*	90
slices:	
(Velveeta), ³/₄ oz.	60
(Velveeta), ⁴/₅ oz.	70
(Velveeta), 1.2 oz.	100

COTTAGE CHEESE, ½ cup, except as noted	

	calories
(Breakstone's Dry Curd), ¼ cup	45
4% fat, creamed:	
(Breakstone's)	120
(Friendship California Style)	115
(Knudsen Large Curd)	130
(Knudsen Small Curd)	120
(Sealtest)	120
pineapple *(Friendship)*	140
2% fat:	
(Breakstone's)	90
(Friendship Pot Style)	90
(Knudsen)	100
(Sealtest)	90
(Weight Watchers)	90
1% fat, low-fat:	
(Friendship)	90
(Light n' Lively)	80
(Weight Watchers)	90
garden salad *(Light 'n Lively)*	90
peach, pineapple, or strawberry, 1.5% *(Knudsen)*, 4 oz.	110
peach and pineapple *(Light n' Lively)*	120
pineapple *(Friendship)*	120
tropical fruit *(Knudsen)*, 4 oz.	120
nonfat:	
(Friendship)	80
(Knudsen Free)	80
(Light n' Lively Free)	80
peach *(Friendship)*	110

Chapter 5

FRUIT AND FRUIT PRODUCTS

FRUIT, FRESH
See also "Fruit, Canned or in Jars," "Fruit, Frozen," and "Fruit, Dried"

	calories
apple *(Dole)*, 1 fruit	80
apricot *(Dole)*, ½ cup	37
atemoya *(Frieda's)*, 3.5 oz.	94
avocado *(Dole)*, ⅕ medium, 1.1 oz.	60
banana *(Dole)*, 1 fruit	120
banana, manzano *(Frieda's)*, 1 oz.	24
cactus pear, peeled *(Frieda's)*, 3.5 oz.	42
cantaloupe *(Dole)*, ¼ fruit	50
carambola *(Frieda's)*, 3.5 oz.	35
cherimoya *(Frieda's)*, 3.5 oz.	94
cherry *(Dole)*, 1 cup	90
coconut *(Dole)*, 1 cup, not packed	283
crabapple, with peel *(Frieda's)*, 1 oz.	19
cranberry, whole *(Dole)*, ½ cup	23
fig, Calimyrna *(Frieda's)*, 1 oz.	23
grape *(Dole)*, 1½ cups	85
grapefruit *(Dole)*, ¼ fruit	50
honeydew melon *(Dole)*, ⅒ fruit	50
kiwi *(Dole)*, 2 fruits	90
kiwi, fuzzless *(Frieda's)*, 1 oz.	10
lemon or lime *(Dole)*, 1 medium	20
loquat *(Frieda's)*, 3.5 oz.	48
lychee, shelled, peeled *(Frieda's)*, 1 oz.	18
mango, peeled *(Frieda's)*, 1 oz.	19
mango, peeled, sliced *(Dole)*, ½ cup	54
nectarine *(Dole)*, 1 fruit	70
orange *(Dole)*, 1 fruit	50
papaya, peeled *(Frieda's)*, 1 oz.	11
papaya, peeled, cubed *(Dole)*, ½ cup	27
passion fruit, purple *(Frieda's)*, 3.5 oz.	90

peach *(Dole)*, 2 fruits 70
pear *(Dole)*, 1 fruit 100
persimmon:
   (Dole), 1 medium 32
   fuyu *(Frieda's)*, 1 oz. 22
   hachiya, trimmed *(Frieda's)*, 1 oz. 36
pineapple, baby, trimmed *(Frieda's Sugarloaf)*, 1 oz. . . .14
pineapple, sliced *(Dole)*, 2 slices 90
plantain *(Frieda's)*, 1 oz. 34
plum *(Dole)*, 2 fruits 70
pomegranate *(Dole)*, 1 medium 104
pomegranate *(Frieda's)*, 1 oz. 18
prickly pear *(Frieda's)*, 3½ oz. 42
pummelo *(Frieda's)*, 3.5 oz. 38
quince, pineapple, pulp *(Frieda's)*, 3.5 oz. 57
raspberry *(Dole)*, 1 cup .45
rhubarb, regular or hothouse *(Frieda's)*, 1 oz. 5
strawberry *(Dole)*, 8 fruits 50
tangerine *(Dole)*, 2 fruits 70
watermelon *(Dole)*, ¹/₁₈ medium, 10 oz. 90
watermelon, seedless *(Frieda's)*, 1 oz. 7

FRUIT, CANNED OR IN JARS, ½ cup, except as noted
See also "Fruit, Fresh," "Fruit, Frozen," "Fruit, Dried," and "Pie Fillings, Canned"

                                          calories

apple:
   baked *(Seneca)*, 1 apple 70
   baked, Dutch *(Lucky Leaf/Musselman's)* 170
   escalloped *(White House)* 160
   fried *(Apple Time/Lucky Leaf)* 170
   sliced *(Comstock Original)*, ⅓ cup 30
   sliced *(Lucky Leaf/Musselman's)* 50
   sliced *(Musselman's Home Style)* 170
   sliced *(Seneca Sweetened)* 50
   sliced *(Seneca Unsweetened)* 45
   sliced *(White House)* 100
   sliced *(Wilderness)* .30
   spiced rings *(Lucky Leaf/Musselman's)*, 1.1-oz. ring 35
   spiced rings *(S&W)*, 2 rings 25
   spiced rings *(White House)*, ½-oz. ring 30

Fruit, Canned or in Jars, apple *(cont.)*

spiced rings, red *(Comstock/Wilderness)*, 2 rings, 1.1 oz.   . .25

applesauce:

(Apple Time Regular/Granny Smith/Red Delicious/McIntosh) . .90

(Apple Time/Lucky Leaf/Musselman's Lite) 50

(Lincoln) 90

(Lucky Leaf), 4-oz. jar .80

(Lucky Leaf Cinnamon) 100

(Lucky Leaf Regular/Chunky/Delicious) 90

(Lucky Leaf Regular/Cinnamon), 6-oz. jar 120

(Mott's/Mott's Chunky) 110

(Mott's Cinnamon) 120

(Musselman's), 6 oz. 120

(Musselman's Chunky/Cinnamon) 100

(Musselman's Cinnamon), 6 oz. 130

(Musselman's Regular/Cinnamon), 4 oz. 80

(Musselman's Regular/Delicious/McIntosh/Premium) 90

(S&W Gravenstein) 90

(Seneca Regular/Cinnamon/McIntosh/Golden Delicious) 100

(Tree Top Original/Cinnamon) 100

(Tree Top Original/Cinnamon), 4 oz. 90

(White House) 90

(White House Cinnamon) 100

applesauce, unsweetened/natural:

(Apple Time/Apple Time 4 oz./*Lincoln)* 50

(Eden) 50

(Lucky Leaf), 6 oz. 70

(Lucky Leaf Regular/Cinnamon/Regular 4 oz./Cinnamon
4 oz.)* 50

(Musselman's), 6 oz. 70

(Musselman's Regular/Cinnamon/Regular 4 oz./Cinnamon
4 oz.)* 50

(S&W Gravenstein) 50

(Santa Cruz Regular/Gravenstein) 45

(Seneca) 60

(Tree Top/Tree Top 4 oz.)* 70

(White House) 70

applesauce blends:

with apricot *(Musselman's Fruit 'N Sauce)* 100

with cherry *(Musselman's Fruit 'N Sauce)* 90

with fruit, all varieties *(Santa Cruz)* 45

with peach *(Musselman's Fruit 'N Sauce)* 90

apricot:
    (Del Monte Lite) 60
    in juice *(Libby's* Lite) 60
    in heavy syrup *(Del Monte)* 100
    in heavy syrup *(S&W)* 110
blackberries *(Allens/Wolco),* ²/₃ cup 60
blackberries, in heavy syrup *(Comstock/Wilderness)* 110
blueberries, in heavy syrup:
    (Comstock/Wilderness) 110
    (Lucky Leaf/Musselman's) 120
    (S&W Wild Maine), ¹/₃ cup 70
boysenberries, in heavy syrup *(Comstock/Wilderness)* 120
cherries, pitted:
    sour, red, in water *(Lucky Leaf/Musselman's)* 60
    sweet, dark, in heavy syrup *(Del Monte)* 120
    sweet, dark, in heavy syrup *(S&W)* 140
    sweet, dark, in heavy syrup *(Comstock/Wilderness)* 110
    sweet *(Comstock/Wilderness* Royal Anne) 110
    sweet *(S&W* Royal Anne) 140
    tart red, in water *(Comstock/Wilderness)* 50
    tart red, in heavy syrup *(Comstock/Wilderness* Dessert) . . . 140
citrus salad, in light syrup *(Sunfresh)* 70
crabapple:
    (S&W), 1 piece 35
    in heavy syrup *(Wilderness),* 1 piece, .9 oz. 35
    spiced *(Apple Time),* 1 piece, 1.1 oz. 40
    spiced *(Comstock),* 1 piece, .9 oz. 35
cranberry sauce:
    (Ocean Spray), 2 oz. 80
    (R. W. Knudsen), 1 tbsp. 25
    (S&W), ¹/₄ cup 100
    with orange, raspberry, or strawberry *(Ocean Spray*
      Cran · Fruit), 2 oz. 90
figs, kadota in syrup, *(S&W),* 5 figs 140
fruit, mixed:
    in juice *(Del Monte* Naturals Snack Cup), 4-oz. cup 50
    in juice, chunky *(Del Monte* Naturals) 60
    in juice, chunky *(Libby's* Lite) 60
    in juice, chunky *(S&W* Natural) 70
    in extra light syrup, chunky *(Del Monte* Lite) 60
    in light syrup *(Del Monte* Lite Snack Cup), 4-oz. cup 50
    in heavy syrup *(Del Monte* Snack Cup), 4-oz. cup 80

Fruit, Canned or in Jars, fruit, mixed *(cont.)*
   in heavy syrup, chunky *(Del Monte)* 100
fruit cocktail:
   (Del Monte Very Cherry) 90
   (Hunt's) 90
   in juice *(Del Monte* Naturals) 60
   in juice *(Libby's* Lite) 60
   in juice *(S&W* Natural) 80
   in extra light syrup *(Del Monte* Lite) 60
   in heavy syrup *(Del Monte)* 100
   in heavy syrup *(S&W)* 90
   honey flavor *(Del Monte* Natural) 80
fruit salad:
   in light syrup *(Sunfresh/Sunfresh* Ambrosia) 70
   tropical, in light syrup *(Del Monte)* 80
   tropical, in light syrup *(Dole)* 80
   tropical, in light syrup *(Sunfresh)* 80
gooseberries, in light syrup *(Comstock/Wilderness)* 70
grapefruit *(S&W* Natural Style), ⅔ cup 50
grapefruit, pink or white, in juice *(Sunfresh)* 45
grapes, seedless:
   in heavy syrup *(Comstock)* 100
   in heavy syrup *(S&W)* 100
   in heavy syrup *(S&W* Fancy Jubilee) 130
mango slices, in light syrup *(Sunfresh)* 100
melon salad, in extra light syrup *(Sunfresh* Lite) 45
melon salad, in light syrup *(Sunfresh)* 90
orange sections, in light syrup *(Sunfresh)* 70
papaya slices, in light syrup *(Sunfresh)* 70
peach:
   (Hunt's) 100
   (S&W Ready-Cut California Sun/Ready-Cut Tropical Sun) 80
   with cinnamon *(S&W Sweet Memory* Ready-Cut Sun) 70
   in juice, cling *(Del Monte* Naturals) 60
   in juice, cling *(Libby's* Lite) 60
   in juice, cling *(S&W* Natural) 80
   in juice *(Del Monte* Naturals Snack Cup), 4-oz. cup 50
   in extra light syrup *(Del Monte* Snack Cup), 4-oz. cup 50
   in extra light syrup, cling or freestone *(Del Monte* Lite) 60
   in heavy syrup, cling *(Del Monte/Del Monte* Melba) 100
   in heavy syrup, cling *(Del Monte* Snack Cup), 4-oz. cup 80
   in heavy syrup, cling *(S&W)* 100

in heavy syrup, cling or freestone *(Del Monte)* 100
in heavy syrup, freestone *(S&W)* 100
raspberry flavor, cling, in heavy syrup *(Del Monte)* 80
spiced *(Del Monte* Natural Harvest) 80
spiced, in heavy syrup *(Del Monte)* 100
spiced, in heavy syrup *(S&W),* 4.3-oz. piece 100
pear:
  (S&W Ready-Cut California Sun) 80
  in juice *(Libby's* Lite) 60
  in juice or extra light syrup *(Del Monte* Naturals/Lite) 60
  in extra light syrup *(Del Monte* Snack Cup), 4-oz. cup 50
  in heavy syrup *(Del Monte)* 100
  in heavy syrup *(Del Monte* Snack Cup), 4-oz. cup 80
  Bartlett, in juice *(S&W* Natural) 80
  Bartlett, in heavy syrup *(S&W)* 90
  ginger flavor *(Del Monte* Natural) 90
pineapple:
  in juice, all varieties, except sliced, spears, and wedges
    (Del Monte) 70
  in juice, chunks or tidbits *(Dole)* 60
  in juice, crushed *(Dole)* 70
  in juice, sliced *(Del Monte),* 2 slices 60
  in juice, sliced *(Dole),* 2 slices, 4 oz. 60
  in juice, spears or wedges *(Del Monte)* 70
  in juice, tidbits *(Del Monte* Snack Cup), 4-oz. cup 50
  in light syrup, chunks *(Sunfresh)* 90
  in heavy syrup, crushed or chunks *(Del Monte)* 90
  in heavy syrup, sliced *(Del Monte),* 2 slices 90
  in heavy syrup, sliced *(S&W)* 90
  in syrup, chunks, crushed, or tidbits *(Dole)* 90
  in syrup, sliced *(Dole)* 90
plum, in heavy syrup, whole *(S&W)* 130
plum, purple, in heavy syrup *(Comstock/Wilderness)* 110
prune, in heavy syrup *(Sonoma),* 3–4 pieces, 1.4 oz. 110
prune, stewed, in heavy syrup *(S&W),* 8 pieces, 4.9 oz. 210
raspberries, in heavy syrup *(Comstock/Wilderness)* 100
strawberries, in heavy syrup *(Comstock/Wilderness)* 140
tangerine:
  in juice *(S&W* Mandarin), ⅔ cup 70
  in light syrup *(Del Monte)* .80
  in light syrup *(S&W* Mandarin), ⅔ cup 100

FRUIT, FROZEN
See also "Fruit, Fresh" and "Fruit, Canned or in Jars"

---

	calories
apple fritters, *see "Miscellaneous Desserts," page 307*	
apples, escalloped *(Stouffer's)*, about ⅔ cup, 6 oz.	180
bar, *see "Ice & Sherbet Bars & Cones," page 356*	
berries, mixed *(Big Valley* Burst O' Berries*)*, ¾ cup	70
blackberries *(Schwan's)*, 1¼ cups	60
blackberries *(Stilwell)*, 1 cup	100
blueberries:	
(Cascadian Farm Organic*)*, 1 cup	50
(Schwan's), ⅔ cup	70
(Stilwell), 1 cup	90
cherries, unsweetened:	
dark, sweet *(Big Valley)*, ¾ cup	90
dark, sweet *(Schwan's)*, ⅔ cup	120
tart, red *(Stilwell)*, 1 cup	60
fruit, mixed:	
(Big Valley), ⅔ cup	60
(Schwan's), 1¼ cups	70
(Stilwell), 1 cup	50
mammy apple, chunks *(Goya)*, ⅓ pkg.	140
melon balls *(Stilwell)*, 1 cup	50
papaya, sliced *(Goya)*, ⅓ pkg.	50
passion fruit, chunks *(Goya)*, ⅓ pkg.	70
peach, sliced:	
(Big Valley), ⅔ cup	50
(Schwan's), 1⅓ cups	60
(Stilwell), 1 cup	60
plantain, fried *(Goya* Tostone*)*, 3 pieces	170
raspberries, red:	
(Big Valley), ⅔ cup	60
(Birds Eye Deluxe*)*, ½ cup	90
(Schwan's), 1¼ cups	60
rhubarb *(Stilwell)*, 1 cup	30
strawberries, ⅔ cup, except as noted:	
(Big Valley)	50
(Birds Eye), ½ cup	70
(Schwan's), 1¼ cups	50
(Stilwell)	50
tamarind, chunks *(Goya)*, ⅓ pkg.	70

FRUIT, DRIED, uncooked
See also "Fruit, Fresh," "Fruit, Canned or in Jars," and "Fruit Snacks"

calories

apple:
    (Sonoma), 1.4 oz. 110
    chips *(Smart Snackers),* ¾ oz. 70
    chips, all varieties *(Seneca),* 1 oz. 140
    slices *(Del Monte),* ⅓ cup, 1.4 oz. 80
apricot:
    (Dole Sun Giant Turkish), 6 pieces, 1.4 oz. 90
    (Sonoma), 1.4 oz. 120
    sun-dried *(Del Monte),* ⅓ cup, 1.4 oz. 80
banana *(Sonoma),* 2 pieces 140
blueberries *(Sonoma),* ¼ cup 140
carambola *(Frieda's),* 1 oz. 77
carambola *(Sonoma),* 1.4 oz. 140
cherries, bing *(Frieda's),* 1 oz. 79
cherries, pitted *(Sonoma),* ¼ cup 140
cranberries *(Craisins),* ⅓ cup 130
cranberries *(Sonoma),* ⅓ cup 120
currant, Zante *(S&W),* ¼ cup 130
date:
    (Del Monte), 5–6 pieces., 1.4 oz. 120
    (Dole), ½ cup 280
    (Sonoma), 5–6 pieces, 1.4 oz. 110
    chopped *(Del Monte),* ¼ cup, 1.4 oz. 120
    chopped *(Dole),* ½ cup 230
    dehydrated, coarse/fine ground *(Dole),* 1 oz. 110
fig:
    Calamata string *(Agora),* ½ cup 250
    Calimyrna or Mission *(Blue Ribbon/Sun · Maid),* 4 figs,
      1.5 oz. 120
    white/Mission *(Sonoma),* 3–4 figs, 1.4 oz. 110
fruit, mixed:
    (Del Monte), ⅓ cup, 1.4 oz. 110
    (Dole Sun Giant), 1.5 oz. 100
    (Sonoma), 1.4 oz. 120
    diced *(Sonoma),* ⅓ cup 120
kiwi *(Sonoma),* 7–8 pieces, 1 oz. 90
mango *(Sonoma),* 2 oz. 180

Fruit, Dried *(cont.)*

with nuts, *see "Trail Mix," page 365*

papaya *(Sonoma)*, 2 pieces, 2 oz.	200
peach *(Sonoma)*, 3–5 pieces, 1.4 oz.	120
peach, sun-dried *(Del Monte)*, ⅓ cup, 1.4 oz.	90
pear *(Sonoma)*, 3–4 pieces, 1.4 oz.	120
persimmon *(Sonoma)*, 6–8 pieces, 1.4 oz.	140
pineapple *(Sonoma)*, 1.4 oz.	140

prune:

(Del Monte), ¼ cup	120
(Dole), 2 oz.	140
pitted *(Sonoma)*, ¼ cup	120

raisins, ¼ cup, except as noted:

golden seedless *(Del Monte)*	120
golden seedless *(Dole)*, ½ cup	250
golden seedless *(S&W)*	130
golden seedless *(Sun · Maid)*	130
monukka/Thompson *(Sonoma)*	130
muscat *(Sun · Maid)*	130
seedless *(Del Monte)*	120
seedless *(Del Monte)*, 1.5-oz. box	130
seedless *(Dole)*, ½ cup	250
seedless *(S&W)*	130
seedless *(Sun · Maid)*	130

FRUIT SNACKS, all varieties
See also "Fruit, Dried" and "Trail Mix"

	calories
(Betty Crocker Tazmanian Devil), 1 pouch	90
(Fruit By the Foot), 1 roll	80
(Fruit Roll-Ups), 2 rolls	110
(Fruit Roll-Ups Pouch), 1 roll	50
(Gushers), 1 pouch	90
(Smart Snackers), .5 oz.	50
(Stretch Island), 1 oz.	90

FRUIT JUICES, eight fluid ounces, except as noted
See also "Fruit & Fruit-Flavored Drinks"

---

                                                                    calories

apple:
(After the Fall) 90
(Apple & Eve) 110
(Apple Time/Lincoln/Lucky Leaf/Speas Farm Regular/Cider) . 120
(Apple Time/Lucky Leaf/Musselman's), 5.5 fl. oz. 80
(Dole), 10 fl. oz. 160
(Goya) 120
(Heinke's Organic/Gravenstein) 120
(R. W. Knudsen Clear/Aseptic) 110
(R. W. Knudsen Natural/Organic/Gravensten) 120
(Minute Maid Box), 8.45 oz. 120
(Mott's Natural) 120
(Musselman's Premium Natural) 130
(Musselman's Regular/Natural/Cider) 120
(Red Cheek) 120
(S&W) 120
(Santa Cruz Organic) 120
(Season's Best), 11.5 fl. oz. 160
(Seneca) 110
(Snapple), 10 fl. oz. 140
(Tree Top/Tree Top Box/Country Style/Cider) 120
(Tree Top), 5.5 fl oz. 80
(Tree Top), 10 fl. oz. 140
(Tree Top), 11.5 fl. oz. 170
(Tree Top Fiber Rich) 150
(Veryfine) 120
(Veryfine), 11.5 fl. oz. 170
(White House) 120
sparkling cider (Apple Time/Lucky Leaf/Musselman's) 150
spiced (Apple & Eve Cider & Spice) 110
frozen, diluted (Minute Maid) 110
frozen, diluted (R. W. Knudsen) 120
frozen, diluted (Schwan's) 120
frozen, diluted (Tree Top/Tree Top Country Style) 120
frozen (Seneca), 2 oz. 120
apple blends, all flavors except cherry cider (R. W. Knudsen) . 120
apple-apricot (After the Fall) 100
apple-apricot (Tree Top Fiber Rich) 160

Fruit Juices *(cont.)*

apple-boysenberry or apple-raspberry *(Heinke's)* 120
apple-cherry *(After the Fall)* 100
apple-cherry cider, bottled or frozen and diluted
   (R. W. Knudsen) 130
apple-cranberry:
   (Apple & Eve) 120
   (R. W. Knudsen Aseptic) 110
   frozen, diluted *(Tree Top)* 130
apple-grape:
   (Apple & Eve), 8.45 fl. oz. 130
   (Juicy Juice) 130
   (Tree Top) 130
   (Tree Top), 5.5 fl. oz. 90
   (Tree Top), 10 fl. oz. 170
   (Tree Top), 11.5 fl. oz. 190
   frozen, diluted *(Tree Top)* 130
apple-orange-banana *(Tree Top Fiber Rich)* 170
apple-pear:
   (Tree Top/Tree Top Box) 120
   (Tree Top), 5.5 fl. oz. 80
   (Tree Top), 10 fl. oz. 140
   frozen, diluted *(Tree Top)* 120
apple-raspberry:
   (After the Fall) 90
   (Tree Top), 5.5 fl. oz. 80
   (Tree Top), 11.5 fl. oz. 160
   (Tree Top Box) 120
   frozen, diluted *(Tree Top)* 110
apple-strawberry *(After the Fall)* 100
apricot nectar:
   (Goya) 160
   (Libby's/Kern's) 150
   (Libby's/Kern's), 11.5 fl. oz. 220
   (R. W. Knudsen) 120
   (S&W) 140
   (S&W), 12-oz. can 210
   (Santa Cruz) 120
apricot-pineapple nectar *(Kern's)*, 11.5 fl. oz. 220
banana nectar *(Libby's/Kern's)*, 11.5-fl.-oz. can 190
banana nectar *(Libby's Quanabana)*, 11.5-fl.-oz. can 210
banana-pineapple nectar *Kern's)* 220

berry:
    (Apple & Eve Nothin' But Juice) 120
    (Heinke's Berry Patch) 120
    (Juicy Juice) 130
    (Veryfine Juice-Ups) 140
blueberry *(After the Fall)* 90
cherry:
    (Juicy Juice) 130
    (Minute Maid Box), 8.45 oz. 130
    black *(Heinke's)* 180
    black *(R. W. Knudsen)* 180
    blend *(Apple & Eve Nothin' But Juice)* 120
    blend *(Dole Mountain)* 120
    blend *(Veryfine Juice-Ups)* 150
    blend, black *(R. W. Knudsen Concentrate)* 130
    blend, cider *(Heinke's)* 115
    blend, cider *(R. W. Knudsen)* 130
    blend, cider *(R. W. Knudsen Aseptic)* 120
    nectar *(Santa Cruz)* 110
    concentrate, diluted *(R. W. Knudsen)* 130
coconut nectar *(R. W. Knudsen)* 140
cranberry:
    (After the Fall Cape Cod) 100
    (After the Fall Nantucket) 60
    (Apple & Eve Naturally Cranberry) 120
    (Heinke's 100%) 60
    (Ocean Spray Cocktail), 6 fl. oz. 100
    (R. W. Knudsen Just Cranberry) 60
    (R. W. Knudsen Yankee) 120
    (Season's Best Medley) 120
    (Snapple), 10 fl. oz. 150
    concentrate, diluted *(R. W. Knudsen)* 70
cranberry nectar:
    (Heinke's) 120
    (Santa Cruz) 110
    bottled or frozen and diluted *(R. W. Knudsen)* 150
cranberry punch blend *(Crantastic)* 150
cranberry-apple *(Cranapple)* 160
cranberry-apricot *(Cranicot)* 160
cranberry-blueberry *(Cran · Blueberry)* 160
cranberry-grape *(Apple & Eve)*, 10 fl. oz. 175
cranberry-grape *(Cran · Grape)* 170

Fruit Juices *(cont.)*

grapefruit:
    (Dole), 10 fl. oz. 120
    (Goya) 160
    (Ocean Spray) 100
    (S&W), 6 fl. oz. .80
    (S&W) 100
    (Tree Top) 100
    (Tree Top), 10 fl. oz. 130
    (Tree Top), 11.5 fl. oz. 140
    (Veryfine) 90
    blend *(Dole* Sunripe) 130
    blend *(Dole* Sunripe), 10 fl. oz. 160
    golden *(Tropicana)* 90
    pink or white *(R. W. Knudsen)* 100
    red *(R. W. Knudsen* Rio) 140
    ruby red *(Tropicana* Carton/Plastic) 100
    frozen, diluted *(Minute Maid)* 100
grapefruit-cranberry *(Apple & Eve* Ruby Red) 120
guava juice *(After the Fall* Maya), 8 fl. oz. 110
guava nectar:
    (Goya), 12 fl. oz. 240
    (Kern's), 8 fl. oz. 150
    (Libby's/Kern's), 11.5 fl. oz. 220
lemon *(ReaLemon)*, 1 tsp. 0
lemon *(Seneca)*, 1 tsp. 0
lime *(ReaLime)*, 1 tsp. 0
lime, sweetened *(Rose's)*, 1 tsp. 10
mango *(After the Fall* Montage) 110
mango nectar *(Goya)*, 12 fl. oz. 230
mango nectar *(Libby's/Kern's)* 150
mango-orange nectar *(Kern's)* 140
mango-peach *(R. W. Knudsen)* 120
orange:
    (Apple & Eve), 10 fl. oz. 130
    (Dole), 10 fl. oz. 140
    (Minute Maid Box), 8.45 fl. oz. 120
    (Tree Top) 120
    (Tree Top), 5.5 fl. oz. 80
    (Tree Top), 10 fl. oz. 150
    (Tree Top), 11.5 fl. oz. 170
    (Tropicana Pure Premium) 110
    (Tropicana Pure Premium + Fiber/Ruby Red Pure Premium) . 120

Fruit Juices, orange *(cont.)*

(S&W), 6-fl.-oz. can 90
(Seneca). 120
(Veryfine) 120
(Veryfine), 11.5 fl. oz. 170
bottled or frozen and diluted *(R. W. Knudsen)* 100
chilled or frozen and diluted, all varieties, except calcium
   rich *(Minute Maid* Premium) 110
chilled or frozen and diluted, calcium rich *(Minute Maid*
   Premium) 120
frozen *(Seneca TreeSweet),* 2 oz. 110
frozen, diluted *(Schwan's)* 120
orange-kiwi-passion fruit or orange-pineapple *(Tropicana*
Tropics) 100
orange-mango *(R. W. Knudsen)* 120
orange-peach-mango *(Tropicana* Tropics) 110
orange punch *(Juicy Juice)* 120
orange punch *(Veryfine* Juice-Ups) 140
papaya, creamed *(R. W. Knudsen),* 2 fl. oz. 40
papaya nectar *(R. W. Knudsen)* 130
passion fruit *(Snapple),* 10 fl. oz. 160
peach juice blend *(Dole* Orchard), 8 fl. oz. 140
peach juice blend *(Dole* Orchard), 10 fl. oz. 170
peach nectar:
  (Goya), 8 fl. oz. 150
  (Goya), 12 fl. oz. 220
  (Libby's), 8 fl. oz. 150
  (Libby's/Kern's), 11.5 fl. oz. 210
  (R. W. Knudsen), 8 fl. oz. 120
pear:
  (After the Fall Harvest) 90
  (After the Fall Rouge River) 100
  (Heinke's Organic/*R. W. Knudsen* Organic) 120
pear nectar:
  (Libby's) 150
  (Libby's/Kern's), 11.5 fl. oz. 220
  (Santa Cruz) .120
pineapple juice:
  (Del Monte), 6 fl. oz. 80
  (Del Monte) .130
  (Del Monte Not from Concentrate) 110
  (Dole Not from Concentrate 46-oz. Can) 110

    (Dole Reconstituted 46-oz. Can) 120
    (Dole Reconstituted/Single Strength) 110
    (Dole Reconstituted/Single Strength), 6 oz. 80
    (Goya), 12 fl. oz. 190
    (S&W) 110
    (S&W), 6 fl. oz. 90
    (S&W), 12 fl. oz. 180
    chilled or frozen and diluted *(Dole)* 130
    frozen, diluted *(Minute Maid)* 129
pineapple-coconut *(R. W. Knudsen)* 130
pineapple-grapefruit *(Dole)*, 6 fl. oz. 100
pineapple-grapefruit, frozen, diluted *(Dole)* 130
pineapple-orange:
    (Dole) 120
    frozen, diluted *(Dole)* 120
    frozen, diluted *(Minute Maid)* 120
pineapple-orange-banana:
    (Dole) 130
    (Dole), 6 fl. oz. 100
    (Dole), 10 fl. oz. 160
pineapple-orange-berry or pineapple-orange-strawberry *(Dole)* . 130
pineapple-orange-guava *(Dole)* 120
pineapple–passion fruit–banana *(Dole)* 120
pineapple–passion fruit–banana *(Dole)*, 10 fl. oz. 160
pomegranate *(R. W. Knudsen)* 150
prune:
    (Del Monte) 170
    (Goya) 180
    (Lucky Leaf/Musselman's) 160
    (R. W. Knudsen Organic) 170
    (S&W) 180
raspberry *(Heinke's)* 120
raspberry, frozen, diluted *(R. W. Knudsen)* 120
raspberry blend *(Dole* Country) 140
raspberry nectar *(Santa Cruz)* 100
raspberry-cranberry *(Apple & Eve)* 120
raspberry-peach *(R. W. Knudsen)* 120
strawberry *(Veryfine* Juice-Ups) 140
strawberry nectar *(R. W. Knudsen)* 120
tamarind nectar *(Goya)*, 12 fl. oz. 240
tangerine, frozen, diluted *(Minute Maid* Beverage) 120
tangerine, blend *(Dole* Mandarin) 140
watermelon *(After the Fall)* 90

FRUIT & FRUIT-FLAVORED DRINKS, eight fluid ounces, except as noted
See also "Fruit Juices," "Soft Drinks," and "Sports Drinks"

	calories
all flavors *(Shasta Plus)*, 12 fl. oz.	170
all flavors, mix, diluted *(Kool-Aid)*	100
apple:	
(Lincoln)	130
frozen, diluted *(Schwan's Vita-Sun)*	100
punch *(Minute Maid)*	120
apple-berry:	
(Dole Burst), 16 fl. oz.	250
white grape *(Veryfine Quenchers)*	120
frozen, diluted *(Dole* Burst)	120
apple-berry-cherry, frozen, diluted *(Schwan's Vita-Sun)*	100
apple-cranberry:	
(Dole), 10 fl. oz.	160
(Tree Top), 10 fl. oz.	200
(Tree Top), 11.5 fl. oz.	230
frozen, diluted *(Schwan's Vita-Sun)*	100
apple-cranberry-tangerine *(Veryfine Quenchers)*	120
apple-peach-kiwi *(Veryfine Quenchers)*	130
apple-peach-plum *(Veryfine Quenchers)*	130
apple–pear–passion fruit *(Veryfine Quenchers)*	120
apple-raspberry *(Tree Top)*, 10 fl. oz.	190
apple-raspberry *(Tree Top)*, 11.5 fl. oz.	220
apple-raspberry-blackberry *(Tropicana Twister)*	130
apple-raspberry-blackberry *(Tropicana Twister)*, 11.5 fl. oz.	180
apple-raspberry-cherry *(Veryfine Quenchers)*	120
apple-raspberry-lime *(Veryfine Quenchers)*	120
apple-strawberry-banana *(Veryfine Quenchers)*	120
banana *(After the Fall* Casablanca)	80
berry:	
(After the Fall Oregon)	100
(Capri Sun Yo Yogi Berry), 6.75 fl. oz.	100
(Hi-C Boppin'/Hi-C Boppin' Box)	120
(R. W. Knudsen Razzleberry)	130
(R. W. Knudsen Razzleberry Aseptic)	110
berry nectar *(Santa Cruz)*	110
berry punch:	
(Minute Maid/Minute Maid Box)	120

(Tropicana) 130
red *(Juice Rivers* Box) 130
frozen, diluted *(Minute Maid)* 120
berry-citrus *(Five Alive)* 110
boysenberry *(Farmer's Market)* 120
boysenberry cider *(Heinke's)* 120
cantaloupe cocktail *(Snapple)* 130
cherry:
(After the Fall Very Cherry) 100
(Farmer's Market) 120
wild *(Capri Sun)*, 6.75 fl. oz. 110
cherry-apple *(Schwan's Vita-Sun)* 100
citrus:
(Five Alive) 120
frozen, diluted *(Five Alive)* 110
frozen, diluted *(Schwan's Vita-Sun)* 110
punch *(Goya)* 130
punch *(Juice Rivers* Box) 130
punch *(Minute Maid)* 120
punch *(Tropicana)* 140
punch, tropical *(Five Alive)* 110
punch, frozen, diluted *(Minute Maid)* 120
tropical, frozen, diluted *(Five Alive)* 110
cranberry:
(Farmer's Market) 120
(Tropicana Punch) 140
(Tropicana Punch), 11.5 fl. oz. 200
(Tropicana Ruby Red) 120
juice cocktail *(Seneca)* 140
juice cocktail, frozen, diluted *(Schwan's)* 140
juice cocktail, frozen *(Seneca)*, 2 oz. 140
spiced *(J.M.S.* Cooler) 120
cranberry-hibiscus *(Heinke's/R. W. Knudsen)* 120
cranberry-lemon *(Santa Cruz)* 120
cranberry-raspberry *(After the Fall)* 90
cranberry-raspberry *(R. W. Knudsen)* 140
cranberry-raspberry-strawberry *(Tropicana Twister)* 120
cranberry-raspberry-strawberry *(Tropicana Twister* Light) 45
fruit:
(Capri Sun Mountain Cooler), 6.75 fl. oz. 100
(Capri Sun Pacific Cooler), 6.75 fl. oz. 100
(Capri Sun Surfer Cooler), 6.75 fl. oz. 100

Fruit & Fruit-Flavored Drinks, fruit *(cont.)*
   (Dole Fruit Fiesta), 16 fl. oz. 270
   (Dole Lanai/Tropical Breeze), 16 fl. oz. 240
   (Hi-C Ecto Cooler) 120
   (Hi-C Ecto Cooler Box), 8.45 fl. oz. 130
   (Lincoln Party) 140
   (Snapple Bali Blast/Samoan Splash) 120
   (Tropicana) 130
   (Veryfine Avalanche) 110
   (Veryfine Tropical Breeze) 120
   frozen, diluted *(Dole* Fruit Fiesta) 140
   frozen, diluted *(Dole* Lanai/Tropical Breeze) 120
fruit nectar *(Kern's* Tropical), 11.5 fl. oz. 210
fruit punch:
   (Capri Sun), 6.75 fl. oz. 100
   (Capri Sun Maui/Safari), 6.75 fl. oz. 100
   (Dole Paradise), 10 fl. oz. 150
   (Dole Tropical), 10 fl. oz. 130
   (Farmer's Market Tropical) 120
   (Heinke's California/Paradise) 110
   (Heinke's Macchu Pichu) 120
   (Hi-C) 110
   (Hi-C Box) 120
   (Hi-C Blue Cooler) 120
   (Hi-C Blue Cooler Box), 8.45 fl. oz. 130
   (Hi-C Tropical Box) 120
   (R. W. Knudsen Rain Forest/Tropical) 120
   (R. W. Knudsen Tropical Aseptic) 120
   (Snapple) 110
   (Tree Top/Juice Rivers Box) 130
   frozen, diluted *(R. W. Knudsen* Tropical) 120
   frozen, diluted *(Schwan's Vita-Sun)* 100
   regular or tropical *(Minute Maid/Minute Maid* Box) 120
   regular or tropical, frozen, diluted *(Minute Maid)* 120
ginger *(Santa Cruz* Hawaiian) 110
grape:
   (Capri Sun), 6.75 fl. oz. 110
   (Dole), 10 fl. oz. 150
   (Hi-C) 120
   (Hi-C Box), 8.45 fl. oz. 130
   (Lincoln) 130
   (Veryfine Glacial) 110

    frozen, diluted *(Bright & Early)* 140
    frozen, diluted *(Minute Maid)* 120
    frozen, diluted *(Schwan's Vita-Sun)* 110
    juice cocktail, frozen, diluted *(Schwan's)* 110
    mix, diluted *(Kool-Aid* with Sugar) 60
    white, cocktail, frozen, diluted *(Seneca)* 130
grape punch:
    (Juice Rivers Box) 140
    (Minute Maid), 8 fl. oz. 120
    or drink, frozen, diluted *(Minute Maid),* 8 fl. oz. 120
grapeade *(Snapple)* 110
grapefruit:
    pink *(Ocean Spray)* 110
    pink *(Tree Top* Desert Ice) 120
    pink *(Tropicana Twister)* 120
    pink *(Tropicana Twister),* 11.5 fl. oz. 160
    pink *(Tropicana Twister* Light) 35
    pink, frozen, diluted *(Schwan's)* 110
    ruby red *(Ocean Spray)* 130
    ruby red and tangerine *(Ocean Spray)* 130
guava *(Mauna La'i)* 130
guava *(Snapple* Guava Mania) 110
kiwi punch *(After the Fall* Bear) 100
kiwi-strawberry *(Snapple)* 120
kiwi-strawberry *(Snapple* Diet) 20
lemonade:
    (After the Fall) 90
    (Heinke's Old Fashion/*R. W. Knudsen)* 120
    (R. W. Knudsen Aseptic) 110
    (Santa Cruz) 120
    (Snapple) 110
    (Tropicana) 120
    (Tropicana), 11.5 fl. oz. 160
    (Veryfine Chillers), 11.5 fl. oz. 180
    chilled or frozen and diluted *(Minute Maid)* 110
    pink *(Minute Maid)* 110
    pink *(Snapple)* 120
    pink *(Snapple* Diet) 20
    pink *(Veryfine* Chillers), 11.5 fl. oz. 180
    frozen, diluted *(R. W. Knudsen* Natural/Organic) 120
    frozen, diluted *(Schwan's)* 140
    frozen, diluted *(Schwan's* Lite) 50

Fruit & Fruit-Flavored Drinks, lemonade *(cont.)*
    mix, diluted *(Country Time/Country Time* Punch) 70
    mix, diluted *(Country Time/Kool-Aid* Sugar Free) 5
    mix, diluted *(Crystal Light)* 5
    mix, diluted *(Kool-Aid* Presweetened) 70
lemonade blends, all fruit flavors:
    (Minute Maid) 120
    (R. W. Knudsen) 120
    (Santa Cruz) 120
    except tropical, frozen, diluted *(Minute Maid)* 110
lemonade-cherry *(Snapple)* 130
lemonade-cherry *(Veryfine* Chillers) 120
lemonade, cranberry *(Heinke's)* 120
lemonade, ginger *(R. W. Knudsen* Echinacea) 100
lemonade, lime *(Veryfine* Chillers) 120
lemonade, peach *(Snapple)* 120
lemonade, peach *(Veryfine* Chillers) 120
lemonade, strawberry *(Snapple)* 120
lemonade, strawberry *(Veryfine* Chillers) 120
lemonade, tangerine *(Veryfine* Chillers) 120
lemonade, tropical, frozen, diluted *(Minute Maid)* 120
lime:
    (After the Fall Key West) 100
    (R. W. Knudsen Cactus Cooler) 120
    frozen, diluted *(Minute Maid* Limeade) 100
mango:
    (Snapple Madness) 110
    (Snapple Madness Diet) 20
    (Tree Top More Mango) 120
mango-tangerine *(Veryfine)* 110
melonberry juice cocktail *(Snapple)* 120
orange:
    (Capri Sun), 6.75 fl. oz. 100
    (Hi-C/Hi-C Box) 120
    (Lincoln) 130
    punch *(Kool-Aid Bursts)*, 6.75 fl. oz. 100
    tropical *(Farmer's Market)* 120
    chilled or frozen and diluted *(Bright & Early)* 120
    frozen, diluted *(Schwan's Vita-Sun)* 90
    mix, diluted *(Kool-Aid* with Sugar) 60
    mix, diluted *(Tang)* 100
    mix, diluted *(Tang* Sugar Free) 5

orange-cranberry *(Tropicana Twister)* 130
orange-cranberry *(Tropicana Twister* Light) 30
orange-guava nectar *(Kern's)* 150
orange-peach drink *(Tropicana Twister)* 120
orange-pineapple drink *(Lincoln)* 130
orange-raspberry *(Tropicana Twister)* 120
orange-raspberry *(Tropicana Twister* Light) 35
orange-strawberry-banana *(Tropicana Twister)* 120
orange-strawberry-banana *(Tropicana Twister* Light) 35
orange-strawberry-guava *(Tropicana Twister)* 120
orangeade *(Snapple)* 120
papaya:
   (Farmer's Market) 130
   juice drink *(After the Fall* Pele's) 100
   nectar *(Goya)*, 12 fl. oz. 220
   nectar *(Libby's/Kern's)*, 11.5 fl. oz. 210
   nectar *(R. W. Knudsen)* 130
   nectar *(Santa Cruz)* 110
   punch *(Lincoln)* 130
papaya colada *(Snapple)* 120
passion fruit–mango *(Heinke's)* 130
peach:
   (After the Fall) 100
   (Farmer's Market) 120
   (Tree Top Quake) 120
pineapple *(Tropicana* Punch, 16 oz.) 120
pineapple *(Tropicana* Punch), 10 fl. oz. 160
pineapple-coconut:
   (Farmer's Market) 120
   nectar *(Kern's)* 200
   nectar *(Kern's)*, 11.5 fl. oz. 290
pineapple-grapefruit, pink *(Dole)*, 6 fl. oz. 100
pineapple-grapefruit, pink *(Dole* 46-oz. Can) 130
pineapple-orange, frozen, diluted *(Schwan's Vita-Sun)* 100
raspberry:
   (Farmer's Market) 120
   hibiscus *(R. W. Knudsen)* 90
   lemon *(Santa Cruz)* 120
   black, frozen, diluted *(Schwan's Vita-Sun)* 110
strawberry:
   (Capri Sun Cooler), 6.75 fl. oz. 100
   (Farmer's Market) 120

Fruit & Fruit-Flavored Drinks, strawberry *(cont.)*
   nectar *(Kern's)* 150
   nectar *(Libby's/Kern's)*, 11.5 fl. oz. 210
   mix, diluted *(Kool-Aid* with Sugar) 60
strawberry nectar blend *(Kern's)* 150
strawberry-banana or strawberry-banana-cactus
   (R. W. Knudsen) 120
strawberry-guava *(R. W. Knudsen)* 110
strawberry-guava *(Santa Cruz)* 100
strawberry-kiwi *(R. W. Knudsen)* 120
strawberry-melon *(Veryfine* Shivering Chillers) 120
strawberry-orange-banana *(Tree Top)* 120
watermelon *(Hi-C Watermelon Rapids* Box), 8.45 fl. oz. 120
watermelon *(R. W. Knudsen* Cooler) 120

Chapter 6

VEGETABLES AND VEGETABLE PRODUCTS

VEGETABLES, FRESH
See also "Vegetable Salad Blends, Fresh"

---

	calories
artichoke, globe *(Dole)*, 1 medium, 4.5 oz.	60
artichoke, Jerusalem *(Frieda's Sunchoke)*, 1 oz.	75
arugula, trimmed *(Frieda's)*, 3.5 oz.	23
asparagus *(Dole)*, 5 spears	25
bean, broad, mature, dry *(Frieda's Fava Beans)*, 1 oz.	15
bean sprouts, *see "sprouts," below*	
broccoli *(Dole)*, 1 medium stalk, 5.3 oz.	45
brussels sprouts *(Dole)*, 1 cup	40
cabbage:	
(Dole), 1/12 medium head	25
Napa *(Frieda's)*, 1 oz.	4
red, shredded *(Dole)*, 3 oz.	25
cactus leaves *(Frieda's)*, 3/4 cup, 3 oz.	20
carrot:	
(Dole), 1 medium, 7" long, 1 1/4" diameter	35
mini *(Frieda's)*, 1 oz.	12
mini, peeled *(Dole)*, 3 oz.	40
shredded *(Dole)*, 3 oz.	40
cauliflower *(Dole)*, 1/6 medium head, 3.2 oz.	25
celery *(Dole)*, 2 medium stalks, 3.9 oz.	20
chayote *(Frieda's)*, 3.5 oz.	28
corn, sweet *(Dole)*, 1 medium ear, 3.2 oz.	80
cucumber *(Dole)*, 1/3 medium	15
cucumber, hothouse, unpeeled *(Frieda's)*, 1 oz.	4
eggplant, Japanese, raw, with peel *(Frieda's)*, 3.5 oz.	25
garlic sprouts *(Jonathan's)*, 1 cup, 4 oz.	70
jicama, peeled *(Frieda's)*, 3.5 oz.	45
lettuce:	
iceberg *(Dole)*, 1/6 head, 3.2 oz.	15
iceberg, precut *(Dole Classic)*, 3 oz.	15
leaf, shredded *(Dole)*, 1 1/2 cups, 3 oz.	15

Vegetables, Fresh *(cont.)*
mushroom:
    (Dole), 5 medium, 3 oz. 20
    Japanese honey, trimmed *(Frieda's)*, 1 oz. 9
    oyster *(Frieda's)*, 1 oz. 7
    portobello *(Frieda's)*, 1 oz. 8
    shiitake, raw *(Frieda's)*, 1 oz. 24
    yamabiko honshimeji *(Frieda's)*, 1 oz. 3
onion:
    (Dole), 1 medium 60
    green, chopped *(Dole)*, ¼ cup 10
    raw, chopped *(Dole Vidalia)*, ½ cup 30
peas, edible-podded, sugar snap *(Frieda's)*, 1 oz. 15
peas, sugar *(Dole)*, ½ cup 30
pepper, bell *(Dole)*, 1 medium, 5.3 oz. 30
potato *(Dole)*, 1 medium, 5.3 oz. 100
potato, boiled in skin, baby *(Frieda's)*, 4 oz. 86
spinach, chopped *(Dole)*, 1 cup 15
sprouts:
    alfalfa *(Arrowhead Mills)*, 1 cup 30
    alfalfa *(Jonathan's)*, 1 cup 25
    alfalfa, with dill or radish sprouts *(Jonathan's)*, 1 cup 30
    alfalfa, with garlic *(Jonathan's)*, 1 cup 27
    alfalfa, with onion *(Jonathan's)*, 1 cup 25
    bean *(Frieda's)*, 1 oz. 10
    bean *(Jonathan's)*, 1 cup .30
    clover *(Jonathan's)*, 1 cup, 3 oz. 25
    clover seed *(Shaw's)*, 2 oz. 7
    hot and spicy *(Jonathan's)*, 1 cup, 4 oz. 25
    mixed *(Jonathan's Gourmet)*, 1 cup, 3 oz. 20
    mixed *(Shaw's)*, 2 oz. 9
    lentil, adzuki, and pea *(Jonathan's)*, 3 oz. 100
    onion *(Jonathan's)*, 1 cup 30
    onion *(Shaw's Premium Salad)*, 2 oz. 11
    radish *(Jonathan's)*, 1 cup 57
    snow pea *(Jonathan's)*, 1 cup 40
    soybean *(Jonathan's)*, 1 cup, 3 oz. 100
    sunflower *(Jonathan's)*, 1 cup 45
squash:
    banana, baked *(Frieda's)*, 1 oz. 18
    Hubbard, raw *(Frieda's)*, 1 oz. 14
    summer *(Dole)*, ½ medium, 3.5 oz. 20

sunburst, raw *(Frieda's)*, 1 oz. 4
taro or taro root, cooked *(Frieda's)*, 5 oz. 150
tomato *(Dole)*, 1 medium, 5.3 oz. 35
water chestnut, Chinese *(Frieda's)*, 1 oz. 22
wheat grass *(Pines)*, 3 servings 29
yam bean tuber, raw *(Frieda's)*, 3.5 oz. 45
yuca, boiled, drained *(Frieda's)*, 4 oz. 77

VEGETABLE SALAD BLENDS, FRESH
See also "Vegetables, Fresh"

calories

with dressing/condiments:
   Caesar *(Dole Complete)*, 3.5 oz. 170
   Caesar *(Dole Complete Lowfat)*, 3.5 oz. 60
   Caesar *(Dole Lunch for One)*, 5.75 oz. 300
   Caesar *(Dole Lunch for One Lowfat)*, 6 oz. 120
   herb ranch *(Dole Complete Lowfat)*, 3.5 oz. 50
   Italian *(Dole Lunch for One Lowfat)*, 7 oz. 110
   Italian, zesty *(Dole Complete Lowfat)*, 3.5 oz. 60
   Oriental *(Dole Complete)*, 3.5 oz. 120
   ranch, classic *(Dole Lunch for One)*, 7 oz. 340
   romaine, raspberry *(Dole Complete Lowfat)*, 3.5 oz. 60
   Romano *(Dole Complete)*, 3.5 oz. 150
   spinach bacon *(Dole Complete)*, 3.5 oz. 160
   sunflower ranch *(Dole Complete)*, 3.5 oz. 170
without dressing:
   America, European, Italian, or romaine blend *(Dole)*, 3 oz. . . .15
   coleslaw blend mix *(Dole Classic)*, 3 oz. 25
   French blend *(Dole)*, 3 oz. 20

VEGETABLES, CANNED OR IN JARS, ½ cup, except as noted
*See also "Vegetables, Frozen," "Vegetables, Dried," "Tomato
Paste, Puree, & Sauce," and "Entrees, Canned or Packaged"*

calories

artichoke bottoms *(S&W)*, 3 pieces 25
artichoke hearts *(S&W)*, 3 pieces 30
asparagus:
   (S&W Blended), 6 pieces .15
   (S&W Colossal), 3 pieces .10
   (Seneca) 20

Vegetables, Canned or in Jars, asparagus *(cont.)*
   (Stokely/Stokely No Salt) 25
   all varieties *(Del Monte)* .20
   spears, extra large *(Green Giant LeSueur)*, 4.5 oz. 20
   spears, regular or extra long *(Green Giant)*, 4.5 oz. 20
   cuts *(Green Giant/Green Giant* 50% Less Sodium) 20
bamboo shoots *(La Choy)*, ¼ cup 5
bean salad, *see "Appetizers & Snacks, Canned or in Jars,"*
   page 151
bean sprouts *(La Choy)*, 1 cup .10
beans, adzuki *(Eden Aduki)* 110
beans, baked:
   (Allens) 150
   (Campbell's New England Style/Old Fashioned) 180
   (Eden Organic) 150
   (Friend's) 170
   (Grandma Brown's) 160
   (Heartland Iron Kettle) 150
   (S&W Brick Oven) 160
   (Van Camp's Fat Free) 130
   (Van Camp's Premium) 140
   all varieties except pork, bacon and onion, and yellow eye
     (B&M) 170
   with bacon *(Grandma Brown's* Saucepan) 150
   bacon and brown sugar *(Bush's* Best Original) 150
   bacon and brown sugar *(Campbell's)* 170
   bacon and brown sugar *(S&W)* 140
   bacon, brown sugar, and onion *(B&M)* 190
   barbecue *(Campbell's/Campbell's* Old Fashioned) 170
   barbecue *(Green Giant/Joan of Arc)* 140
   barbecue, Texas style *(S&W)* 140
   brown sugar *(Van Camp's)* 170
   with franks, *see "Entrees, Canned or Packaged," page 159*
   honey *(Health Valley/Health Valley* No Salt) 110
   honey, bacon *(Green Giant/Joan of Arc)* 160
   honey, mustard *(S&W)* 130
   kidney, red *(Friend's)* 170
   maple sugar *(S&W)* 150
   Mexican style, *see "beans, Mexican," below*
   with onion *(Green Giant/Joan of Arc)* 150
   with pork *(B&M)* 180
   with pork *(Campbell's)* 130

with pork *(Crest Top)* 130
with pork *(Green Giant/Joan of Arc)* 120
with pork *(Hunt's)* 130
with pork *(Stokely* Sugar*)* 150
with pork *(Stokely* Tomato*)* 140
with pork *(Van Camp's)* 110
with pork *(Wagon Master/Trappey's)* 110
with pork *(Wagon Master/Trappey's* 42 oz.*)* 130
with pork, jalapeño *(Trappey's)* 130
with pork, peas *(East Texas Fair* Peas 'n Pork*)* 110
vegetarian *(Heinz)* 140
vegetarian *(Stokely)* 140
vegetarian *(Van Camp's)* 110
vegetarian, brown sugar sauce *(Stokely)* 150
yellow eye *(B&M)* 180
beans, black:
  (Eden Organic*)* 100
  (Goya) 90
  (Green Giant/Joan of Arc) 100
  (Old El Paso) 110
  (Progresso) 110
  (S&W/S&W 50% Less Salt*)* 70
  (Stokely) 110
  (Sun-Vista) 70
  with ginger and lemon *(Eden* Organic*)* 120
  seasoned *(Allens/Trappey's)* 120
beans, broad, mature *(Progresso* Fava Beans*)* 110
beans, chili:
  (Eden Organic*)* 130
  (Gebhardt) 135
  (Hunt's) 85
  (S&W) 110
  (Stokely) 120
  (Sun-Vista) 110
  (Van Camp's Mexican*)* 110
  hot *(S&W* Chipotle*)* .90
  spicy *(Green Giant/Joan of Arc)* 110
  zesty *(Campbell's)* 130
beans, garbanzo, *see "chickpeas," below*
beans, great northern:
  (Allens) 100
  (Eden Organic*)* 120

Vegetables, Canned or in Jars, beans, great northern *(cont.)*
  (Goya) 80
  (Green Giant/Joan of Arc) 100
  (Seneca) 150
  (Stokely) 110
  (Sun-Vista) 70
  with sausage *(Trappey's)* 100
beans, green:
  (Allens Shells Out) .30
  (Goya) 20
  (Green Giant Kitchen Sliced) 20
  (Seneca) 25
  (Stokely/Stokely No Salt) 20
  all varieties except Italian cut *(Del Monte/Del Monte* No
    Salt) 20
  whole *(Green Giant)* .25
  whole, cut, or French *(S&W)* 20
  cut *(Allens* No Salt) 15
  cut *(Allens/Sunshine/Alma/Crest Top)* 30
  cut *(Green Giant/Green Giant* Less Sodium) 20
  cut, with wax beans *(S&W)* 20
  dilled *(S&W)*, 1 oz. .20
  French style *(Allens)* 25
  French style *(Green Giant)* 20
  Italian cut *(Allens/Sunshine)* 35
  Italian cut *(Del Monte)* 30
  with potatoes *(Allens/Sunshine)* 35
beans, kidney:
  red *(Eden* Organic) 100
  red *(Hunt's)* 95
  red *(Seneca)* 110
  red, dark *(Allens/East Texas Fair/Trappey's)* 130
  red, dark *(Goya)* 90
  red, dark *(Van Camp's)* 90
  red, dark or light *(Green Giant/Joan of Arc)* 110
  red, dark or light *(Progresso)* 110
  red, dark or light *(Stokely)* 120
  red, dark or light *(Stokely* No Sugar) 110
  red, light *(Allens/Trappey's)* 120
  red, light *(Van Camp's)* 90
  red, with bacon, light *(Trappey's* New Orleans) 110
  red, with chili gravy *(Trappey's)* 110

red, with jalapeños, light *(Trappey's)* 110
white *(Progresso* Cannellini) 100
beans, lima:
    (Goya) 76
    (Green Giant/Joan of Arc Butterbeans) 90
    (S&W Butterbeans) 70
    (Seneca) 70
    (Stokely/Stokely No Salt) 100
    (Stubb's Harvest Butter Beans) 120
    (Van Camp's Butterbeans) 110
    baby *(Allens* Butterbeans) 120
    green *(Allens/East Texas Fair/Sunshine* Limas/Butterbeans) . 120
    green *(Del Monte)* 80
    green *(Goya)* 90
    green and white *(Allens)* 110
    large *(Allens* Butterbeans) 120
    mature, baby, green, or butter beans *(Stokely)* 110
    with bacon, baby green *(Trappey's* Limas) 120
    with bacon, baby white *(Trappey's* Limas) 130
    with ham and sauce *(Nalley)*, 1 cup 240
    with sausage, large white *(Trappey's* Butterbeans) 110
beans, lupin *(Canto Lupinin)*, ¼ cup 30
beans, Mexican:
    (Allens/Brown Beauty) 120
    (Chi-Chi's Ranchero) 100
    (Old El Paso Mexe Beans) 110
    (Stokely Red) 110
    with jalapeños *(Brown Beauty)* 120
    with jalapeños *(Trappey's* Mexi-Beans) 130
beans, mixed *(Stokely* Chulent) 110
beans, navy:
    (Allens) 110
    (Eden Organic) 110
    (Stokely) 110
    bacon or bacon/jalapeño *(Trappey's)* 110
beans, pink *(Goya)* 120
beans, pink, in tomato sauce *(Goya* Guisadas) 100
beans, pinquito *(S&W)* 80
beans, pinto:
    (Allens/East Texas Fair/Brown Beauty) 110
    (Eden Organic) 100
    (Gebhardt) 90

Vegetables, Canned or in Jars, beans, pinto *(cont.)*
   (Goya) 80
   (Green Giant/Joan of Arc) 110
   (Las Palmas) 100
   (Old El Paso) 100
   (Progresso) 110
   (Stokely) 110
   (Sun-Vista) 80
   with bacon *(Trappey's/Trappey's* Jala-pinto) 120
   spicy *(Eden* Organic) 125
   in tomato sauce *(Goya* Guisadas) 100
beans, red *(see also "beans, kidney," above):*
   (Allens) 160
   (Goya), ¼ cup 160
   (Green Giant/Joan of Arc) 100
   (Stokely) 110
   (Van Camp's) 90
   small *(Hunt's)* 90
beans, refried:
   (Allens) 150
   (Chi-Chi's) 130
   (Chi-Chi's Fat Free) 80
   (Gebhardt) 110
   (Gebhardt No Fat) 90
   (Goya) 110
   (Las Palmas) 110
   (Old El Paso) 110
   (Rosarita) 125
   (Rosarita No Fat) 110
   all varieties *(Old El Paso* Fat Free) 100
   all varieties *(Las Palmas* Fat Free) 100
   bacon *(Rosarita)* .115
   black beans *(Las Palmas)* 110
   black beans *(Old El Paso)* 120
   black beans *(Rosarita* Low Fat) 105
   with cheese *(Old El Paso)* 130
   with cheese, nacho *(Rosarita)* 135
   with green chilies *(Old El Paso)* 100
   with green chilies *(Rosarita)* 110
   with green chilies and lime *(Rosarita* No Fat) 100
   with jalapeño *(Gebhardt)* 105
   with onion *(Rosarita)* 115

with salsa, zesty *(Rosarita* No Fat) 100
with sausage *(Old El Paso)* 200
spicy *(Old El Paso)* 140
spicy *(Rosarita)* 120
vegetarian *(Chi-Chi's)* 80
vegetarian *(Gebhardt)* 120
vegetarian *(Old El Paso)* 100
vegetarian *(Rosarita)* 120
beans, Roman *(Goya)*, ¼ cup 90
beans, shellie *(Stokely)* 45
beans, soy, black *(Eden* Organic) 90
beans, wax:
   (S&W) 20
   (Seneca/Seneca No Salt) 25
   (Stokely/Stokely No Salt) 20
   golden *(Del Monte)* 20
beans, white:
   (Goya) 80
   small *(S&W)* 80
   in tomato sauce *(Goya* Guisados) 110
beets:
   all varieties, except Harvard and pickled *(Seneca)* 35
   whole *(Stokely)*, 4.5 oz. 80
   whole, baby *(Green Giant LeSueur)* 35
   whole or sliced *(Del Monte)* 35
   whole or sliced *(Green Giant)* 35
   whole, sliced or julienne *(S&W)* 30
   sliced *(Goya)* 45
   sliced *(Green Giant* No Salt) 35
   sliced *(Stokely)* 40
   Harvard *(Green Giant)*, ⅓ cup 60
   Harvard *(Greenwood)* 100
   Harvard *(Seneca)* 90
   Harvard *(Stokely)*, ⅓ cup 80
   pickled *(S&W)*, 1 oz. .15
   pickled *(Stokely* Can/Jar), 1 oz. 25
   pickled, all varieties *(Seneca)*, 2 tbsp. 15
   pickled, crinkle *(Del Monte)* 80
   pickled, sliced *(Greenwood)*, 4 slices, 1 oz. 25
   pickled, small whole *(Greenwood)*, 2 beets, 1 oz. 25
black-eyed peas:
   fresh *(Goya* Cowpeas) .90

Vegetables, Canned or in Jars, black-eyed peas *(cont.)*
fresh *(Green Giant/Joan of Arc)* 90
fresh *(Stokely)* 110
fresh *(Sun-Vista)* 70
fresh, with or without snaps *(Allens/East Texas Fair/
    Homefolks)* 120
fresh, with jalapeño *(Homefolks)* 120
fresh, with jalapeño *(Stubb's Harvest)* 120
dry *(Allens/East Texas Fair)* 110
dry, with bacon *(Allens)* 105
dry, with bacon *(Trappey's)* 120
dry, with bacon and jalapeño *(Trappey's)* 110
cabbage, red:
    (Seneca) 80
    sweet and sour *(Greenwood)* 100
    sweet and sour *(S&W)*, 2 tbsp. 15
cactus, marinated *(Goya* Napolitos), 2–3 pieces 20
carrot:
    all varieties *(S&W)* 25
    all varieties *(Seneca)* .25
    baby, whole *(Green Giant LeSueur)* 35
    whole or sliced *(Stokely)*, 4.5 oz. 30
    sliced *(Allens/Crest Top)* 35
    sliced *(Del Monte)* 35
    sliced *(Goya)* 30
    sliced *(Green Giant)* 25
    sliced *(Stokely* No Salt) 30
cauliflower, pickled, sweet *(Vlasic)*, 1 oz. 35
chickpeas:
    (Allens/East Texas Fair) 120
    (Eden Organic) 120
    (Goya) 100
    (Green Giant/Joan of Arc) 110
    (Old El Paso) 100
    (Progresso) 120
    (Progresso Garbanzo) 100
    (Seneca Garbanzo) 110
    (Stokely) 110
collard greens:
    (Allens/Sunshine) 30
    (Stubb's Harvest) 30
    seasoned *(Sylvia's Restaurant)* 45

corn, baby *(Haddon House)*	.30
corn, baby *(Roland)*	.25
corn, kernel:	
golden *(Del Monte)*	.90
golden *(Del Monte* Fiesta)	.50
golden *(Del Monte* Supersweet No Salt/Sugar)	.60
golden *(Del Monte* Supersweet Vac Pack)	.70
golden *(Del Monte* Supersweet Vac Pack No Salt)	.70
golden *(Goya)*	100
golden *(Green Giant/Green Giant* Less Salt)	.80
golden *(Green Giant Niblets),* ⅓ cup	.70
golden *(Green Giant Niblets* Extra Sweet), ⅓ cup	.50
golden *(Green Giant Niblets* 50% Less Sodium), ⅓ cup	.60
golden *(Green Giant Niblets* No Added Salt/Sugar), ⅓ cup	.60
golden *(S&W)*	.90
golden *(S&W* Sweet 'n Crisp), ⅓ cup	.70
golden *(Seneca)*	.90
golden *(Seneca),* ⅓ cup	.80
golden *(Seneca* Super Sweet)	100
golden *(Seneca* Water Pack)	.80
golden *(Stokely)*	.90
golden *(Stokely* No Salt)	.90
golden *(Stokely* Vac Pack), ⅓ cup	.80
golden *(Stokely* Vac Pack No Salt), ⅓ cup	.70
golden and white *(Del Monte* Supersweet)	.80
white *(Del Monte)*	.80
white *(Green Giant),* ⅓ cup	.80
white *(Stokely)*	.90
white *(Stokely* No Salt)	.90
with peppers *(Green Giant Mexicorn),* ⅓ cup	.60
with peppers *(Stokely),* ⅓ cup	.80
corn, cream style:	
(Del Monte/Del Monte No Salt)	.90
(Del Monte Supersweet/Supersweet No Salt)	.60
(Green Giant)	100
(S&W)	100
(Seneca)	.80
(Stokely)	100
white *(Del Monte)*	100
garlic:	
crushed *(Christopher Ranch),* 1 tsp.	.10
crushed *(Frieda's),* 1 oz.	.39

Vegetables, Canned or in Jars, garlic *(cont.)*
   pickled *(Christopher Ranch)*, 3 pieces, ¼ oz. 5
grape leaves *(Krinos)*, 1 leaf 5
greens, mixed *(Allens/Sunshine)* 30
kale *(Allens/Sunshine)* .25
kale *(Stubb's Harvest)* .25
lentils *(Eden* Organic) .90
lentils, spiced *(Patak's* Moong Dhal) 160
mushrooms:
   (Seneca Jars) 30
   (Seneca/Seneca No Salt) 25
   all varieties, except with garlic *(B in B)*, 4¼-oz. can 30
   all varieties *(Green Giant)* 30
   with garlic, sliced *(B in B)*, 4¼-oz. can 35
   pickled *(Seneca)*, 1 oz. 5
   shiitake *(Seneca)* 25
   teriyaki, sliced *(Seneca)* 80
mustard greens *(Allens/Sunshine)* 30
mustard greens *(Stubb's Harvest)* 30
okra:
   cut *(Allens/Trappey's)* 25
   cut *(Stubb's Harvest)* 25
   Creole gumbo *(Trappey's)* 35
   with tomatoes *(Allens/Trappey's)* 25
   with tomatoes and corn *(Allens/Trappey's)* 30
onion, whole *(Green Giant)* 35
onion, whole *(S&W)* 40
palm, hearts of *(Haddon House)*, 4.5 oz. 20
peas, cream *(Allens/East Texas Fair)* 100
peas, crowder *(Allens/East Texas Fair/Homefolks)* 110
peas, field:
   fresh shell *(Sunshine)* 120
   fresh shell, with snaps *(Allens/East Texas Fair/Homefolks)* . 120
   fresh shell, with snaps *(Goya)* 110
   dry, with bacon *(Trappey's)* 90
   dry, with snaps and bacon *(Trappey's)* 110
peas, green:
   (Del Monte/Del Monte No Salt) 60
   (Goya) 95
   (Goya Tender Sweet) 70
   (S&W Petit Pois/Sweet) 70
   (Seneca/Seneca No Salt) 70

(Stokely/Stokely No Salt) .60
all varieties *(Green Giant* 50% Less Sodium) 60
all varieties *(Green Giant LeSueur)* 60
all varieties *(Green Giant LeSueur* 50% Less Sodium) 60
all varieties except peas and carrots *(Green Giant)* 60
early June *(Sun-Vista)* 80
early June, dry *(Crest Top)* 100
early or sweet *(Green Giant/Green Giant* Less Sodium) 60
very young, small *(Del Monte)* 60
and carrots *(Del Monte)* .60
and carrots *(Goya)* 60
and carrots *(Green Giant)* 50
and carrots *(S&W)* 50
and carrots *(Seneca)* 60
and carrots *(Stokely)* 60
and carrots *(Stokely* No Salt/Sugar) 50
with pearl onions *(S&W)* .40
peas, lady *(Sunshine)* 100
peas, lady, with snaps *(East Texas Fair)* 100
peas, pepper *(Allens/East Texas Fair/Homefolks)* 120
peas, pigeon, dried *(El Jib)* 80
peas, pigeon, green *(Tupi)* 70
peas, purple hull *(East Texas)* 120
peas, purple hull *(Stubb's Harvest)* 120
peas, white acre *(East Texas Fair)* 100
pepper, banana *(Nalley)*, 1 oz. 5
pepper, banana, hot or mild *(Vlasic)*, 1 oz. 5
pepper, cherry:
   (Trappey's), 2 pieces .10
   hot *(B&G)*, 1 oz. 10
   hot *(Hebrew National)*, 1⅓ pieces 25
   hot *(Progresso)*, 1 piece 10
   hot or mild *(Vlasic)*, 1 oz. 10
   hot, sliced, drained *(Progresso)*, 2 tbsp. 25
   sweet *(Nalley)*, 1 oz. .10
pepper, chili:
   green, whole *(Chi-Chi's)*, ¾ chili 10
   green, whole *(Nalley)*, 1 oz. 10
   green, whole *(Rosarita)*, 1.2 oz. 5
   green, whole, peeled *(Old El Paso)*, 1 chili 10
   green, chopped *(Old El Paso)*, 2 tbsp. 5
   green, diced *(Chi-Chi's)*, 2 tbsp. 10

Vegetables, Canned or in Jars, pepper, chili *(cont.)*
  green, diced *(Pancho Villa)*, 2 tbsp. 5
  green, diced *(Rosarita)*, 2 tbsp. 5
  yellow, hot *(Del Monte)*, 4 pieces, 1 oz. 10
pepper, jalapeño:
  all varieties *(Clemente Jacques)*, 1 oz. 10
  whole *(Goya)*, 2 pieces 10
  whole *(Nalley)*, 1 oz. 5
  whole *(Rosarita)*, 1.2 oz. .10
  whole *(Trappey's)*, 2 pieces 10
  whole, peeled *(Old El Paso)*, 3 pieces, 1.1 oz. 5
  whole or wheels *(Chi-Chi's)* 10
  diced *(La Victoria)*, 1.1 oz. 10
  diced *(Rosarita)*, 1.1 oz. 5
  hot *(Vlasic)*, 1 oz. 10
  marinated *(La Victoria)*, 1.1 oz. 10
  nacho, sliced *(La Victoria)*, 1.1 oz. 0
  nacho, sliced *(Rosarita)*, 1.1 oz. 5
  pickled *(La Victoria)*, 1.1 oz. 10
  pickled *(Old El Paso)*, 2 pieces 5
  pickled, sliced *(Old El Paso)*, 2 tbsp., 1.1 oz. 10
  sliced *(Nalley)*, 1 oz. 5
pepper, nacho, pickled *(Goya)*, 14 slices 10
pepper, serrano, *(Stubb's Legendary)*, 1 oz. 5
pepper, sweet:
  (B&G), 1 oz. 10
  filet *(Hebrew National/Rosoff/Shorr's)*, 1 oz. 9
  fire-roasted, with garlic and oil *(Paesana)*, 2 tbsp. 20
  fried, drained *(Progresso)*, 2 tbsp. 60
  red *(B&G)*, 1 oz. 20
  rings *(Vlasic)*, 1 oz. 25
  roasted *(Progresso)*, 1 piece 10
pepper, pepperoncini:
  (Krinos), ¼ cup 5
  (Nalley), 1 oz. 5
  (Progresso Tuscan), 3 peppers 10
  (Vlasic Salad), 1 oz. 5
  (Zorba), 5 pieces, 1.1 oz. .15
pimiento *(Goya)*, ¼ pepper 0
pimiento, drained *(S&W)*, 2¼ oz. 20
poke greens *(Allens)* 35

potato:
  (Seneca), ⅔ cup 80
  whole *(Butterfield/Sunshine)*, 2½ pieces, 5.6 oz. 90
  whole *(Stokely/Stokely No Salt)*, 5.5 oz. 80
  whole, new *(Del Monte)*, 2 medium with liquid 60
  whole, new *(S&W)* .60
  sliced *(Butterfield)* .100
  sliced *(Del Monte)*, ⅔ cup 60
  diced *(Butterfield)*, ⅔ cup 100
  mashed *(Idahoan Complete)*, ⅓ cup 100
  mashed *(Idahoan Real)*, ⅓ cup 80
pumpkin:
  (Comstock) 50
  (Libby's) 60
  (Stokely) 50
rutabaga *(Sunshine)* .30
sauerkraut:
  (Boar's Head), 2 tbsp. 5
  (Claussen), ¼ cup 5
  (Del Monte), 2 tbsp. 0
  (Eden Organic) 25
  (Frank's/Snowfloss), 2 tbsp. 5
  (Hebrew National), 2 tbsp. 5
  (Hebrew National) .25
  (Hebrew National/Shorr's New) 50
  (Pickle Eater's Kozmic Kraut/Reduced Sodium), 2 tbsp. 0
  (Rosoff Home Style) 50
  (S&W), 2 tbsp. 5
  (Seneca), 2 tbsp. 5
  (Silver Floss), 2 tbsp. 5
  (Stokely), 2 tbsp. 5
  (Stokely) 25
  Bavarian style *(Del Monte)*, 2 tbsp. 15
  Bavarian style *(Frank's/Snowfloss)*, 2 tbsp. 15
  Bavarian style *(Seneca)*, 2 tbsp. 10
  Bavarian style *(Silver Floss)*, 2 tbsp. 10
  Bavarian style *(Stokely)*, 2 tbsp. 10
  Bavarian style *(Stokely)*, ...35
  sweet and sour *(Stokely)*, 2 tbsp. 20
  sweet and sour *(Stokely)* 80
spinach:
  (Allens Popeye) 45

Vegetables, Canned or in Jars, spinach *(cont.)*
    (Allens Popeye Low Sodium) 35
    (Del Monte/Del Monte No Salt) 30
    (S&W) 30
    chopped *(Allens Popeye/Sunshine)* 40
squash *(Stokely)* 50
squash, yellow *(Allens/Sunshine)* 25
succotash:
    kernel *(S&W)* 100
    kernel *(Seneca)* 90
    kernel *(Stokely)* 100
sweet potato:
    (Seneca Yams) 150
    whole *(Royal Prince/Trappey's)*, 4 pieces 200
    halves *(Royal Prince)*, 5.7 oz., 3 pieces 190
    cut or pieces *(Allens/Sugary Sam/Princella* Yams), ⅔ cup . 160
    mashed *(Princella/Sugary Sam)*, ⅔ cup 120
    candied *(Royal Prince)* 210
    candied *(S&W)* 170
    orange-pineapple *(Royal Prince)* 210
tomatillo *(La Victoria* Entero), 5 pieces 40
tomatillo, crushed *(La Victoria)*, 4½ oz. 45
tomato:
    (Contadina Pasta Ready) 40
    (Contadina Recipe Ready) 25
    (Hunt's) 30
    whole *(Del Monte)* 25
    whole *(Hunt's/Hunt's* No Salt), 2 pieces 20
    whole, Italian pear *(Contadina)* 25
    whole, Italian pear, with basil *(S&W)* 25
    whole, pear *(Hunt's)* 20
    whole, peeled *(Contadina)* 25
    whole, peeled *(Progresso)* 20
    whole, peeled *(S&W)* 25
    whole, peeled *(S&W* No-Salt) 20
    whole, with basil *(Progresso/Progresso* Imported) 20
    whole, with green chilies *(Ro*Tel)* 20
    aspic *(S&W)* 50
    with cheeses, three *(Contadina* Pasta Ready) 70
    chunky, chili *(Del Monte)* 30
    chunky, pasta *(Del Monte)* 45
    chunky, salsa *(Del Monte)* 35

crushed *(Contadina)*, ¼ cup 20
crushed *(Eden* Organic) 20
crushed *(Hunt's/Hunt's* Angela Mia) 30
crushed *(Progresso)* 20
crushed *(S&W)*, ¼ cup 20
cut *(Hunt's* Choice Cut) 20
cut, in juice *(S&W* Ready-Cut/Ready-Cut No Salt) 25
cut, in juice, Italian style *(S&W* Ready-Cut) 25
cut, in puree *(S&W* Ready-Cut) 30
diced *(Del Monte)* 25
diced *(Eden* Organic) 30
wedges *(Del Monte)* 35
diced, with basil *(Master Choice)* 40
diced, with basil, garlic, and oregano *(Del Monte)* 50
diced, with green chilies *(Eden* Organic) 30
diced, with green chilies *(Hunt's* Choice Cut), 2 tbsp. 0
diced, with onion, garlic *(Del Monte)* 35
diced, with roasted garlic or Italian herb *(Hunt's* Choice
  Cut) 25
with green chilies, whole or diced *Ro*Tel)* 20
with green chilies or jalapeños, *(Old El Paso)*, ¼ cup 10
with green chilies, diced *(Chi-Chi's)*, ¼ cup 20
with mushrooms or primavera *(Contadina* Pasta Ready) 50
with olives *(Contadina* Pasta Ready) 60
paste or puree, *see "Tomato Paste, Puree & Sauce,"*
  page 120
with red pepper, crushed *(Contadina* Pasta Ready) 60
stewed *(Contadina)* 40
stewed *(Del Monte/Del Monte* No Salt) 35
stewed *(Green Giant* Classic) 35
stewed *(Hunt's)* 35
stewed *(S&W/S&W* No-Salt) 35
stewed, Cajun or Mexican *(Del Monte)* 35
stewed, Italian *(Contadina)* .40
stewed, Italian *(Del Monte)* .30
stewed, Italian *(Green Giant)* 30
stewed, Italian *(S&W)* 35
stewed, Mexican *(Contadina)* 40
stewed, Mexican *(Green Giant)* 35
tomato sauce, *see "Tomato Paste, Puree & Sauce," page 120,*
  and "Pasta Sauces," page 263

Vegetables, Canned or in Jars *(cont.)*
turnip greens:
    (Allens/Sunshine) 25
    (Stubb's Harvest) 25
    chopped, with diced turnip *(Allens/Sunshine)* 30
vegetables, mixed:
    (Del Monte/Del Monte No Salt) 40
    (Green Giant) 60
    (Green Giant Garden Medley) 40
    (S&W) 35
    (Seneca/Seneca No Salt) .45
    (Stokely/Stokely No Salt) 35
    and sauce *(House of Tsang* Cantonese Classic) 70
    and sauce, hot and spicy *(House of Tsang* Szechuan) 70
    and sauce, sweet and sour *(House of Tsang* Hong Kong) . . . 160
    and sauce, teriyaki *(House of Tsang* Tokyo) 100
    stew *(Seneca)* 45
    stew *(Stokely)* 45
water chestnuts *(La Choy)*, 2 whole or 2 tbsp. slices 10
water chestnuts, sliced *(Sun Luck)*, ¼ cup 15
zucchini, Italian style *(Del Monte)* 30
zucchini, Italian style *(Progresso)* 40

VEGETABLES, FROZEN
See also "Vegetables, Canned or in Jars," "Vegetable Dishes, Frozen," and "Entrees, Frozen"

---

                                                        calories
artichoke hearts *(Birds Eye)*, ½ cup 40
asparagus:
    cuts *(Birds Eye)*, ½ cup .25
    cuts *(Green Giant Harvest Fresh)*, ⅔ cup 25
    spears *(Birds Eye)*, 3 oz. 20
beans, green:
    (Seabrook), 1 cup 25
    whole *(Birds Eye)*, 3 oz. 20
    cut or French cut *(Birds Eye)*, ½ cup 25
    cut *(Green Giant)*, ¾ cup 25
    cut *(Green Giant Harvest Fresh)*, ⅔ cup 25
    cut *(Schwan's)*, ⅔ cup .20
    Italian *(Birds Eye)*, ½ cup 35
    sliced *(Stilwell)*, ⅔ cup 25

and almonds *(Green Giant Harvest Fresh)*, ²/₃ cup 60
with potatoes, onions, peppers *(Green Giant American
Mixtures)*, ³/₄ cup 45
beans, lima:
baby *(Birds Eye)*, ¹/₂ cup 130
baby *(Green Giant Harvest Fresh)*, ¹/₂ cup 80
baby *(Seabrook)*, ¹/₂ cup 110
baby *(Stilwell)*, ¹/₂ cup 110
baby, butter sauce *(Green Giant)*, ²/₃ cup 120
Fordhook *(Birds Eye)*, ¹/₂ cup 100
Fordhook *(Stilwell)*, ¹/₂ cup 90
plain or speckled *(Stilwell* Butterbeans)*, ¹/₂ cup 100
beans, wax *(Seabrook)*, ²/₃ cup 25
black-eyed peas *(Stilwell)*, ¹/₂ cup 110
broccoli:
spears *(Green Giant)*, 3 oz. 25
spears *(Green Giant Harvest Fresh)*, 3.5 oz. 25
spears *(Schwan's)*, 1 spear 20
spears or baby spears *(Birds Eye)*, 3 oz. 25
florets *(Birds Eye)*, 3 oz. 25
florets *(Green Giant)*, 1¹/₃ cups 25
florets *(Stilwell)*, 4 florets 25
chopped *(Birds Eye)*, ¹/₃ cup 25
chopped *(Green Giant)*, ³/₄ cup 25
chopped *(Seabrook)*, ³/₄ cup, 3 oz. 25
cut *(Birds Eye)*, ¹/₂ cup .25
cut *(Green Giant)*, 1 cup .25
cut *(Green Giant Harvest Fresh)*, ²/₃ cup 25
cut *(Stilwell)*, ¹/₂ cup .25
in butter sauce, spears *(Green Giant)*, 4 oz. 50
in cheese sauce *(Freezer Queen* Family Side Dish)*, ²/₃ cup . .50
in cheese sauce *(Green Giant)*, ²/₃ cup 70
carrots and cauliflower *(Green Giant American Mixtures)*,
³/₄ cup 25
carrots and water chestnuts *(Birds Eye)*, ¹/₂ cup 30
carrots and water chestnuts *(Green Giant American
Mixtures)*, ³/₄ cup 30
cauliflower *(Birds Eye)*, ¹/₂ cup 20
cauliflower *(Stilwell)*, ¹/₂ cup 25
cauliflower and carrots *(Birds Eye)*, ¹/₂ cup 25
cauliflower and carrots *(Green Giant Harvest Fresh)*, 1 cup . .30
cauliflower and carrots *(Schwan's)*, 1 cup 25

Vegetables, Frozen, broccoli *(cont.)*

    cauliflower and carrots, cheese sauce *(Green Giant)*, ⅔ cup . . .80
    cauliflower and red peppers *(Birds Eye)*, ½ cup 20
    cauliflower, carrots, corn, and peas, in butter sauce *(Green Giant)*, ¾ cup 60
    cauliflower, peas, peppers *(Green Giant American Mixtures)*, ¾ cup 30
    corn and red peppers *(Birds Eye)*, ½ cup 50
    green beans, onions, and red peppers *(Birds Eye)*, ½ cup . .25
    pasta, peas, corn, and peppers, in butter sauce *(Green Giant)*, ¾ cup 70
    red peppers, onions, and mushrooms *(Birds Eye)*, ½ cup . .25
    stir-fry *(Birds Eye)*, 1 cup 30
Brussels sprouts:
    (Birds Eye), 11 sprouts 35
    (Stilwell), 6 sprouts 35
    baby, in butter sauce *(Green Giant)*, ⅔ cup 60
    cauliflower and carrots *(Birds Eye)*, ½ cup 30
carrot:
    baby, whole *(Birds Eye)*, ½ cup 40
    baby, whole *(Schwan's)*, 13 pieces 35
    baby, whole *(Stilwell)*, ⅔ cup 35
    baby cut *(Green Giant)*, ¾ cup 30
    baby cut *(Green Giant Harvest Fresh)*, ⅔ cup 20
    crinkle *(Stilwell)*, ⅔ cup .35
    sliced *(Birds Eye)*, ½ cup 35
    and green beans, cauliflower *(Green Giant American Mixtures)*, ¾ cup 25
cauliflower:
    (Birds Eye), ½ cup 20
    (Stilwell), 1 cup 20
    florets *(Green Giant)*, 1 cup 25
    in cheese sauce *(Green Giant)*, ½ cup 60
    carrots and snow pea pods *(Birds Eye)*, ½ cup 30
    carrots and sugar snap and sweet peas *(Green Giant American Mixtures)*, ¾ cup 35
corn:
    on the cob *(Birds Eye Big Ears)*, 1 ear 120
    on the cob *(Birds Eye Little Ears)*, 2 ears 110
    on the cob *(Green Giant Extra Sweet)*, 1 ear 120
    on the cob *(Green Giant Nibblers)*, 1 ear 70
    on the cob *(Green Giant Niblets)*, 1 ear 160

on the cob *(John Cope's)*, 1 ear 120
on the cob *(Ore-Ida Mini-Gold)*, 1 ear 80
on the cob *(Schwan's)*, 1 ear 180
on the cob, white *(John Cope's)*, 1 ear 150
kernel, golden *(Birds Eye)*, ¹/₃ cup 70
kernel, golden *(Birds Eye* Sweet/Tendersweet)*, ¹/₃ cup 60
kernel, golden *(Green Giant Harvest Fresh Niblets)*, ²/₃ cup . .80
kernel, golden *(Green Giant Niblets)*, ²/₃ cup 80
kernel, golden *(Green Giant Niblets* Extra Sweet)*, ²/₃ cup 70
kernal, golden *(Schwan's)*, ²/₃ cup 80
kernel, golden *(Stilwell)*, ²/₃ cup 80
kernel, white *(Green Giant)*, ³/₄ cup 100
kernel, white *(Green Giant* Extra Sweet)*, ²/₃ cup 50
kernel, white *(Green Giant Harvest Fresh)*, ¹/₂ cup 70
kernel, white *(John Cope's)*, ¹/₃ cup 80
cream-style *(Green Giant)*, ¹/₂ cup 110
cream-style, white *(John Cope's Sweet 'N Creamy)*, ¹/₃ cup . 100
in butter sauce *(Green Giant Niblets)*, ²/₃ cup 130
in butter sauce, white *(Green Giant)*, ³/₄ cup 120
corn, broccoli, and peppers *(Green Giant American Mixtures)*,
    ³/₄ cup 60
kale *(Seabrook)*, 3 oz. 30
mustard greens, chopped *(Seabrook)*, 3 oz. 30
okra:
    whole *(Seabrook)*, 9 pods, 3 oz. 25
    whole *(Stilwell)*, 9 pods, 3 oz. 35
    cut *(Stilwell)*, ³/₄ cup .25
    and tomatoes *(Stilwell)*, ²/₃ cup 25
onion, whole, small *(Birds Eye)*, 17 pieces 30
onion, chopped *(Ore-Ida)*, ³/₄ cup 25
peas, butter *(Stilwell)*, ¹/₂ cup 110
peas, crowder *(Stilwell)*, ¹/₂ cup 120
peas, edible-podded, sugar snap:
    (Birds Eye), ¹/₂ cup .40
    (Green Giant), ³/₄ cup 35
    (Green Giant Harvest Fresh), ²/₃ cup 50
    (Schwan's), ²/₃ cup .45
    stir-fry *(Birds Eye)*, ³/₄ cup 35
peas, field, with snaps *(Stilwell)*, ¹/₂ cup 110
peas, green, ²/₃ cup, except as noted:
    (Birds Eye) 70
    (Schwan's) 70

Vegetables, Frozen, peas, green *(cont.)*

(Seabrook) 70
(Stilwell) 70
early June or baby sweet *(Green Giant LeSueur)* 60
sweet *(Green Giant)* 70
sweet *(Green Giant Harvest Fresh)* 60
tiny *(Birds Eye)* 60
in butter sauce, baby, early *(Green Giant LeSueur)*, ¾ cup . 100
in butter sauce, sweet *(Green Giant)*, ¾ cup 100
and carrots *(Stilwell)*, ½ cup 50
and mushrooms *(Green Giant LeSueur)*, ¾ cup 60
and pearl onions *(Green Giant)* 60
and pearl onions *(Green Giant Harvest Fresh)*, ½ cup 50
and potatoes and carrots *(Green Giant American Mixtures)* . .70
peas, purple hull *(Stilwell)*, ½ cup 110
pepper stir-fry *(Birds Eye)*, 3 oz. 25
potato, 3 oz., except as noted:
whole *(Stilwell)*, 3 pieces 50
curls *(Schwan's)* 160
fried *(Ore-Ida Deep Fries/Deep Fries Crinkle Cuts)* 160
fried *(Ore-Ida Shoestrings)* 150
fried *(Ore-Ida Steak Fries)* 110
fried *(Ore-Ida Crispers!)* 220
fried *(Ore-Ida Crispy Crowns!)* 190
fried *(Ore-Ida Crispy Crunchies!/Ore-Ida Zesties)* 160
fried *(Ore-Ida Fast Fries/Ore-Ida Golden Twirls)* 150
fried *(Ore-Ida Golden Crinkles)* 140
fried *(Ore-Ida Golden Fries)* 120
fried *(Ore-Ida Golden Pixie Crinkles)* 130
fried *(Ore-Ida Homestyle Wedges with Skin)* 110
fried *(Ore-Ida Snackin' Fries)*, 5-oz. pkg. 340
fried *(Ore-Ida Texas Crispers!)* 170
fried *(Ore-Ida Waffle Fries)* 150
fried *(Schwan's)* 150
fried, cottage fries *(Ore-Ida)* 130
fried, country fries *(Ore-Ida)* 120
fried, crinkle cut *(Empire Kosher)*, ½ cup 90
fried, ranch flavor *(Ore-Ida Fast Fries)* 150
fried, zesty *(Ore-Ida Snackin' Fries)*, 5-oz. pkg. 340
hash brown *(Ore-Ida Microwave)*, 4-oz. pkg. 220
hash brown *(Ore-Ida Golden Patties)*, 1 piece 160
hash brown *(Schwan's)*, 1 patty 60

hash brown, with cheddar *(Ore-Ida Cheddar Browns)*,
1 piece 80
hash brown, country *(Ore-Ida)*, 1 cup 60
hash brown, shredded *(Ore-Ida)*, 1 piece 70
hash brown, Southern style *(Ore-Ida)*, ¾ cup 80
hash brown, toaster *(Ore-Ida)*, 2 pieces 190
mashed *(Ore-Ida)*, ⅔ cup .90
O'Brien *(Ore-Ida)*, ¾ cup .60
puffs *(Hot Tots)* 160
puffs *(Schwan's Quik Taters)*, 13 pieces 160
puffs *(Tater Tots)* 160
puffs *(Tater Tots* Microwave), 4-oz. pkg. 180
spinach:
(Green Giant), ¾ cup 25
(Green Giant Harvest Fresh), ½ cup 25
leaf *(Seabrook)*, 1 cup 20
leaf or chopped *(Birds Eye)*, ⅓ cup 20
chopped *(Seabrook)*, ⅓ cup 20
in butter sauce, cut *(Green Giant)*, ½ cup 40
squash *(Stilwell)*, ½ cup 15
squash, winter *(Birds Eye)*, ½ cup 50
turnip greens, with diced turnips *(Seabrook)*, ½ cup 30
vegetables, mixed:
(Goya), ⅔ cup 60
(Green Giant), ¾ cup 50
(Green Giant Harvest Fresh), ⅔ cup 50
(Stilwell), ½ cup 60
in butter sauce *(Green Giant)*, ¾ cup 70
California or Capri *(Stilwell)*, ½ cup 25
soup *(Birds Eye)*, ⅔ cup .45
stew *(Ore-Ida)*, ⅔ cup 50
stir-fry *(Birds Eye)*, 1 cup 30
stir-fry *(Schwan's)*, 1 cup 35
tropical *(Goya* Pasteles de Masa), 1 pouch 280
tropical *(Goya* Viando Sancocho), 3 oz. 100
tropical *(Goya* Yautia Malanga), ⅛ pkg. 130
yuca *(Goya)*, ½ cup 191

> **VEGETABLES, DRIED,** ¼ cup, except as noted
> *See also "Vegetables, Canned or in Jars," "Vegetable Dishes,*
> *Mixes," and "Seasonings, Dry & Mixes"*

	calories
beans, adzuki *(Arrowhead Mills)*	160
beans, anasazi *(Arrowhead Mills)*	150
beans, black:	
(Frieda's), 1 oz.	40
(Goya)	70
turtle soup *(Arrowhead Mills)*	150
beans, canary *(Goya)*	190
beans, great northern, boiled *(Goya)*	70
beans, green, freeze-dried *(Mountain House)*, ⅔ cup	25
beans, kidney *(Arrowhead Mills)*	160
beans, mung *(Arrowhead Mills)*	160
beans, pinto *(Arrowhead Mills)*	150
beans, pinto *(Goya)*	60
beans, Roman *(Goya)*	80
chickpeas *(Arrowhead Mills)*	170
corn:	
(John Cope's)	130
freeze-dried *(AlpineAire)*, ½ cup	85
freeze-dried *(Mountain House)*, ½ cup	80
lentil, green or red *(Arrowhead Mills)*	150
mixed, freeze-dried *(AlpineAire)*, ½ cup	71
mixed, garden, freeze-dried *(AlpineAire)*, ½ cup	79
mushroom, oyster *(Frieda's)*, 1 oz.	7
mushroom, portobello *(Frieda's)*, .5 oz.	13
peas, green *(Goya)*	100
peas, green, freeze-dried *(Mountain House)*, ½ cup	80
peas, pigeon *(Goya)*	140
peas, split:	
(Goya)	110
green, dry *(Arrowhead Mills)*	170
yellow *(Goya)*	110
seaweed:	
arame *(Eden)*, ½ cup	30
agar flakes *(Eden)*, 1 tbsp.	10
hiziki *(Eden)*, ½ cup	30
kombu *(Eden)*, ½ of 7" piece	10
nori *(Eden/Eden Sushi)*, 1 sheet	10

wakame, regular or flakes *(Eden)*, ½ cup 25
soybean *(Arrowhead Mills)*. 170
tomato:
    (Frieda's No Salt), 1 oz. .86
    bits *(Sonoma)*, 2–3 tsp. .15
    flakes *(Christopher Ranch)*, 3 tbsp. 80
    halves *(Sonoma)*, 2–3 pieces 15
    julienne *(Sonoma)*, 7–9 strips 15
    in oil, drained *(Sonoma* Spice Medley), 1 tbsp. 50
    pasta toss *(Sonoma)*, ½ cup 70
    seasoning *(Sonoma* Season It), 2–3 tsp. 20

VEGETABLE DISHES, FROZEN
See also "Vegetables, Frozen," "Entrees, Frozen," and "Rice Dishes, Frozen"

                                             calories

broccoli, pasta, cauliflower, and carrots, in cheese sauce
    (Freezer Queen Family Side Dish), ⅔ cup 70
corn, scalloped *(Schwan's)*, ½ cup 140
corn fritter *(Mrs. Paul's)*, 1 piece 130
corn soufflé *(Stouffer's)*, about ½ cup, 4.8 oz. 170
green bean mushroom casserole *(Stouffer's)*, approx. ½ cup,
    3.8 oz. 140
mushrooms, breaded *(Empire* Kosher), 7 pieces, 2.9 oz. 90
mushrooms, breaded *(Schwan's)*, 1 cup 210
onion rings:
    (Mrs. Paul's), 7 rings, 3 oz. 230
    (Ore-Ida Classic/Gourmet), 4 rings 220
    (Ore-Ida Onion Ringers), 6 rings 230
    (Schwan's), 3 oz. 160
pepper, stuffed:
    (Stouffer's), 10 oz. 200
    (Stouffer's), ½ of 15½-oz. pkg. 180
    jalapeño *(Schwan's)*, 3 pieces 250
pierogi, frozen or refrigerated:
    (Schwan's), 3 pieces 180
    potato cheese *(Empire* Kosher), 4 oz. 214
    potato onion *(Empire* Kosher), 4 oz. 165
    potato onion *(Giorgio)*, 3 pieces 230
potato:
    (Goya Rellenos de Papa), 2 pieces 280

Vegetable Dishes, Frozen, potato *(cont.)*
   (Goya Rellenos de Papa Cocktail), 6 pieces 260
   au gratin *(Schwan's)*, ½ cup 180
   au gratin *(Stouffer's* Side Dish), about ½ cup, 4.6 oz. 130
   baked, broccoli and cheese *(Ore-Ida* Twice Baked), 1 pkg. . 150
   baked, broccoli and cheese *(Weight Watchers)*, 10 oz. 250
   baked, butter flavor *(Ore-Ida* Twice Baked), 5 oz. 200
   baked, cheddar *(Ore-Ida* Twice Baked), 5 oz. 190
   baked, sour cream and chive *(Ore-Ida* Twice Baked), 5 oz. . 200
   blintz, *see "Entrees, Frozen," page 168*
   cheddar *(Lean Cuisine* Deluxe), 1 pkg. 230
   cheddar broccoli *(Healthy Choice)*, 1 pkg. 310
   garden casserole *(Healthy Choice)*, 1 pkg. 210
   roasted, with broccoli, cheese sauce *(Lean Cuisine Lunch*
     Classics), 1 pkg. 210
   scalloped *(Stouffer's* Side Dish), approx. ½ cup, 4.6 oz. . . . 140
   scalloped, and ham *(Swanson)*, 1 pkg. 290
   stuffed *(Schwan's)*, 1 potato 220
potato pancake *(Empire* Kosher), 2-oz. cake 80
potato pancake, mini *(Empire* Kosher), 2 cakes, 2 oz. 90
spinach:
   creamed *(Green Giant)*, ½ cup 80
   creamed *(Seabrook)*, ½ cup 120
   creamed *(Schwan's)*, ½ cup . . . . : 120
   creamed *(Stouffer's* Side Dish), ½ of 9-oz. pkg. 160
   creamed *(Tabatchnick)*, 7.5 oz. 60
   Indian *(Deep* Palak Paneer), 5 oz. 230
   soufflé *(Stouffer's* Side Dish), approx. ½ cup, 4 oz. 150
sweet potato, candied:
   (Mrs. Paul's), 5 oz. 300
   (Mrs. Paul's Sweets 'n Apples), 1¼ cups 270
   (Ore-Ida), 5 pieces 170
vegetable samosa *(Deep* Indian Cuisine), 2 pieces 130
vegetables, with pasta, *see "Pasta Side Dishes, Frozen," page*
   221
zucchini, breaded *(Empire)*, 1 piece 100

VEGETABLE DISHES, MIXES
*See also "Vegetables, Dried," "Pasta & Noodle Dishes, Mixes,"
and "Rice Dishes, Mixes"*

calories

beans, black:
   with fusilli *(Bean Cuisine)*, ½ cup* 174
   instant *(Fantastic Foods)*, ½ cup* 160
   Jamaican, and brown rice *(Fantastic* One Pot Meals),
      ⅜ cup 140
   zesty, and penne *(Fantastic* One Pot Meals), ⅜ cup 150
beans, Florentine, with bow ties *(Bean Cuisine)*, ½ cup* 199
beans, French, country, with gemelli *(Bean Cuisine)*, ½ cup* . 214
beans, Italian *(Knorr* Cup), 1 pkg. 230
beans, red, Barcelona, with radiatore *(Bean Cuisine)*, ½ cup* . 170
beans, red, New Orleans, and brown rice
   (Fantastic One Pot Meals), ½ cup 150
beans, refried *(Fantastic Foods)*, ½ cup* 160
hummus *(Casbah)*, 1 oz. 120
lentils:
   burgoo, spicy *(Buckeye Beans)*, 2½ tbsp. 110
   cassoulet, sausage *(Buckeye Beans)*, 2½ tbsp. 110
   hearty, and wild rice *(Spice Islands* Quick Meal), 1 pkg. . . 190
   and herb *(Eastern Traditions)*, 2 oz. 160
   honey baked *(Buckeye Beans)*, 4 tbsp. 180
   pilaf *(Casbah)*, 1 oz. 100
   pilaf *(Near East)*, 1 cup* 210
   pilaf, almond *(Spice Islands* Quick Meal), 1 pkg. 190
potatoes:
   (Betty Crocker Potato Shakers), 3 tsp. 25
   (Betty Crocker Potato Shakers), ⅔ cup* 140
   (Betty Crocker Potato Buds), ⅓ cup 80
   (Betty Crocker Potato Buds), ⅔ cup* 160
   all varieties *(Hungry Jack)*, ½ cup 110
   all varieties, except sour cream and chive *(Hungry Jack)*,
      ⅛ pkg.* 150
   au gratin *(Betty Crocker)*, ½ cup 100
   au gratin *(Betty Crocker)*, ½ cup* 110
   au gratin *(Idahoan)*, ⅓ cup 110
   au gratin, broccoli *(Betty Crocker)*, ½ cup 90

* Prepared according to package directions

Vegetable Dishes, Mixes, potatoes *(cont.)*

* Prepared according to package directions

cheese, three *(Betty Crocker)*, ½ cup* 120
French country *(Good Harvest)*, ⅓ cup 100
hash brown *(Betty Crocker)*, ½ cup 130
hash brown *(Betty Crocker)*, ½ cup* 200
garlic *(Betty Crocker Potato Shakers)*, 2 tsp. 20
garlic *(Betty Crocker Potato Shakers)*, ⅔ cup* 130
garlic, low-fat recipe *(Betty Crocker Potato Shakers)*,
   ⅔ cup* 110
garlic and herbs *(Fantastic* Potato Cup), 1.7 oz. 180
Italian, southern *(Good Harvest)*, ⅓ cup 110
julienne *(Betty Crocker)*, ½ cup 90
julienne *(Betty Crocker)*, ½ cup* 110
mashed *(Barbara's)*, ⅓ cup .70
mashed *(Hungry Jack* Flakes), ⅓ cup 80
mashed *(Hungry Jack* Flakes), ½ cup* 160
mashed *(Idahoan)*, ⅓ cup 80
mashed *(Martha White Spudflakes)*, ⅓ cup 80
mashed *(Pillsbury* Idaho Flakes), ⅓ cup 80
mashed *(Pillsbury* Idaho Flakes), ½ cup* 150
mashed, all flavors *(Hungry Jack)*, ⅓ cup 80
mashed, all flavors *(Hungry Jack)*, ½ cup* 150
mashed, granules *(Pillsbury* Idaho), 2 tbsp. 90
mashed, granules *(Pillsbury* Idaho), ½ cup* 160
ranch *(Betty Crocker)*, ½ cup 110
ranch *(Betty Crocker)*, ½ cup* 130
reduced-fat recipe *(Betty Crocker Potato Buds)*, ⅔ cup* . . . 120
scalloped *(Betty Crocker)*, ½ cup 100
scalloped *(Betty Crocker)*, ½ cup* 130
scalloped *(Idahoan)*, ⅓ cup 110
scalloped, cheesy *(Betty Crocker)*, ⅔ cup 100
scalloped, cheesy *(Betty Crocker)*, ½ cup* 120
scalloped, cheesy, stove-top recipe *(Betty Crocker)*,
   ½ cup* 140
scalloped, and ham *(Betty Crocker)*, ½ cup 100
scalloped, and ham *(Betty Crocker)*, ½ cup* 120
sour cream and chive *(Betty Crocker)*, ½ cup 100
sour cream and chive *(Betty Crocker)*, ½ cup* 120
sour cream and chive *(Betty Crocker Potato Buds)*, ⅓ cup . 120
sour cream and chive *(Betty Crocker Potato Buds)*, ⅔ cup* . 190
sour cream and chive *(Fantastic* Potato Cup), 1.7 oz. 180

* Prepared according to package directions

Vegetable Dishes, Mixes, potatoes *(cont.)*
  sour cream and chive *(Hungry Jack)*, ⅛ pkg.* 160
  sour cream and chive, reduced-fat recipe *(Betty Crocker
    Potato Buds)*, ⅔ cup* .160
  vegetable and herb *(Good Harvest)*, ⅓ cup 110
  Western *(Idahoan)*, ¼ cup 100
potato pancake:
  (Hungry Jack), 2 tbsp. 70
  (Hungry Jack), 3 cakes*, 3″ 90
  (Knorr), 2 tbsp. 80

TOMATO PASTE, PUREE & SAUCE
*See also "Vegetables, Canned or in Jars," "Condiments &
Sauces," and "Pasta Sauces"*

---

                                                            calories
tomato paste, 2 tbsp.:
  (Contadina) 30
  (Del Monte) 30
  (Goya) 30
  (Hunt's/Hunt's No Salt) .30
  (Progresso) 30
  (S&W) 30
  with garlic or Italian *(Hunt's)* 30
  Italian *(Contadina)* 40
tomato puree, ¼ cup:
  (Contadina) 20
  (Hunt's) 25
  regular or thick style *(Progresso)* 25
tomato sauce, ¼ cup, except as noted:
  (Contadina/Contadina Thick & Zesty) 20
  (Del Monte/Del Monte No Salt) 20
  (Goya) 20
  (Hunt's/Hunt's No Salt) .15
  (Progresso) 20
  (S&W) 20
  chili, chunky *(Hunt's Ready Sauce)* 20
  chunk, chunky Mexican or salsa *(Hunt's Ready Sauce*
    Special) 20
  chunky *(Hunt's Ready Sauce)* 15

* Prepared according to package directions

garden *(S&W)* Original) 20
garden, Italian herb *(S&W)*, ½ cup 35
garden, mild Mexican *(S&W)* 20
garlic *(Hunt's Ready Sauce)* 30
garlic and herb *(Hunt's Ready Sauce)* 25
herb *(Hunt's)* 30
herb, country *(Hunt's Ready Sauce)* 35
herb and garlic *(S&W* Cooking Sauce)*, 1 tbsp. 15
Italian *(Contadina)* 15
Italian *(Hunt's/Hunt's Ready Sauce)* 30
Italian, chunky *(Hunt's Ready Sauce)* 25
meat loaf *(Hunt's Ready Sauce Meatloaf Fixin's)* 20
seasoned, lightly *(Eden)* 25

PICKLES, CUCUMBER, one ounce, except as noted
*See also "Vegetables, Canned or in Jars," "Pickle Relish,
Cucumber," "Olives," and "Condiments & Sauces"*

calories

bread and butter:
   (B&G Sandwich Toppers) 30
   (Mrs. Fanning's), 3 slices 25
   (Shorr's) 12
   chips *(B&G)* 30
   chips *(Claussen)*, 4 slices 20
   chips, unsalted *(B&G)* 25
   chips or sandwich stackers *(Vlasic)* 30
   chunks *(Nalley* Banquet) .25
   sandwich *(Claussen)*, 2 slices, 1.2 oz. 25
   slices *(Nalley)* 25
chips *(Nalley* Cucumber) 35
chips, with honey *(Pickle Eater's)* 25
dill:
   (Vlasic Milwaukee) 5
   all varieties *(Del Monte)* 5
   all varieties *(Nalley)* 5
   baby *(Pickle Eater's)* 0
   hamburger chips/slices *(Claussen)*, 10 slices, 1.1 oz. 5
dill, kosher:
   (Claussen Halves/*Claussen* Whole) 5
   (Claussen Mini)*, .8-oz. piece 5
   (Hebrew National Barrel/Hot), 1 pickle 23

Pickles, Cucumber, dill, kosher *(cont.)*

(Heinz), ½ pickle 0
(Nalley) 5
(Pickle Eater's/Pickle Eater's No Salt) 0
all varieties (B&G/B&G Sandwich Toppers) 0
all varieties (Vlasic) 5
chips (Claussen), 4 slices 5
slices (Claussen), 2 slices, 1.1 oz. 5
spears (Claussen), 1.2-oz. spear 5
spears (Pickle Eater's) 0
dill, Polish or zesty, spears (Vlasic) 5
kosher:
(Shorr's Deli) 4
whole (Rosoff/Shorr's) 4
halves (Hebrew National/Rosoff/Shorr's) 4
spears (Hebrew National/Shorr's) 4
sour:
(Claussen New York Deli/New York Garlic Deli), ½ pickle 5
(Claussen New York Garlic Deli), 2 slices, 1.2 oz. 5
kosher (Hebrew National/Rosoff/Shorr's New Half Sours) 4
kosher, garlic (Hebrew National/Shorr's) 3
kosher, spears (Rosoff/Shorr's Half Sour) 4
sweet:
(B&G Mixed) 30
(Nalley) 30
all varieties (Del Monte) 40
all varieties (Vlasic) .40
gherkins (B&G) 35
gherkins (Nalley) 25
midgets (Nalley) 30
nubbins (Nalley) 25

PICKLE RELISH, CUCUMBER one tablespoon
*See also "Vegetables, Canned or in Jars," "Pickles,
Cucumber," and "Condiments & Sauces"*

	calories
dill, chunky (Nalley)	0
emerald (B&G)	15
hamburger (B&G)	15
hamburger (Nalley)	15
hamburger or sweet (Del Monte)	20

hot dog:
    (B&G) 20
    (Del Monte) 15
    (Nalley) 15
India *(B&G)* 15
India *(Heinz)* 20
piccalilli *(B&G)* 20
piccalilli, tomato *(Pickle Eater's)* 10
red hot *(Ron's)* 15
sweet:
    (B&G) 15
    (Claussen) 15
    (Del Monte) 20
    (Hebrew National) 18
    (Nalley) 20
    honey *(Pickle Eater's)* .15
    unsalted *(B&G)* 20

OLIVES
See also "Pickles, Cucumber"

calories

black, *see "ripe," below*
Calamata:
    (Krinos), 3 olives 45
    (Zorba), 5 olives 90
green, cracked *(Krinos)*, ½ oz. 20
green, queen/Spanish:
    (B&G), 2 olives 20
    (S&W), 2 olives 20
    (Zorba), 2 olives 25
ripe, pitted:
    (Lindsay), 6 small, 5 medium, 4 large, or 1⅓ tbsp.
      chopped 25
    (S&W), 3 extra large or 3 jumbo 25
    (Vlasic), 4 large or 6 small 25
    California *(Vlasic)*, 1 tsp. chopped or 4–6 pieces 25
    Spanish *(Vlasic)*, 8 small 20
ripe, with pits *(Lindsay)*, 5 medium or 4 large 25
ripe, with pits *(S&W)*, 1 super colossal 15
ripe, oil-cured *(Progresso)*, 3 olives 50
ripe, oil-cured *(Krinos)*, ½ oz. 70

Olives *(cont.)*
ripe, Greek:
    (Krinos), ½ oz. 35
    (Krinos Alfonso), ½ oz. .30
    (Krinos Nafplion), ½ oz. 20
    (Zorba), 1.7-oz. olive 60
royal *(Krinos)*, ½ oz. 30
salad:
    (B&G), 2 tbsp. 25
    (Goya), ¼ cup 25
    (Progresso), 2 tbsp. 25
stuffed, Manzanilla:
    (B&G), 5 olives 25
    (Goya), 4 olives 25
    (Lindsay), 5 olives 25
    (S&W), 3 olives 25
stuffed, queen:
    (B&G), 2 olives 15
    (Goya), 2 olives 20
    (Lindsay), 2 olives 15
    (S&W, 4¾ oz.), 2 olives 15
    (S&W, 7 oz.), 2 olives .20
    (S&W, 10 oz.), 1 olive .10
    queen *(Vlasic)*, ½ oz. 20
    stuffed with tuna *(Goya)*, 4 olives 25

VEGETABLE JUICES

	calories
sauerkraut *(S&W)*, 10-oz. can	35
sauerkraut *(Stokely)*, 8 fl. oz.	20

tomato:
    (Campbell's/Campbell's Enhanced Flavor Low Sodium),
      8 fl. oz. 50
    (Campbell's), 5.5 oz. 30
    (Campbell's), 10.75 oz. .60
    (Campbell's), 11.5 oz. 70
    (Del Monte), 8 fl. oz. 50
    (Del Monte Not from Concentrate), 8 fl. oz. 40
    (Hunt's/Hunt's No Salt), 8 fl. oz. 35
    (S&W), 8 fl. oz. 40
    (Sacramento), 8 fl. oz. .35

plain or garlic *(R.W. Knudsen)*, 8 fl. oz. 60
tomato-beef cocktail *(Beefamato)*, 8 fl. oz. 80
tomato-chile cocktail *(Snap-E-Tom)*, 6 fl. oz. 40
tomato-chile cocktail *(Snap-E-Tom)*, 10 fl. oz. 60
tomato-clam cocktail *(Clamato)*, 8 fl. oz. 100
tomato-clam cocktail, Caesar *(Clamato)*, 8 fl. oz. 100
vegetable:
   (V-8 Plus 100%), 5.5 fl. oz. 40
   (V-8 Plus 100%), 8 fl. oz. .50
   (V-8 Plus 100%), 10 fl. oz. 70
   all flavors *(R.W. Knudsen Very Veggie)*, 8 fl. oz. 50
   low-sodium *(V-8)*, 5.5 fl. oz. 40
   low-sodium *(V-8)*, 8 fl. oz. 60
   original or spicy hot *(V-8 100%)*, 5.5 fl. oz. 35
   original or spicy hot *(V-8 100%)*, 8 fl. oz. 50
   original or spicy hot *(V-8 100%)*, 10.75 fl. oz. 60
   original or spicy hot *(V-8 100%)*, 11.5 fl. oz. 70
   picante *(V-8)*, 5.5 fl. oz. 35
   picante *(V-8)*, 8 fl. oz. .50
   picante *(V-8)*, 10.75 fl. oz. 60
   picante *(V-8)*, 11.5 fl. oz. 70
   tangy *(V-8 100%)*, 8 fl. oz. 60
   tangy *(V-8 100%)*, 11.5 fl. oz. 80

Chapter 7

VEGETARIAN FOODS

Although vegetarian foods can be found throughout this book (most specifically in the previous two chapters), this chapter primarily contains food products especially formulated for vegetarians.

VEGETARIAN FOODS, CANNED
See also "Vegetarian Foods, Dry & Mixes" and "Nondairy 'Milk' Beverages"

	calories
(Loma Linda Swiss Stake), 1 piece	120
(Worthington Numete), ⅜" slice	130
(Worthington Protose), ⅜" slice	130
"beef":	
slices *(Worthington Savory Slices)*, 3 slices	150
steak *(Worthington Prime Stakes)*, 1 piece	140
steak *(Worthington Vegetable Steaks)*, 2 slices	80
stew *(Worthington Country)*, 1 cup	210
"burger":	
(LaLoma Redi-Burger), ⅝" slice	170
(Loma Linda Vege-Burger), ¼ cup	70
(Worthington), ¼ cup	60
"chicken":	
diced *(Worthington Chik)*, ¼ cup	60
fried *(Worthington FriChik)*, 2 pieces	120
fried *(Worthington FriChik Low Fat)*, 2 pieces	80
fried, with gravy *(Loma Linda Chik'n)*, 2 pieces	210
sliced *(Worthington Chik)*, 3 slices	90
choplet *(Worthington)*, 2 pieces	90
cutlet:	
(Worthington), 1 piece	70
cuts, dinner *(Loma Linda)*, 2 pieces	90
multi-grain *(Worthington)*, 2 pieces	100

"frankfurter," 1 link:
 (Loma Linda Big) 110
 (Loma Linda Linketts) 70
 (Worthington Veja-Links) 50
 (Worthington Veja-Links Low Fat) 40
 (Worthington Super-Links) 110
"hamburger," *see " 'burger,' " above*
lunch "meat" *(Loma Linda* Nuteena), 3/8" slice 160
"meatball," with gravy *(Loma Linda* Tender Rounds), 6 pieces . 120
sandwich spread *(Loma Linda)*, 1/4 cup 80
"sausage" *(Loma Linda* Little Links), 2 links 90
"sausage" *(Worthington* Saucettes), 1 link 90
"scallop" *(Loma Linda* Tender Bits), 6 pieces 110
"scallop" *(Worthington* Vegetable Skallops), 1/2 cup 90
"turkey" *(Worthington* Turkee), 3 slices 190

VEGETARIAN FOODS, FROZEN OR REFRIGERATED
See also "Tofu, Fresh," "Eggs, Substitute," "Cheese, Substitute or Imitation," and " 'Ice Cream,' Nondairy"

                calories
(Worthington FriPats), 1 patty 130
(Worthington Stakelets), 1 piece 140
"bacon" *(Morningstar Farms* Breakfast Strips), 2 strips 60
"bacon" *(Worthington* Stripples), 2 strips 60
bean loaf *(Natural Touch)*, 1" slice 160
"beef":
 (Worthington Meatless), 3/8" slice 110
 corned, slices *(Worthington* Slices), 4 slices 140
 smoked, slices *(Worthington* Slices), 6 slices 120
"bologna" *(Worthington* Bolono), 3 slices 80
"burger," ground:
 (Green Giant Harvest Burger For Recipes), 2/3 cup 90
 (Morningstar Farms Burger Style Recipe Crumbles), 2/3 cup . .90
 (Natural Touch Vegan Crumbles), 1/2 cup 60
 (NewMenu VegiBurger), 3 oz. 110
 (Worthington), 1/2 cup 80
"burger" patty, 1 patty:
 (Amy's California), 2.5 oz. 100
 (Amy's Chicago), 2.5 oz. 160
 (Green Giant Harvest Burger Original) 140
 (Hempeh Burger) 140

Vegetarian Foods, Frozen or Refrigerated, "burger" patty *(cont.)*
  (Ken & Robert's Veggie Burger) 110
  (Morningstar Farms Better'n Burger) 70
  (Morningstar Farms Grillers) 140
  (Morningstar Farms Prime Patties) 110
  (Natural Touch Vegan Burger) 70
  (Natural Touch Vege Burger) 140
  (Yves Veggie Cuisine) 83
  black bean, Southwestern *(Fantastic Nature's Burger)*,
    2.5 oz. 110
  black bean, spicy *(Morningstar Farms/Natural Touch)* 100
  garden grain *(Morningstar Farms)* 120
  garden vegetable *(Morningstar Farms)* 100
  garden vegetable *(Natural Touch)* 100
  grilled *(Fantastic Nature's Burger)*, 2.5 oz. 120
  Italian or Southwestern *(Green Giant Harvest Burger)* 140
  red pepper and garlic *(Fantastic Nature's Burger)*, 2.5 oz. . 110
  tofu *(Natural Touch Okara)* 110
"chicken":
  (Worthington Chik Stiks), 1 piece 110
  fried *(Loma Linda Chik'n)*, 1 piece 180
  nuggets *(Loma Linda)*, 5 pieces 240
  nuggets *(Morningstar Farms)*, 4 pieces 160
  patties *(Morningstar Farms Chik)*, 1 patty 170
  patties *(Worthington Crispy Chik)*, 1 patty 170
  roll *(Worthington Chic-ketts)*, 2 slices, ³⁄₈″ 120
  roll or sliced *(Worthington)*, 2 slices 80
croquettes *(Worthington Golden)*, 4 pieces 210
dinner entree *(Natural Touch)*, 3-oz. patty 220
"egg" roll *(Worthington)*, 1 roll 180
"fish" *(Worthington)*, 2 fillets 180
"frankfurter," 1 link:
  (Morningstar Farms Deli Franks) 110
  (Natural Touch Vege) 100
  (NewMenu VegiDog) 45
  (Worthington Leanies) 110
  chili *(Yves Veggie Cuisine Dogs)* 70
  corn battered *(Loma Linda Corn Dog)* 220
  tofu *(Yves Veggie Cuisine Wieners)* 57
"ham," sliced *(Worthington Wham)*, 2 slices 80
"hamburger," *see " 'burger,' " above*
lentil rice loaf *(Natural Touch)*, 1″ slice 170
"meat," ground *(Morningstar Farms Ground Meatless)*, ½ cup . .60

noodles *(Morningstar Farms* Homestyle), ½ cup 160
nuggets, with rice *(Hain* Hawaiian), 10 oz. 310
"pepperoni" *(Yves Veggie Cuisine),* 3½ slices 78
"roast," dinner *(Worthington),* ¾″ slice 180
"salami" *(Worthington),* 3 slices 130
"sausage":
    (Green Giant Harvest Burger Breakfast), 3 links 120
    (Green Giant Harvest Burger Breakfast), 2 patties 100
    (Morningstar Farms Breakfast), 2 links 60
    (Morningstar Farms Breakfast), 1 patty 70
    (Worthington Prosage Links), 2 links 60
    (Worthington Prosage Patties), 1 patty 100
    ground *(Morningstar Farms* Recipe Crumbles), ⅔ cup 90
    ground *(Natural Touch* Vegan Crumbles), ½ cup 60
    ground *(Worthington* Vegetarian), ½ cup 110
    roll *(Worthington Prosage),* ⅝″ slice 140
"tuna" *(Worthington Tuno),* drained, ½ cup 80
"turkey," smoked *(Worthington), 3 slices* 140
"veal" *(Worthington Veelets),* 1 patty 180

VEGETARIAN FOODS, DRY & MIXES
See also "Vegetarian Foods, Canned"

                                 calories

"burger":
    (Morningstar Farms Garden Grille Veggie Kit), ¼ pkg. 80
    (Morningstar Farms Southwestern Veggie Kit), ¼ pkg. 90
    (Natural Touch Original Veggie Kit), ¼ pkg. 80
    (Natural Touch Southwestern Veggie Kit), ¼ pkg. 90
    (Worthington Granburger), 3 tbsp. 60
    chunks *(Loma Linda Vita-Burger),* ¼ cup 70
    granules *(LaLoma Vita-Burger),* 3 tbsp. 70
    patty *(Fantastic Nature's Burger* Original/BBQ), 1 patty* . . . 170
"chicken" *(Loma Linda* Supreme), ⅓ cup 90
"fish" *(Loma Linda* Ocean Platter), ⅓ cup 90
loaf, dinner *(Loma Linda),* ⅓ cup 90
"meat" loaf *(Natural Touch),* ¼ cup 100
patty *(Loma Linda),* ⅓ cup .90
"sausage" *(Fantastic Nature's Sausage),* 1 patty* 65
taco *(Natural Touch),* 3 tbsp. 60

* *Prepared according to package directions*

NONDAIRY "MILK" BEVERAGES, eight fluid ounces, except as noted
See also "Milk" and "Vegetarian Foods, Canned"

---

calories

rice beverage:
    (Rice Dream Original/*Rice Dream* Original Enriched) 120
    carob *(Rice Dream)* 150
    chocolate *(Rice Dream/Rice Dream* Enriched) 170
    vanilla *(Rice Dream/Rice Dream* Enriched) 130
rice and soy *(EdenBlend)* 120
soy beverage:
    (EdenSoy/EdenSoy Extra) 130
    (Soy Moo Fat Free) 110
    carob *(EdenSoy)* 150
    vanilla *(EdenSoy/EdenSoy* Extra) 150
soy beverage mix, all varieties *(Loma Linda Soyagen)*, ¼ cup . . 130

TOFU, FRESH
See also "Vegetarian Foods, Frozen or Refrigerated"

---

calories

5-spice or French *(Nasoya)*, ¼ block 70
extra firm *(Nasoya)*, ⅕ of 1-lb. block 90
firm *(Nasoya)*, ⅕ of 1-lb. block 80
pasturized *(Frieda's)*, 4.2 oz. 86
silken *(Nasoya)*, ⅕ of 1-lb. block 50
soft *(Nasoya)*, ⅙ of 1-lb. block .60

Chapter 8

SOUPS, BROTHS, AND CHOWDERS

SOUPS, CANNED, READY-TO-SERVE, one cup, except as noted
See also "Soups, Canned, Condensed," "Soups, Canned, Semi-Condensed," "Soups, Frozen," and "Soups, Mixes"

	calories
bean:	
(Grandma Brown's)	190
black (Goya)	210
black (Progresso)	170
black, with bacon (Old El Paso)	160
black, and vegetable (Health Valley)	110
salsa (Campbell's Home Cookin')	160
bean with bacon (Campbell's Microwave), 10½ oz.	280
bean and ham:	
(Campbell's Chunky)	190
(Campbell's Chunky), 11 oz.	260
(Campbell's Home Cookin')	180
(Healthy Choice)	185
(Progresso)	160
beef:	
barley (Progresso)	130
barley (Progresso 99% Fat Free)	140
chowder, chunky (Nalley), 7½-oz. can	110
hearty (Old El Paso)	120
minestrone or noodle (Progresso)	140
pasta (Campbell's Chunky)	150
pasta (Campbell's Chunky), 10¾ oz.	190
potato (Healthy Choice)	120
Stroganoff (Campbell's Chunky), 10¾ oz.	310
beef broth:	
(College Inn/College Inn Low Sodium)	20
(Health Valley)	20
(Swanson)	20

Soups, Canned, Ready-to-Serve *(cont.)*
beef vegetable:
    (Progresso 99% Fat Free) 160
    country *(Campbell's* Chunky) 160
    country *(Campbell's* Chunky), 10¾ oz. 200
    and rotini *(Progresso)* 130
borscht *(Gold's)* 70
broccoli *(Health Valley* Carotene) 70
broccoli and shells *(Progresso* Pasta Soup) 80
cheddar potato, white *(Progresso* 99% Fat Free) 140
chicken:
    (Progresso Chickarina) 120
    barley or minestrone *(Progresso)* 100
    broccoli cheese *(Campbell's* Chunky) 200
    broccoli cheese *(Campbell's* Chunky), 10¾ oz. 250
    hearty *(Healthy Choice)* 130
    rotisserie, seasoned *(Progresso)* 100
    with vegetables, hearty *(Campbell's* Chunky) 90
    with vegetables, hearty *(Campbell's* Chunky), 10¾ oz. 110
    with vegetables, homestyle *(Progresso)* 80
chicken, cream of *(Campbell's* Home Cookin')* 210
chicken, cream of, with mushrooms or vegetables *(Healthy
    Choice)* 125
chicken broth:
    (Campbell's Low Sodium), 10¾ oz. 40
    (Campbell's Healthy Request) 20
    (College Inn/College Inn Less Sodium) 25
    (Health Valley) 30
    (Pritikin) 15
    (Progresso) 15
    (Swanson) 30
    (Swanson Natural Goodness) 15
chicken chowder:
    (Nalley), 7½ oz. 120
    corn *(Campbell's* Chunky) 250
    corn *(Campbell's* Chunky), 10¾ oz. 310
    corn *(Healthy Choice)* 175
    mushroom *(Campbell's* Chunky) 210
chicken noodle:
    (Campbell's Chunky Classic) 130
    (Campbell's Chunky Classic), 10¾ oz. 160
    (Campbell's Home Cookin')* 100

(*Campbell's* Home Cookin'), 10¾ oz. 120
(*Campbell's* Low Sodium), 7¼ oz. 80
(*Campbell's* Microwave), 1 container 13
(*Healthy Choice* Old Fashioned) 140
(*Progresso*) 80
(*Progresso* 99% Fat Free) 90
(*Weight Watchers*), 10½ oz. 150
hearty (*Campbell's Healthy Request*) 160
hearty (*Old El Paso*) 110
chicken pasta:
(*Campbell's* Glass Jar) .90
(*Healthy Choice*) 120
(*Pritikin*) 100
with mushrooms (*Campbell's* Chunky) 120
with mushrooms (*Campbell's* Chunky), 10¾ oz. 150
chicken and penne, spicy (*Progresso* Pasta Soup) 110
chicken rice:
(*Campbell's* Chunky) 140
(*Campbell's* Home Cookin') 110
(*Campbell's* Home Cookin'), 10¾ oz. 140
(*Campbell's* Microwave), 10¾ oz. 120
(*Campbell's Healthy Request*) 100
(*Healthy Choice*) 110
(*Old El Paso*) 90
(*Pritikin*) 80
(*Weight Watchers*), 10½ oz. 110
with vegetables (*Progresso*) 100
with vegetables (*Progresso* 99% Fat Free) 90
wild rice (*Progresso*) 90
chicken and rotini (*Progresso* Pasta Soup) 90
chicken vegetable:
(*Campbell's* Chunky) 130
(*Campbell's* Home Cookin') 130
(*Campbell's* Home Cookin'), 10¾ oz. 170
(*Old El Paso*) 110
(*Progresso*) 100
hearty (*Campbell's Healthy Request*) 120
spicy (*Campbell's* Chunky) 90
chili beef with beans (*Campbell's* Chunky), 11 oz. 300
chili beef with beans (*Healthy Choice*) 165
clam chowder, Manhattan (*Campbell's* Chunky) 130
clam chowder, Manhattan (*Progresso*) 110

Soups, Canned, Ready-to-Serve *(cont.)*
clam chowder, New England:
   (Campbell's Chunky) 240
   (Campbell's Chunky), 10¾ oz. 300
   (Campbell's Home Cookin') 200
   (Campbell's Healthy Request) 120
   (Healthy Choice) 125
   (Nalley), 7½ oz. 140
   (Progresso) 200
   (Progresso 99% Fat Free) 130
clam rotini chowder *(Progresso* Pasta Soup) 190
corn, country, and vegetable *(Health Valley)* 70
crab bisque *(Bookbinder's),* ½ cup 120
egg flower *(Rice Road)* 90
escarole, in chicken broth *(Progresso)* 25
hot and sour *(Rice Road)* 90
Italian, carotene *(Health Valley* Fat Free) 80
lentil:
   (Healthy Choice) 145
   (Pritikin) 130
   (Progresso) 140
   (Progresso 99% Fat Free) 130
   and carrots *(Health Valley* Fat Free) 90
   savory *(Campbell's* Home Cookin') 130
   and shells *(Progresso* Pasta Soup) 130
lobster bisque *(Bookbinder's),* ½ cup 90
macaroni and bean *(Progresso)* 160
meatballs and pasta pearls *(Progresso)* 140
minestrone:
   (Campbell's Chunky) 140
   (Campbell's Glass Jar/*Campbell's* Home Cookin') 120
   (Healthy Choice) 110
   (Pritikin) 90
   (Progresso) 120
   (Progresso 99% Fat Free) 130
   (Weight Watchers), 10½ oz. 130
   hearty *(Campbell's Healthy Request)* 120
   Italian *(Health Valley)* 80
   Parmesan *(Progresso)* 100
   Tuscany *(Campbell's* Home Cookin') 160
mushroom, cream of:
   (Campbell's Glass Jar) 260

   (Campbell's Home Cookin') 170
   (Campbell's Low Sodium), 10¾ oz. 200
   (Healthy Choice) 75
   (Progresso) 130
mushroom chicken, creamy (Progresso 99% Fat Free) 90
mushroom rice (Campbell's Home Cookin') 80
Oriental broth (Swanson) 15
oyster stew (Bookbinder's), ½ can 90
pasta:
   Bolognese (Health Valley Healthy Pasta) 70
   cacciatore (Health Valley Healthy Pasta) 90
   Chinese (Rice Road) 70
   fagioli or primavera (Health Valley Healthy Pasta) 80
   Romano (Health Valley Healthy Pasta) 140
pea, split:
   (Campbell's Low Sodium), 10¾ oz. 240
   (Grandma Brown's) 210
   (Pritikin) 140
   (Progresso 99% Fat Free) 170
   and carrots (Health Valley) 110
   green (Progresso) 170
pea, split, with ham:
   (Campbell's Chunky) 190
   (Campbell's Chunky), 10¾ oz. 240
   (Campbell's Home Cookin'/Campbell's Healthy Request) . . .170
   (Healthy Choice) 155
   (Progresso) 150
penne, hearty, in chicken broth (Progresso Pasta Soup) 90
penne, zesty (Campbell's Healthy Request) 90
pepper steak (Campbell's Chunky) 140
potato, with roasted garlic (Campbell's Home Cookin') 180
potato ham chowder (Campbell's) 220
potato ham chowder (Campbell's Chunky), 10¾ oz. 270
seafood bisque (Bookbinder's), ½ cup 140
shrimp bisque (Bookbinder's), ½ cup 120
sirloin burger, with vegetable (Campbell's Chunky) 190
sirloin burger, with vegetable (Campbell's Chunky), 10¾ oz. . . .230
snapper (Bookbinder's), ½ cup 110
steak and potato (Campbell's Chunky) 160
steak and potato (Campbell's Chunky), 10¾ oz. 200
tomato:
   (Campbell's Low Sodium), 10½ oz. 170

Soups, Canned, Ready-to-Serve, tomato *(cont.)*
    garden *(Campbell's* Home Cookin'), 10¾ oz. 150
    garden *(Healthy Choice)* 105
    hearty, and rotini *(Progresso* Pasta Soup) 130
    tortellini *(Progresso* Pasta Soup) 120
    vegetable *(Campbell's* Glass Jar) 80
    vegetable *(Health Valley)* 80
    vegetable *(Progresso)* 90
    vegetable, garden *(Progresso* 99% Fat Free) 100
    vegetable, with pasta *(Campbell's Healthy Request)* 120
tortellini in chicken broth *(Progresso)* 70
tortellini with chicken and vegetables *(Campbell's)* 110
turkey with wild rice *(Healthy Choice)* 100
turkey with wild rice and vegetables *(Campbell's Healthy*
    Request) 120
vegetable:
    (Campbell's Chunky) 130
    (Campbell's Chunky), 10¾ oz. 160
    (Progresso) 90
    (Progresso 99% Fat Free) 80
    (Weight Watchers), 10½ oz. 130
    5-bean *(Health Valley)* 140
    14-garden *(Health Valley* Fat Free) 80
    barley *(Health Valley* Fat Free) 90
    carotene *(Health Valley* Fat Free) 70
    country *(Campbell's* Home Cookin') 110
    country *(Campbell's* Home Cookin'), 10¾ oz. 130
    country *(Healthy Choice)* 105
    garden *(Healthy Choice)* 130
    garden *(Old El Paso)* 110
    harborside *(Campbell's* Home Cookin') 80
    hearty *(Campbell's Healthy Request)* 100
    hearty *(Pritikin)* 90
    hearty, with pasta *(Campbell's* Chunky) 130
    hearty, with rotini *(Progresso* Pasta Soup) 110
    Italian *(Campbell's* Home Cookin') 100
    and pasta *(Campbell's* Glass Jar) 110
    Southwestern *(Campbell's* Home Cookin') 130
    Southwestern, with black bean *(Campbell's Healthy*
      Request) 140
    vegetarian *(Pritikin)* 100

vegetable beef:
   (Campbell's Chunky) 150
   (Campbell's Chunky), 10¾ oz. 180
   (Campbell's Home Cookin') 120
   (Campbell's Home Cookin'), 10¾ oz. 150
   (Campbell's Low Sodium), 10¾ oz. 160
   (Campbell's Microwave), 1 container 140
   (Healthy Choice) 130
   hearty *(Campbell's Healthy Request)* 140
vegetable broth *(Pritikin)* 10
vegetable broth *(Swanson)* 20

SOUPS, CANNED, CONDENSED, undiluted, ½ cup
*See also "Soups, Canned, Ready-to-Serve," "Soups, Canned,
Semi-Condensed," "Soups, Frozen," and "Soups, Mixes"*

---

                                                  calories

asparagus, cream of *(Campbell's)* 90
bean:
   with bacon *(Campbell's)* 180
   with bacon *(Campbell's Healthy Request)* 150
   black *(Campbell's)* 120
beef:
   broth, double rich *(Campbell's)* 15
   consommé *(Campbell's)* 25
   noodle *(Campbell's)* .70
   with vegetables, barley *(Campbell's)* 80
broccoli:
   cream of *(Campbell's)* 100
   cream of *(Campbell's Healthy Request)* 70
   cream of or cheese *(Campbell's 98% Fat Free)* 80
   creamy *(Campbell's Healthy Request Creative Chef)* 70
   cheese *(Campbell's)* 110
celery, cream of:
   (Campbell's) 110
   (Campbell's 98% Fat Free) 70
   (Campbell's Healthy Request) 70
cheese, cheddar *(Campbell's)* 90
cheese, nacho *(Campbell's)* 140
chicken:
   alphabet, with vegetables *(Campbell's)* 80
   broth *(Campbell's)* 30
   cream of *(Campbell's)* 130

Soups, Canned, Condensed, chicken (cont.)
    cream of *(Campbell's 98% Fat Free)* 80
    cream of *(Campbell's Healthy Request)* 70
    cream of *(Campbell's Healthy Request Creative Chef)* 80
    cream of, and broccoli *(Campbell's)* 120
    cream of, and broccoli *(Campbell's Healthy Request)* 80
    dumplings *(Campbell's)* .80
    gumbo *(Campbell's)* 60
    mushroom, creamy *(Campbell's)* 130
    noodle *(Campbell's/Campbell's Healthy Request)* 70
    noodle, creamy *(Campbell's)* 130
    noodle, curly or noodle O's *(Campbell's)* 80
    noodle, homestyle *(Campbell's)* 70
    with rice *(Campbell's)* .70
    with rice *(Campbell's Healthy Request)* 60
    and stars *(Campbell's)* .70
    vegetable *(Campbell's/Campbell's Healthy Request)* 80
    vegetable, Southwestern *(Campbell's)* 110
    wild rice *(Campbell's)* .70
chili beef with beans *(Campbell's)* 170
clam chowder:
    Manhattan *(Campbell's)* 60
    New England *(Campbell's)* 100
    New England *(Doxsee)* .90
corn, golden *(Campbell's)* .120
minestrone *(Campbell's)* 100
minestrone *(Campbell's Healthy Request)* 90
mushroom:
    beefy *(Campbell's)* 70
    cream of *(Campbell's)* 110
    cream of *(Campbell's 98% Fat Free/Campbell's Healthy
      Request)* 70
    cream of *(Campbell's Healthy Request Creative Chef)* 70
    golden *(Campbell's)* 80
noodle, double, chicken broth *(Campbell's)* 100
noodle and ground beef *(Campbell's)* 100
onion, creamy *(Campbell's)* 110
onion, French, with beef stock *(Campbell's)* 70
oyster stew *(Campbell's)* 90
pea, green, or split, with ham and bacon *(Campbell's)* 180
pepper, cream of, Mexican *(Campbell's)* 110
pepper pot *(Campbell's)* .100
potato, cream of *(Campbell's)* 90

potato, cream of *(Campbell's Healthy Request Creative Chef)* . .80
Scotch broth *(Campbell's)* .80
shrimp, cream of *(Campbell's)* 100
tomato:
    (Campbell's) 100
    (Campbell's Healthy Request) 90
    bisque *(Campbell's)* 130
    cream of *(Campbell's* Homestyle) 110
    fiesta *(Campbell's)* .70
    Italian, with basil, oregano *(Campbell's)* 100
    rice *(Campbell's* Old Fashioned) 120
    with herbs *(Campbell's Healthy Request Creative Chef)* 100
turkey, noodle or vegetable *(Campbell's)* 80
vegetable:
    (Campbell's 10¾ oz.) 80
    (Campbell's 26¼ oz./*Campbell's Healthy Request)* 90
    (Campbell's Old Fashioned) 70
    beef *(Campbell's/Campbell's Healthy Request)* 80
    California style *(Campbell's)* 60
    hearty, and pasta *(Campbell's/Campbell's Healthy Request)* . .90
    vegetarian *(Campbell's)* 70
won ton *(Campbell's)* 45

SOUPS, CANNED, SEMI-CONDENSED, undiluted, ⅔ cup
*See also "Soups, Canned, Ready-to-Serve" and "Soups,
Canned, Condensed"*

                                        calories
bacon, lettuce, tomato with chicken broth *(Pepperidge Farm)* . 130
bean, black, with sherry *(Pepperidge Farm)* 120
broccoli, cream of *(Pepperidge Farm)* 90
chicken curry *(Pepperidge Farm)* 170
chicken with rice *(Pepperidge Farm)* 80
clam chowder, Manhattan *(Pepperidge Farm)* 80
clam chowder, New England *(Pepperidge Farm)* 160
consommé, madrilene *(Pepperidge Farm)* 50
corn chowder *(Pepperidge Farm)* 140
crab *(Pepperidge Farm)* .80
gazpacho *(Pepperidge Farm)* 70
hunter's, with turkey and beef *(Pepperidge Farm)* 130
lobster bisque *(Pepperidge Farm)* 160
minestrone *(Pepperidge Farm)* 100

Soups, Canned, Semi-Condensed *(cont.)*

mushroom, shiitake *(Pepperidge Farm)* 80
onion, French *(Pepperidge Farm)* 50
oyster stew *(Pepperidge Farm)* 160
pea, green, with ham *(Pepperidge Farm)* 210
vichyssoise *(Pepperidge Farm)* 120
watercress *(Pepperidge Farm)* 80

SOUPS, FROZEN, 7.5 oz., except as noted
See also "Soups, Canned, Ready-to-Serve" and "Soups, Canned, Condensed"

	calories
barley mushroom or barley mushroom, no salt *(Tabatchnick)*	.70
bean, Yankee *(Tabatchnick)*	160
broccoli, cream of *(Schwan's)*, 1 cup	180
broccoli, cream of *(Tabatchnick)*	.90
cabbage *(Tabatchnick)*	.60
cheese, cheddar vegetable *(Tabatchnick)*	140
cheese, Wisconsin *(Schwan's)*, 1 cup	210
chicken with noodles and dumplings *(Tabatchnick)*	.70
chicken with noodles and vegetables *(Tabatchnick)*	.35
clam chowder, Boston *(Schwan's)*, 1 cup	180
corn chowder or minestrone *(Tabatchnick)*	150
lentil, Tuscany *(Tabatchnick)*	140
pea or pea, no salt *(Tabatchnick)*	180
potato, New England *(Tabatchnick)*	150
potato, old-fashioned *(Tabatchnick)*	.70
spinach, cream of *(Tabatchnick)*	.90
vegetable or vegetable, no salt *(Tabatchnick)*	110

SOUPS, MIXES, one package, except as noted
See also "Soups, Canned, Ready-to-Serve," "Soups, Canned, Condensed," "Condiments & Sauces," "Sauces, Mixes," and "Seasonings, Dry & Mixes"

	calories
barley:	
beef *(Buckeye Beans)*, 2 tbsp.	.70
beef *(Buckeye Beans)*, 1 cup*	170

* *Prepared according to package directions*

better *(Aunt Patsy's Pantry)*, 2 tbsp. 90
vegetable, hearty *(Fantastic Foods)*, 1.5 oz. 150

bean:
  (Bean Cuisine Bouillabaisse), 1 serving 99
  (Buckeye Beans), 3 tbsp. 100
  (Buckeye Beans), 1 cup* 170
  5, hearty *(Fantastic Foods)*, 2.3 oz. 230
  black *(Aunt Patsy's Pantry)*, 1/6 pkg. 190
  black *(Bean Cuisine* Island), 1 serving 126
  black *(Knorr* Cup) 190
  black *(Smart Soup)* 190
  black, hearty *(Fantastic Foods)* 210
  black, spicy, with couscous *(Health Valley)*, 1/3 cup 130
  black, zesty, with rice *(Health Valley)*, 1/3 cup 100
  navy *(Aunt Patsy's Pantry)*, 3 tbsp. 120
  navy *(Knorr* Cup) 130
  pasta, *see "pasta and bean," below*
  rice, *see "rice and beans," below*
  vegetable *(Buckeye Beans)*, 3 tbsp. 100
  vegetable *(Buckeye Beans)*, 1 cup* 150
  white *(Bean Cuisine* Provençal), 1 serving 103

bean and ham *(Hormel* Micro Cup) 190

beef, ground, vegetable:
  (Soup Starter), 1/8 pkg. .80
  (Soup Starter Quick Cook), 1/4 pkg. 80

beef stew, hearty *(Soup Starter)*, 1/7 pkg. 80

beef vegetable:
  (Hamburger Helper), 1/4 cup 80
  (Hamburger Helper), 1 cup* 190
  (Hormel Micro Cup) 90
  (Soup Starter), 1/8 pkg. .90
  barley *(Soup Starter)*, 1/8 pkg. 100

bouillon, 1 tsp., cube, or packet, except as noted:
  beef or chicken *(Herb-Ox/Herb-Ox* Instant) 10
  beef or chicken *(Knorr)* .20
  beef or chicken *(MBT/Wyler's* Instant/Low Sodium) 15
  beef or chicken *(Wyler's/Steero/Steero* Reduced Sodium) 5
  fish *(Knorr)*, 1/2 cube 10
  onion *(MBT* Instant) 15
  vegetable *(Herb-Ox)* 10

* Prepared according to package directions

Soups, Mixes, bouillon *(cont.)*

vegetable *(MBT* Instant) 10
vegetable *(Wyler's)* 5
vegetarian *(Knorr)*, ½ cube 15
broccoli, cream of *(Knorr* Chef's), 2 tbsp. 60
broccoli-cheese:
    cheddar, creamy *(Fantastic Foods)*, ⅓ oz. 130
    creamy *(Cup-a-Soup)* 70
    with ham *(Hormel* Micro Cup) 170
    and rice *(Uncle Ben's* Hearty) 160
broth, beef or chicken *(Weight Watchers* Instant), .16 oz. 10
broth concentrate, see *"Condiments & Sauces,"* page 251
chicken:
    broth *(Cup-a-Soup)* 20
    broth, with pasta *(Cup-a-Soup)* 45
    cream of *(Cup-a-Soup)* 70
    creamy, flavor *(Cup-a-Soup)* 80
    noodle *(Campbell's* Real Chicken Broth), 3 tbsp. 100
    noodle *(Campbell's* Soup and Recipe), 3 tbsp. 90
    noodle *(Cup-a-Soup)* 50
    noodle *(Hormel* Micro Cup) 110
    noodle *(Soup Starter)*, ⅛ pkg. 80
    noodle *(Soup Starter* Quick Cook), ¼ pkg. 80
    noodle, double *(Campbell's)* 170
    noodle, hearty *(Cup-a-Soup)* 60
    'n onion *(Lipton Soup Secrets* Kettle Style), ¼ cup 120
    with pasta and beans *(Lipton Soup Secrets* Kettle Style),
      ¼ cup 110
    with pasta and herbs, country *(Lipton Soup Secrets* Kettle
      Style), ¼ cup 100
    rice *(Hormel* Micro Cup) 110
    rice *(Mrs. Grass)*, ¼ pkg. 80
    rice *(Soup Starter)*, ⅛ pkg. 70
    rice *(Soup Starter* Quick Cook), ¼ pkg. 50
    rice, white and wild *(Soup Starter)*, ⅛ pkg. 70
    thyme *(Aunt Patsy's Pantry)*, 2 tbsp. 100
    thyme *(Buckeye Beans)*, 2 tbsp. 110
    thyme *(Buckeye Beans)*, 1 cup* 180
    vegetable *(Smart Soup)* 130
    vegetable *(Soup Starter)*, ⅐ pkg. 70

* *Prepared according to package directions*

chili:
- (Aunt Patsy's Pantry Cowgirl), 4 tbsp. 160
- black bean (Aunt Patsy's Pantry), 3 tbsp. 100
- black bean (Buckeye Beans), 3 tbsp. 140
- black bean (Buckeye Beans), 1 cup* 180
- chicken (Aunt Patsy's Pantry), 4 tbsp. 180
- chicken, white (Buckeye Beans), 1/4 cup 190
- chicken, white (Buckeye Beans), 1 cup* 290
- hearty (Fantastic Cha-Cha Cup), 2.4 oz. 220
- vegetarian (Fantastic Foods), 1/2 cup 50

clam chowder, New England (Hormel Micro Cup) 130
clam chowder, New England (Knorr Chef's), 3 tbsp. 90

corn chowder:
- (Knorr Cup) 140
- (Smart Soup) 100
- and potato, creamy (Fantastic Foods), 1.7 oz. 170
- with tomatoes (Health Valley), 1/2 cup 90

couscous (Casbah Moroccan Stew Cup) 180
couscous with lentil, hearty (Fantastic Foods), 2/3 oz. 230

herb:
- fiesta, with red pepper (Lipton Recipe Secrets), 1 1/3 tbsp. . .30
- fine (Knorr Box), 2 tbsp. 100
- golden, with lemon (Lipton Recipe Secrets), 1 1/2 tbsp. 35
- Italian, with tomato (Lipton Recipe Secrets), 2 tbsp. 40
- herb with garlic, savory (Lipton Recipe Secrets), 1 tbsp. 30

hot and sour (Knorr Box), 2 tbsp. 45
leek (Knorr Box), 2 tbsp. 70

lentil:
- (Smart Soup) 190
- with couscous (Health Valley), 1/3 cup 130
- hearty (Fantastic Foods), 2/3 oz. 230
- hearty (Knorr Cup) 220
- homestyle (Lipton Soup Secrets Kettle Style), 1/4 cup 130
- red (Aunt Patsy's Pantry), 2 tbsp. 80

minestrone:
- (Lipton Soup Secrets, Kettle Style), 1/4 cup 110
- (Smart Soup) 120
- hearty (Fantastic Foods), 1.5 oz. 150
- hearty (Knorr Cup) 120

* Prepared according to package directions

Soups, Mixes *(cont.)*

mushroom:

beefy *(Lipton Recipe Secrets)*, 1½ tbsp.	.35
creamy *(Fantastic Foods)*, 1.2 oz.	120
creamy, flavor *(Cup-a-Soup)*	.60

noodle:

(Nissin Top Ramen Damae/Oriental)	200
(Nissin Top Ramen Low Fat Oriental)	150
with chicken broth *(Mrs. Grass)*, ¼ pkg.	.60
chicken free *(Fantastic Foods)*, 1.5 oz.	140
extra, with chicken broth *(Lipton Soup Secrets)*, 3 tbsp.	.90
homestyle *(Borden)*, ¼ pkg.	.70
ring noodle *(Cup-a-Soup)*	.50

noodle, beef:

(Campbell's Baked Ramen)	210
(Campbell's Baked Ramen), ½ block	140
(Campbell's Ramen)	290
(Campbell's/Sanwa Ramen), ½ block	170
(Nissin Cup Noodles)	290
(Nissin Cup Noodles Twin), 1.2 oz.	160
(Nissin Top Ramen)	200
(Nissin Top Ramen Low Fat)	150
onion *(Nissin Cup Noodles)*	280
spicy *(Nissin Top Ramen)*	200

noodle, chicken:

(Campbell's Baked Ramen)	210
(Campbell's Ramen)	290
(Knorr Box), 2 tbsp.	.90
(Knorr Cup)	110
(Lipton Soup Secrets Giggle Noodle), 2 tbsp.	.70
(Lipton Soup Secrets Ring-O-Noodle), 2 tbsp.	.70
(Nissin Cup Noodles)	300
(Nissin Cup Noodles Twin), 1.2 oz.	160
(Nissin Top Ramen)	200
(Nissin Top Ramen Low Fat)	150
(Sanwa Ramen Pride), ½ block	170
broth *(Lipton Soup Secrets)*, 2 tbsp.	.60
broth *(Mrs. Grass)*, ¼ pkg.	.60
mushroom *(Nissin Cup Noodles)*	300
mushroom or sesame *(Nissin Top Ramen)*	200
regular or spicy *(Campbell's* Baked Ramen), ½ block	140
spicy *(Campbell's* Ramen), ½ block	170

spicy *(Nissin Cup Noodles)* 300
spicy *(Nissin Cup Noodles* Twin), 1.2 oz. 160
with vegetables *(Health Valley)*, ⅓ cup 80
with white meat chicken *(Lipton Soup Secrets)*, 3 tbsp. 80
noodle, crab *(Nissin Cup Noodles)* 290
noodle, lobster *(Nissin Cup Noodles)* 300
noodle, Oriental *(Campbell's/Sanwa* Ramen), ½ block 170
noodle, pork:
   (Campbell's Ramen), ½ block 170
   (Nissin Cup Noodles) 290
   (Nissin Top Ramen) 200
noodle, shrimp:
   (Sanwa/Campbell's Ramen), ½ block 170
   (Nissin Cup Noodles) 290
   (Nissin Cup Noodles Twin), 1.2 oz. 150
   (Nissin Top Ramen) 200
   picante *(Nissin Cup Noodles)* 290
noodle, vegetable:
   beef *(Mrs. Grass)*, ¼ pkg. 70
   curry *(Fantastic Foods)*, 1.5 oz. 140
   garden *(Nissin Cup Noodles)* 290
   miso *(Fantastic Foods)*, 1.3 oz. 130
   tomato *(Fantastic Foods)*, 1.5 oz. 150
onion:
   (Campbell's Soup and Recipe), 1 tbsp. 20
   (Knorr Box), 2 tbsp. .45
   (Lipton Recipe Secrets), 1 tbsp. 20
   (Mrs. Grass Soup/Recipe), ¼ pkg. 35
   beefy *(Lipton Recipe Secrets)*, 1½ tbsp. 25
   golden *(Lipton Recipe Secrets)*, 1⅔ tbsp. 50
onion mushroom *(Lipton Recipe Secrets)*, 2 tbsp. 30
onion mushroom *(Mrs. Grass* Soup/Recipe), ¼ pkg. 60
oxtail *(Knorr* Box), 2 tbsp. 60
pasta:
   Italiano *(Health Valley* Fat Free), ½ cup 140
   marinara, Parmesan, or Mediterranean *(Health Valley* Pasta
      Cup Fat Free), ½ cup 100
   spiral, with chicken broth *(Lipton Soup Secrets)*, 3 tbsp. . . .60
pasta and bean:
   (Bean Cuisine Ultima), 1 serving 117
   (Casbah Pasta Fasul) 160
   white bean *(Uncle Ben's* Hearty), ⅕ oz. 160

Soups, Mixes *(cont.)*

pea, green *(Cup-a-Soup)* 80
pea, snow, cream of *(Knorr* Chef's), 3 tbsp. 70
pea, split:
   (Aunt Patsy's Pantry), 3 tbsp. 160
   (Bean Cuisine Thick as Fog), 1 serving 116
   (Buckeye Beans), ¼ cup 200
   (Buckeye Beans), 1 cup* 250
   (Knorr Cup) 150
   (Smart Soup) 150
   hearty *(Fantastic Foods),* 2 oz. 190
   with carrots *(Health Valley),* ½ cup 130
potato, with broccoli *(Health Valley),* ⅓ cup 70
potato cheese, with ham *(Hormel* Micro Cup) 190
potato leek *(Knorr* Cup) 120
potato leek *(Smart Soup)* 120
rice *(Casbah Thai Yum)* 160
rice and beans:
   (Casbah La Fiesta) 170
   black *(Uncle Ben's* Hearty) 150
   Cajun *(Casbah* Jambalaya) 128
   red *(Smart Soup)* 180
spinach, cream of *(Knorr* Box), 2 tbsp. 70
tomato:
   (Cup-a-Soup) 100
   basil *(Knorr* Box), 2 tbsp. .80
   basil *(Uncle Ben's* Hearty) 110
   rice Parmesano *(Fantastic Foods),* 1.9 oz. 200
vegetable:
   (Knorr Box), 2 tbsp. 30
   (Lipton Recipe Secrets), 1⅔ tbsp. 30
   (Mrs. Grass Soup/Recipe), ¼ pkg. 35
   barley, hearty *(Fantastic* Cup) 150
   beef *(Mrs. Grass),* ¼ pkg. 70
   chicken flavor *(Cup-a-Soup)* 50
   chicken flavor *(Knorr* Cup) 100
   chicken flavor, creamy *(Cup-a-Soup)* 80
   spring *(Cup-a-Soup)* 45
   spring *(Knorr),* 2 tbsp. 25

* *Prepared according to package directions*

Chapter 9

DIPS AND APPETIZERS

DIPS, two tablespoons
See also "Cheese Spreads," "Dips, Mixes," "Salsa,"
"Condiments & Sauces" and "Dessert Toppings & Syrups"

	calories
artichoke *(Victoria)*	30
avocado *(Kraft)*	60
avocado *(Nalley/Nalley Guacamole)*	120
baba ghanouj, roasted *(Cedar's)*	50
bacon and horseradish:	
(Heluva Good)	60
(Heluva Good Free)	25
(Kraft)	60
(Kraft Premium)	50
bacon and onion:	
(Breakstone's)	60
(Knudsen Premium)	60
(Kraft Premium)	60
(Nalley)	110
barbecue *(Heluva Good)*	60
bean:	
(Chi-Chi's Fiesta)	35
(Frito-Lay's)	40
(Marie's Fiesta)	140
(Old Dutch)	30
black *(Old El Paso)*	20
black, spicy *(Guiltless Gourmet)*	30
jalapeño *(Frito-Lay's)*	40
pinto, spicy *(Guiltless Gourmet)*	35
cheese:	
(Chi-Chi's Fiesta)	40
and bacon *(Nalley)*	110
blue *(Kraft Premium)*	45
cheddar, jalapeño *(Heluva Good Light)*	30
cheddar, mild *(Frito-Lay's)*	50

Dips, cheese *(cont.)*
   cheddar, mild *(Old Dutch)* 30
   cheddar, and mustard *(Heluva Good Pretzel)* 80
   chili *(Fritos)* 45
   hot *(Price's Fiesta)* 80
   nacho *(Knudsen Premium)* 60
   nacho *(Kraft Premium)* 60
   nacho *(Nalley)* 120
   nacho *(Old Dutch)* 35
   Parmesan, garlic *(Marie's)* 140
   salsa *(Heluva Good Cheese 'N Salsa)* 80
   salsa *(Old El Paso)* .40
   salsa *(Tostitos Con Queso/Con Queso Low Fat)* 40
   salsa *(Old El Paso Low Fat)* 30
chili, green *(La Victoria)* 10
clam:
   (Breakstone's Chesapeake) 50
   (Heluva Good New England) 50
   (Kraft) 60
   (Kraft Premium) 45
   (Nalley) 100
cucumber, creamy *(Kraft Premium)* 50
dill:
   (Bernstein's Zesty) 120
   (Heluva Good) 60
   (Marie's) 190
eggplant *(Victoria)* 30
garlic:
   (Nalley) 130
   Italian *(Marie's)* 180
   roasted, and onion *(Marie's Fat Free)* 35
guacamole, *see "avocado," above*
hummus:
   (Casbah) 120
   (Cedar's) 50
   (Cedar's Sports Dip) 34
   pimiento and olive *(Cedar's)* 56
jalapeño:
   (Kraft) 60
   (Old El Paso) 30
   and cheddar *(Breakstone's)* 60
   and cheddar *(Frito-Lay's)* 50

cheese *(Kraft* Premium) 60
nacho, mild *(Guiltless Gourmet)* 25
(Nance's Pretzel) 90
onion:
   creamy *(Kraft* Premium) 45
   French *(Breakstone's)* 50
   French *(Frito-Lay's)* .60
   French *(Heluva* Good) 50
   French *(Heluva* Good Free) 25
   French *(Knudsen* Premium) 50
   French *(Kraft)* 60
   French *(Kraft* Premium) 50
   French *(Nalley)* 100
   French *(Old Dutch)* 50
   French *(Ruffles)* 70
   French *(Ruffles* Low Fat) 40
   French *(Sealtest)* .50
   green *(Kraft)* 60
   toasted *(Breakstone's)* 50
   sour cream and *(Lay's* Low Fat) 40
pickle, dill *(Nalley)* 70
ranch:
   (Heluva Good Classic) 60
   (Heluva Good Fat Free) 25
   (Kraft) 60
   (Marie's Creamy) 190
   (Marie's Homestyle) 150
   (Nalley) 110
   (Old Dutch) 50
   (Ruffles) 70
   (Ruffles Low Fat) 40
   bacon *(Marie's)* 150
   peppercorn *(Marie's* Fat Free) 35
   vegetable *(Bernstein's)* 120
red pepper *(Victoria)* 50
spinach or sun-dried tomato *(Marie's)* 140
tzatziki *(Western Creamy)* 60

DIPS, MIXES, dry, except as noted
See also "Dips"

	calories
bean, black or Mexican *(Knorr)*, 1 tsp.	10
chili, caliente *(Knorr)*, ½ tsp.	5
hummus *(Fantastic Foods)*, 2 tbsp.*	60
onion and chive *(Knorr)*, ½ tsp.	5
ranch, cracked pepper *(Knorr)*, ½ tsp.	5
sour cream *(Durkee)*, 2 tsp.	25

SALSA, two tablespoons, except as noted
See also "Dips" and "Condiments & Sauces"

	calories
(Gracias Original Chunky)	15
(Kaukauna Extra Chunky)	14
(La Victoria Ranchera)	10
(La Victoria Victoria)	5
(Marie's Tomato)	10
all varieties:	
(Clemente Jacques)	10
(Del Monte/Del Monte Traditional/Thick & Chunky/Fire Roasted/Garlic)	10
(Heluva Good Thick & Chunky)	10
(Hunt's Alfresco Homestyle)	10
(Hunt's Homestyle)	30
(La Victoria/La Victoria Jalapena/Thick N Chunky)	10
(Nalley Superba)	10
(Old El Paso Homestyle)	10
(Old El Paso Thick 'n Chunky)	15
(Pace Thick & Chunky)	10
(Progresso)	10
(Rosarita/Rosarita Extra Chunky/Traditional)	10
(S&W Ready-Cut), ¼ cup	20
(Sun-Vista)	5
(Tostitos)	15
except medium *(La Victoria* Suprema)	10
except mild *(Las Palmas* Mexicana)	10
except verde *(Chi-Chi's)*	10

* Prepared according to package directions

and cheese, *see "Dips," page 147*
fajita *(Gracias* Superba) 10
garlic, roasted *(Marie's)* 10
green *(Goya)* 10
green or salsa verde *(Old El Paso)* 10
hot *(Gracias)* 15
hot *(Guiltless Gourmet)* 10
medium *(La Victoria* Suprema) 5
medium *(Porino's)* 10
mild *(Las Palmas* Mexicana) 5
picante *(Old Dutch)* 10
picante, all varieties *(Old El Paso* Thick 'n Chunky) 10
verde, medium or mild *(Chi-Chi's)* 15

APPETIZERS & SNACKS, CANNED OR IN JARS
See also "Appetizers & Snacks, Frozen or Refrigerated," "Meat & Poultry, Canned or in Jars," "Meat, Fish, & Poultry Spreads," "Fish & Seafood, Canned or in Jars," "Sausages," and "Condiments & Sauces"

calories

anchovies, in olive oil:
    flat fillets *(King Oscar)*, 6 pieces, 1/2 oz. 25
    flat fillets *(Reese)*, 6 pieces 25
    rolled, with capers *(Reese)*, 5 pieces 25
artichoke appetizer:
    (Contorno Caponata di Carciofi), 1/3 cup 130
    in brine *(Goya)*, 4.5 oz. 65
    in olive oil *(Goya)*, 3 oz. 210
    hearts, in brine *(Progresso)*, 2 pieces 30
    hearts, marinated *(Progresso)*, 2 pieces with liquid 60
    quarters *(S&W)*, 2 pieces 20
bean salad:
    deli style *(S&W)*, 1/2 cup 80
    marinated *(S&W)*, 1/2 cup 70
    three *(Green Giant)*, 1/2 cup 90
    three *(Hanover)*, 1/3 cup 100
    three *(Seneca)*, 1/3 cup .60
caviar, 1 tbsp.:
    carp roe *(Krinos* Tarama) 20
    lumpfish, black or red *(Romanoff)* 15
    salmon, red *(Romanoff)* .35

Appetizers & Snacks, Canned or in Jars, caviar *(cont.)*

whitefish, black *(Romanoff)*	.25
cucumber salad *(Rosoff/Schorr's)*, 1 oz.	.12
eggplant appetizer:	
(Progresso Caponata), 2 tbsp.	.25
roasted *(Peloponnese)*, 2 tbsp.	.25
stuffed, baby *(Krinos)*, approx. 2 pieces, 1.1 oz.	.20
stuffed, rolettes *(Paesana)*, 3¾ oz.	260
franks, cocktail, see "Frankfurters," page 200	
garden salad, dill *(S&W)*, ½ cup	.50
garden salad, marinated *(S&W)*, ½ cup	.50
grape leaves, stuffed *(Perfecta* Dolmadakia), 4.35 oz.	220
kishke *(Hebrew National)*, 2 oz.	160
mushroom, marinated *(Seneca)*, 1 oz.	.90
mushroom salad, all varieties *(Seneca)*, 1 tbsp.	5
olives or olive salad, see "Olives," page 123	
onions:	
cocktail *(Crosse & Blackwell)*, 1 tbsp.	5
cocktail *(S&W* 4 oz.), 12 pieces, 1.1 oz.	5
cocktail *(S&W* 16 oz.), 8 pieces, 1.1 oz.	5
sweet, in sauce *(Boar's Head* Vidalia), 1 tbsp.	.10
wild, marinated *(Krinos* Volvi), 1 oz.	.15
Oriental noodles:	
chow mein *(La Choy)*, ½ cup	140
chow mein *(Mee Tu)*, ⅔ cup	120
crispy, wide *(La Choy)*, ½ cup	150
pâté, liver *(Sells)*, ¼ cup	160
pâté, vegetarian *(Bonavita* Swiss), 1 oz.	.61
pepper salad *(B&G)*, 1 oz.	.10
pepper salad, drained *(Progresso)*, 2 tbsp.	.15
pickles, see "Pickles, Cucumber," page 121	
pig's feet, pickled *(Hormel)*, 2 oz.	.80
pork hocks, pickled *(Hormel)*, 2 oz.	110
pork tidbits, pickled *(Hormel)*, 2 oz.	100
shrimp cocktail:	
(Sau-Sea), 4-oz. jar	100
(Sau-Sea), 6-oz. jar	150
(Vita), 4-oz. jar	110
tomato, pickled, 1 oz.:	
(Claussen)	5
(Hebrew National/Shorr's)	4
half sour *(Rosoff)*	5

vegetable antipasto *(Paesana)*, 3¾ oz. 260
vegetables, mixed, pickled (gardiniera):
   (Krinos), 3 oz. 0
   (Perfecta), 5.3 oz. 0
   (Zorba), ½ cup 20

APPETIZERS & SNACKS, FROZEN OR REFRIGERATED
See also "Appetizers & Snacks, Canned or in Jars" and "Pizza, Frozen"

---

              calories

burritos, 10 pieces, 6 oz.:
   beef, nacho *(Patio Britos)* 410
   beef and bean *(Patio Britos)* 420
   cheese, nacho *(Patio Britos)* 360
   chicken and cheese, spicy *(Patio Britos)* 400
cheese nuggets, breaded nuggets *(Schwan's)*, ¼ cup 110
cheese sticks, mozzarella, breaded *(Schwan's)*, 2 pieces 100
cheese sticks, with cornmeal coating *(Goya Surullitos)*,
   7 pieces 300
egg rolls:
   (Empire Kosher), 3-oz. roll 190
   (Empire Kosher Mini), 6 rolls 280
   chicken *(Schwan's)*, 2 rolls, 4 oz. 220
   chicken, mini *(Chun King)*, 12 rolls 400
   chicken or pork *(Chun King/La Choy)*, 3-oz. roll 170
   chicken or pork and shrimp, mini *(La Choy)*, 14 rolls 430
   chicken, sweet and sour *(La Choy)*, 3-oz. roll 180
   pork *(Schwan's)*, 2 rolls, 4 oz. 240
   pork, moo shu *(La Choy)*, 3-oz. roll 190
   pork and shrimp, bite size *(La Choy)*, 15 rolls 240
   pork and shrimp, mini *(Chun King)*, 12 rolls 420
   shrimp *(Chun King/La Choy)*, 3-oz. roll 150
   shrimp or vegetable with lobster, mini *(La Choy)*, 14 rolls . 410
   shrimp, mini *(Chun King)*, 12 rolls 370
empanadilla:
   plain *(Goya)*, 2 pieces 380
   plain, cocktail size *(Goya)*, 7 pieces 370
   pizza flavor *(Goya)*, 2 pieces 370
frankfurter, corn dog, mini *(Hormel Quick Meal)*, 5 pieces 250
grape leaves, stuffed *(Cedar's)*, 6 pieces, 5 oz. 180

Appetizers & Snacks, Frozen or Refrigerated *(cont.)*
hors d'oeuvre kit:

    (Pepperidge Farm), 7 sheets 470

    beef Stroganoff *(Pepperidge Farm)*, 1 sheet 420

    chicken à la king *(Pepperidge Farm)*, 1 sheet 400

    shrimp Newburg *(Pepperidge Farm)*, 1 sheet 340

lentil salad, garden *(Cedar's)*, 2 tbsp. 30

pizza snacks:

    cheese, double *(Hot Pockets Pizza Snacks)*, 3 oz. 210

    cheese, three *(Totino's Pizza Rolls)*, 6 pieces 200

    combination or spicy Italian style *(Totino's Pizza Rolls)*,

      6 pieces 220

    hamburger and cheese *(Totino's Pizza Rolls)*, 6 pieces . . . 200

    nuggets *(Hormel Quick Meal)*, 5 pieces, 2.8 oz. 210

    pepperoni *(Hot Pockets Pizza Snacks)*, 3 oz. 220

    pepperoni and cheese *(Totino's Pizza Rolls)*, 6 pieces 230

    pepperoni and sausage *(Hot Pockets Pizza Snacks)*, 3 oz. . 210

    sausage *(Hot Pockets Pizza Snacks)*, 3 oz. 200

    sausage and cheese, supreme or three meat *(Totino's Pizza*

      Rolls), 6 pieces 210

    sausage and mushroom *(Totino's Pizza Rolls)*, 6 pieces . . . 200

tabouli salad *(Cedar's)*, 2 tbsp. 30

Wonton Rolls, pizza flavor *(Schwan's)*, 5 pieces, 5 oz. 390

Chapter 10

DINNERS, ENTREES, & POTPIES

DINNERS, FROZEN
See also "Entrees, Frozen," "Entree Mixes, Frozen," "Potpies, Frozen," "Meat & Poultry, Frozen or Refrigerated," "Fish & Seafood, Frozen or Refrigerated," "Pasta, Frozen," and "Pasta Side Dishes, Frozen"

calories

beef:
barbecue, mesquite *(Healthy Choice)*, 11 oz.	310
and broccoli *(Swanson)*, 1 pkg.	340
and broccoli *(Swanson Hungry Man)*, 1 pkg.	500
and broccoli Beijing *(Healthy Choice)*, 12 oz.	300
chicken fried steak *(Banquet Extra Helping)*, 18.65 oz.	800
chicken fried steak *(Marie Callender's)*, 15 oz.	650
chicken fried steak, with gravy *(Swanson)*, 1 pkg.	450
and gravy *(Swanson)*, 1 pkg.	310
patty, charbroiled *(Freezer Queen Meal)*, 9.5 oz.	230
and peppers Cantonese *(Healthy Choice)*, 11.5 oz.	270
pot roast *(Freezer Queen Meal)*, 9.2 oz.	170
pot roast, homestyle *(Schwan's)*, 1 pkg.	320
pot roast, Yankee *(The Budget Gourmet Light)*, 11 oz.	250
pot roast, Yankee *(Healthy Choice)*, 11 oz.	280
pot roast, Yankee *(Swanson)*, 1 pkg.	260
pot roast, Yankee *(Swanson Hungry Man)*, 1 pkg.	400
roast beef sandwich, smothered *(Swanson)*, 1 pkg.	350
Salisbury steak *(Banquet Extra Helping)*, 19 oz.	740
Salisbury steak *(The Budget Gourmet Light)*, 11 oz.	260
Salisbury steak *(Freezer Queen Meal)*, 9.5 oz.	260
Salisbury steak *(Healthy Choice)*, 11.5 oz.	320
Salisbury steak *(Swanson)*, 1 pkg.	420
Salisbury steak *(Swanson Hungry Man)*, 1 pkg.	590
Salisbury steak, con queso *(Patio)*, 11 oz.	390
sirloin *(The Budget Gourmet Light Special Recipe)*, 11 oz.	270
sirloin, chopped, with gravy *(Swanson)*, 1 pkg.	310

Dinners, Frozen, beef *(cont.)*

   sirloin, meatballs and gravy *(The Budget Gourmet Light)*,
     11 oz. 240
   sirloin, in wine sauce *(The Budget Gourmet Light)*, 11 oz. . 220
   sirloin tips *(Swanson Hungry Man)*, 1 pkg. 450
   sirloin tips, with noodles *(Swanson)*, 1 pkg. 280
   sliced, gravy and *(Freezer Queen Meal)*, 9 oz. 140
   steak patty, charbroiled *(Healthy Choice)*, 11 oz. 280
   Stroganoff *(Healthy Choice)*, 11 oz. 310
   teriyaki *(The Budget Gourmet Light)*, 11 oz. 320
   teriyaki *(Schwan's)*, 10 oz. 370
   tips *(Healthy Choice)*, 11¼ oz. 260
burrito, beef *(Chi-Chi's Burro)*, 15 oz. 570
burrito, chicken *(Chi-Chi's Burro)*, 15 oz. 530
cannelloni *(Amy's)*, 10 oz. 260
chicken:
   barbecue, mesquite *(The Budget Gourmet Light)*, 11 oz. . . . 270
   barbecue, mesquite *(Healthy Choice)*, 10.5 oz. 270
   barbecue, with potato and vegetables *(Tyson BBQ)*, 1 pkg. . 560
   boneless *(Swanson Hungry Man)*, 1 pkg. 690
   breaded, country *(Healthy Choice)*, 10¼ oz. 360
   breast, herb roasted *(Schwan's)*, 1 pkg. 270
   broccoli Alfredo *(Healthy Choice)*, 11.5 oz. 300
   cacciatore *(Healthy Choice)*, 12.5 oz. 250
   Cantonese *(Healthy Choice)*, 10¾ oz. 260
   Dijon *(Healthy Choice)*, 11 oz. 270
   fingers and BBQ sauce *(Freezer Queen Meal)*, 9 oz. 310
   Francesca *(Healthy Choice)*, 12.5 oz. 330
   fried *(Banquet Extra Helping)*, 18 oz. 790
   fried, country, with gravy *(Marie Callender's)*, 14 oz. . . . 610
   fried, dark meat *(Swanson)*, 1 pkg. 550
   fried, dark meat *(Swanson Budget)*, 1 pkg. 460
   fried, dark meat *(Swanson Hungry Man)*, 1 pkg. 810
   fried, Southern *(Banquet Extra Helping)*, 17.5 oz. 750
   fried, white meat *(Banquet Extra Helping)*, 18 oz. 820
   fried, white meat *(Swanson)*, 1 pkg. 560
   fried, white meat, mostly *(Swanson Hungry Man)*, 1 pkg. . . 810
   ginger, Hunan *(Healthy Choice)*, 12.6 oz. 350
   grilled, patties *(Swanson Hungry Man)*, 1 pkg. 580
   grilled, Southwestern *(Healthy Choice)*, 10.2 oz. 200
   grilled, white meat, in garlic sauce *(Swanson)*, 1 pkg. . . . 260
   herb, country *(Healthy Choice)*, 12.15 oz. 310

herbed breast, with fettuccine *(The Budget Gourmet* Light),
11 oz. 260
honey mustard *(The Budget Gourmet* Light), 11 oz. 310
nuggets *(Freezer Queen* Meal), 6 oz. 320
nuggets *(Swanson)*, 1 pkg. 440
parmigiana *(Banquet* Extra Helping), 19 oz. 650
parmigiana *(The Budget Gourmet* Light), 11 oz. 280
parmigiana *(Healthy Choice)*, 11.5 oz. 300
parmigiana *(Marie Callender's)*, 16 oz. 620
parmigiana *(Swanson)*, 1 pkg. 400
parmigiana *(Swanson* Budget), 1 pkg. 340
pasta and *(Swanson* Budget), 1 pkg. 250
patty, breaded *(Freezer Queen* Meal), 7.5 oz. 290
picante *(Healthy Choice)*, 10.75 oz. 260
roasted *(Healthy Choice)*, 11 oz. 220
roasted, with herb gravy *(The Budget Gourmet* Light),
11 oz. 250
roasted, herb *(Swanson)*, 1 pkg. 290
roasted, herb, mashed potatoes *(Marie Callender's)*, 14 oz. . 670
sesame, Shanghai *(Healthy Choice)*, 12 oz. 310
sweet and sour *(Healthy Choice)*, 11 oz. 330
tenders, platter *(Swanson)*, 1 pkg. 320
teriyaki *(The Budget Gourmet* Light), 11 oz. 300
teriyaki *(Healthy Choice)*, 11 oz. 230
teriyaki *(Schwan's)*, 10 oz. 380
chili, with corn bread *(Marie Callender's* Dinner), 16 oz. 350
chimichanga, beef *(Chi-Chi's)*, 15 oz. 630
chimichanga, chicken *(Chi-Chi's)*, 15 oz. 600
enchilada:
(*Amy's)*, 10 oz. 250
(Chi-Chi's Baja), 15.4 oz. 580
beef *(Patio)*, 12 oz. 350
beef *(Swanson)*, 1 pkg. 470
beef, with chili sauce *(Banquet* Family), 1 piece, 4.7 oz. . . . 130
cheese *(Patio)*, 12 oz. 330
chicken *(Chi-Chi's* Suprema), 14.9 oz. 580
chicken *(Healthy Choice* Suprema), 11.3 oz. 270
chicken *(Patio)*, 12 oz. 380
fish *(see also specific fish listings)*:
baked, herb *(Healthy Choice)*, 10.9 oz. 340
battered portions, with chips *(Swanson)*, 1 pkg. 480
breaded sticks *(Swanson* Budget), 1 pkg. 340

Dinners, Frozen, fish *(cont.)*
    lemon pepper *(Healthy Choice)*, 10.7 oz. 290
macaroni and cheese *(Swanson* Budget), 1 pkg. 320
meat loaf:
    (Banquet Extra Helping), 19 oz. 650
    (Freezer Queen Meal), 9.5 oz. 260
    (Healthy Choice), 12 oz. 320
    (Marie Callender's), 14 oz. 540
    (Schwan's), 1 pkg. 320
    (Swanson), 1 pkg. 380
    (Swanson Budget), 1 pkg. 330
    (Swanson Hungry Man), 1 pkg. 610
Mexican:
    (Patio), 13¼ oz. 430
    (Patio Fiesta), 12 oz. 340
    (Patio Ranchera), 13 oz. 410
    style *(Banquet* Extra Helping), 22 oz. 820
    style *(Swanson* Budget), 1 pkg. 400
    style *(Swanson Hungry Man)*, 1 pkg. 780
    style, combination *(Swanson)*, 1 pkg. 470
pasta shells, stuffed, marinara *(Healthy Choice)*, 12 oz. 380
pork, barbecue *(Swanson Hungry Man)*, 1 pkg. 770
pork patty, grilled, glazed *(Healthy Choice)*, 9.6 oz. 280
shrimp:
    marinara *(Healthy Choice)*, 10.5 oz. 220
    Mariner *(The Budget Gourmet Light)*, 11 oz. 270
    and vegetables maria *(Healthy Choice* Maria), 12.5 oz. 270
spaghetti and meatballs, frozen *(Swanson)*, 1 pkg. 300
turkey:
    breast *(Healthy Choice)*, 10.5 oz. 280
    breast, with gravy *(Schwan's)*, 1 pkg. 280
    breast, with pasta *(Swanson)*, 1 pkg. 270
    breast, stuffed *(The Budget Gourmet Light)*, 11 oz. 240
    mostly white meat *(Swanson)*, 1 pkg. 300
    mostly white meat *(Swanson Hungry Man)*, 1 pkg. 510
    and gravy, with dressing *(Banquet* Extra Helping), 18.8 oz. . 560
    and gravy, with dressing *(Freezer Queen* Meal), 9.2 oz. . . . 210
    and gravy, with dressing *(Marie Callender's)*, 14 oz. 530
    roast *(Healthy Choice* Country Inn), 10 oz. 250
veal parmigiana:
    (Freezer Queen Meal), 10.2 oz. 290
    (Swanson), 1 pkg. 400

(Swanson Hungry Man), 1 pkg.	640
vegetable loaf *(Amy's)*, 10 oz.	260
vegetable "Salisbury steak" *(Amy's* Country), 11 oz.	380

ENTREES, CANNED OR PACKAGED
See also "Entrees, Freeze-Dried," "Vegetables, Canned or in Jars," "Meat and Poultry, Canned or in Jars," and "Rice Dishes, Canned"

	calories
amaranth *(Health Valley Fast Menu)*, 1 cup	160
beans and franks:	
(Hormel), 7.5 oz.	290
(Kid's Kitchen), 7.5 oz.	310
(Libby's Diner), 7.75 oz.	330
(Van Camp's Beanee Weenee), 1 cup	320
baked *(Van Camp's Beanee Weenee)*, 1 cup	410
barbecue *(Van Camp's Beanee Weenee)*, 1 cup	340
chili *(Van Camp's Beanee Weenee)*, 1 can	240
beef:	
chow mein *(La Choy* Bi-Pack), 1 cup	110
goulash *(Hormel)*, 7.5-oz. can	230
pepper steak *(La Choy)*, 1/5 pkg.	35
pepper steak Oriental *(La Choy* Bi-Pack), 1 cup	105
pepper steak Oriental, with noodles *(La Choy* Bi-Pack), 1 cup	160
pot roast *(Dinty Moore American Classics)*, 10 oz.	210
roast, with gravy *(Libby's)*, 2/3 cup	140
roast, with gravy *(Hormel)*, 2 oz.	60
roast, with mashed potato *(Dinty Moore American Classics)*, 10 oz.	240
Salisbury steak *(Dinty Moore American Classics)*, 10 oz.	310
stew *(Dinty Moore)*, 1 cup	230
stew *(Dinty Moore* Can/Cup), 7.5 oz.	190
stew *(Dinty Moore American Classics)*, 10 oz.	260
stew *(Hormel* Micro Cup), 7.5 oz.	180
stew *(Hunt's* Homestyle), 1 cup	155
stew *(Libby's Diner)*, 7.75 oz.	290
stew *(Nalley)*, 7.5-oz. can	180
stew *(Nalley* Big Chunk), 1 cup	260
stew *(Nalley* Homestyle), 1 cup	210
stew, burger *(Dinty Moore* Hearty Cup), 7.5 oz.	240

Entrees, Canned or Packaged *(cont.)*
beef, hash *(Broadcast Morning Classics* Original), 1 cup 240
beef, corned, hash:
    (Castleberry's), 1 cup 430
    (Dinty Moore Cup), 7.5 oz. 200
    (Goya), 1 cup 410
    (Libby's), 1 cup 490
    (Mary Kitchen), 7.5 oz. 350
    (Mary Kitchen), 1 cup 390
    (Nalley), 1 cup 490
beef, roast, hash:
    (Libby's), 1 cup 460
    (Mary Kitchen), 7.5 oz. 348
    (Mary Kitchen), 1 cup 390
beef, sausage flavor, hash *(Broadcast Morning Classics)*,
    1 cup 240
chicken:
    à la king *(Swanson* Main Dish), 1 cup 320
    à la king *(Top Shelf)*, 10 oz. 380
    breast, glazed *(Top Shelf)*, 10 oz. 200
    cacciatore *(Top Shelf)*, 10 oz. 210
    chow mein *(La Choy* Bi-Pack), 1 cup 110
    chow mein *(La Choy* Entree), 1 cup 80
    and dumplings *(Dinty Moore* Cup), 7.5 oz. 190
    and dumplings *(Swanson* Main Dish), 1 cup 260
    fiesta *(Top Shelf)*, 10 oz. 420
    with mashed potato *(Dinty Moore American Classics)*,
      10 oz. 220
    and noodles *(Dinty Moore American Classics)*, 10 oz. 260
    Oriental, with noodles *(La Choy)*, 1 cup 150
    and pasta *(Chef Boyardee* Bowl), 7.5 oz. 150
    spicy *(La Choy* Szechwan Bi-Pack), 1 cup 100
    stew *(Dinty Moore)*, 1 cup 220
    stew *(Dinty Moore* Cup), 7.5 oz. 180
    stew *(Swanson* Main Dish), 1 cup 180
    sweet and sour *(La Choy* Bi-Pack), 1 cup 160
    teriyaki *(La Choy* Bi-Pack), 1 cup 110
chili:
    with beans *(Chi-Chi's* San Antonio), 1 cup 340
    with beans *(Gebhardt)*, 1 cup 320
    with beans *(Hormel)*, 7.5-oz. can 250
    with beans *(Hormel)*, 1 cup 340

with beans *(Hormel* Micro Cup), 1 cont. 250
with beans *(Hormel* Micro Cup), 10.5-oz. cont. 410
with beans *(Just Rite),* 1 cup 380
with beans *(Libby's),* 1 cup 420
with beans *(Libby's Diner),* 7.75 oz. 320
with beans *(Nalley* Microwave), 7.5-oz. cont. 260
with beans *(Nalley* Real Hearty), 1 cup 310
with beans *(Nalley* Thick), 1 cup 290
with beans *(Old El Paso),* 1 cup 200
with beans *(Van Camp's),* 1 cup 350
with beans *(Wolf),* 1 cup 330
with beans, beef, and hot dogs *(Nalley* Chili Dog), 1 cup . . . 300
with beans and cheddar *(Nalley),* 1 cup 320
with beans and cheddar *(Nalley* Microwave), 7.5-oz. cont. . 260
with beans, chunky *(Hormel),* 1 cup 330
with beans, hot *(Hormel),* 1 cup 340
with beans, hot *(Hormel/Hormel* Micro Cup), 7.5 oz. 250
with beans, hot *(Nalley* Microwave), 7.5-oz. cont. 240
with beans, jalapeño *(Wolf),* 1 cup 330
with beans, jalapeño hot *(Nalley),* 1 cup 280
without beans *(Hormel),* 7.5-oz. can 390
without beans *(Hormel),* 1 cup 410
without beans *(Hormel* Micro Cup), 1 cont. 290
without beans *(Libby's),* 1 cup 480
without beans *(Nalley Big Chunk),* 1 cup 280
without beans *(Wolf),* 1 cup 420
without beans, hot *(Hormel),* 1 cup 410
without beans, jalapeño *(Wolf),* 1 cup 420
without beans, onion *(Nalley* Walla Walla), 1 cup 300
turkey, with beans *(Hormel),* 1 cup 220
turkey, without beans *(Hormel),* 1 cup 190
vegetarian *(Hormel),* 1 cup 200
vegetarian *(Natural Touch),* 1 cup 270
vegetarian *(Worthington),* 1 cup 290
vegetarian, all varieties *(Health Valley* Nonfat), ½ cup 80
with macaroni *(Hormel* Chili Mac), 7.5-oz. can 200
with macaroni *(Hormel* Chili Mac Micro Cup), 1 cont. 200
chili base:
    (Hunt's Homestyle Fixings), ½ cup 85
    (S&W Chili Makin's), ½ cup 80
    (Stubb's Legendary Chili Fixin's), 1 cup 50
    black bean *(S&W* Chili Makin's), ½ cup 80

Entrees, Canned or Packaged, chili base *(cont.)*
   homestyle *(S&W Chili Makin's)*, ½ cup 80
   Santa Fe *(S&W Chili Makin's)*, ½ cup 80
enchilada *(Gebhardt)*, 2 pieces 260
fajita, beef or chicken *(Nalley Superba)*, 1 cup 230
hash *(see also specific hash listings) (Mary Kitchen Fiesta)*,
   1 cup 210
lasagna:
   (Hormel), 7.5 oz. 250
   (Hormel Micro Cup), 7.5 oz. 250
   (Libby's Diner), 7.75 oz. 200
   (Nalley), 7.5-oz. can 200
   (Nalley), 1 cup 250
   and beef *(Hormel* Micro Cup), 10.5 oz. 359
   cheese, three, with beef *(Nalley* Microwave), 7.5-oz. cont. . . 180
   Italian *(Top Shelf)*, 10 oz. 340
macaroni:
   and beef *(Kid's Kitchen* Beefy), 7.5 oz. 190
   and beef *(Kid's Kitchen* Cheezy Mac & Beef), 7.5 oz. 260
   and beef *(Libby's Diner)*, 7.75 oz. 220
   and beef *(Nalley)*, 1 cup 220
   and cheese *(Chef Boyardee* Bowl), 7.5 oz. 160
   and cheese *(Franco-American)*, 1 cup 200
   and cheese *(Hormel* Micro Cup), 7.5 oz. 260
   and cheese *(Kid's Kitchen)*, 7.5 oz. 260
   and cheese *(Libby's Diner)*, 7.75 oz. 320
   and cheese *(Nalley* Microwave), 7.5-oz. cont. 250
meatball stew *(Dinty Moore)*, 1 cup 270
meatball stew *(Dinty Moore* Cup), 7.5 oz. 250
noodle rings *(Kid's Kitchen)*, 7.5 oz. 150
noodles with beef *(Hunt's* Homestyle), 1 cup 150
noodles with beef *(La Choy* Bi-Pack), 1 cup 150
noodles with chicken:
   (Dinty Moore), 7.5 oz. 200
   (Hormel Micro Cup), 7.5 oz. 200
   (Hormel Micro Cup), 10.5 oz. 270
   (La Choy Bi-Pack), 1 cup 160
   (Nalley Dinner), 1 cup 190
   cacciatore or regular *(Hunt's* Homestyle), 1 cup 175
   with mushrooms *(Hunt's* Homestyle), 1 cup 200
   with vegetables *(Nalley)*, 7.5-oz. can 140
   with vegetables *(Nalley)*, 1 cup 160

noodles with franks *(Van Camp's Noodle Weenee)*, 1 can 230
noodles, sweet and sour, with chicken *(La Choy* Entree), 1 cup . 260
noodles with vegetables:
    (La Choy Entree), 1 cup 130
    and beef *(La Choy* Entree), 1 cup 160
    and chicken *(La Choy* Entree), 1 cup 160
pasta spirals, and chicken *(Libby's Diner)*, 7.75 oz. 130
pasta twists *(Franco-American)*, 1 cup 250
penne, in meat sauce *(Franco-American)*, 1 cup 240
pork chow mein *(La Choy* Bi-Pack), 1 cup 80
potatoes:
    au gratin, and bacon *(Hormel)*, 7.5 oz. 250
    scalloped, and ham *(Hormel)*, 7.5 oz. 260
    scalloped, and ham *(Nalley* Microwave), 7.5-oz. cont. 210
    sliced, and beef *(Dinty Moore)*, 7.5 oz. 230
ravioli, beef, tomato sauce:
    (Franco-American), 1 cup 250
    (Hunt's Homestyle), 1 cup 220
    (Libby's), 7.75 oz. 230
    (Nalley), 7.5-oz. can 230
    (Nalley), 1 cup 280
    (Nalley Microwave), 7.5-oz. cont. 240
    (Progresso), 1 cup 260
    (Top Shelf), 10 oz. 300
    with meat *(Chef Boyardee)*, 1 cup 230
    with meat *(Franco-American)*, 1 cup 300
    mini, with meat *(Chef Boyardee* Bowl), 7.5 oz. 180
    mini, with meat *(Franco-American)*, 1 cup 270
ravioli, cheese, tomato sauce:
    (Chef Boyardee), 1 cup 210
    (Progresso), 1 cup 220
    with cheese *(Chef Boyardee* Bowl), 7.5 oz. 170
    with meat *(Chef Boyardee* Bowl), 7.5 oz. 190
ravioli, tomato sauce:
    (Hormel Micro Cup), 7.5 oz. 270
    mini *(Kid's Kitchen)*, 7.5 oz. 240
rigatoni, Italian garden sauce *(Hunt's* Homestyle), 1 cup 165
sausage hash *(Mary Kitchen)*, 1 cup 410
shrimp chow mein *(La Choy* Bi-Pack), 1 cup 55
spaghetti:
    (Franco-American Garfield Pizzos), 1 cup 190
    with beef *(Franco-American Garfield* Pizzos), 1 cup 260

Entrees, Canned or Packaged, spaghetti *(cont.)*

with franks *(Franco-American SpaghettiO's)*, 1 cup 250
with franks *(Van Camp's Weenee)*, 1 can 230
with franks, rings *(Kid's Kitchen)*, 7.5 oz. 230
with meatballs *(Campbell's Superiore/Franco-American)*,
1 cup 270
with meatballs *(Franco-American SpaghettiO's)*, 1 cup . . . 260
with meatballs *(Hormel Micro Cup)*, 7.5 oz. 210
with meatballs *(Libby's Diner)*, 7.5 oz. 190
with meatballs *(Top Shelf)*, 10 oz. 300
with meatballs, rings *(Kid's Kitchen)*, 7.5 oz. 250
with mini meatballs *(Kid's Kitchen)*, 7.5 oz. 220
rings *(Kid's Kitchen)*, 7.5 oz. 190
tomato-cheese sauce *(Franco-American)*, 1 cup 210
tomato-cheese sauce *(Franco-American SpaghettiO's)*,
1 cup 190
tamale:
(Gebhardt), 2 pieces 270
(Gebhardt Jumbo), 2 pieces 330
(Just Rite), 3 pieces 255
(Nalley), 3 pieces 290
(Van Camp's), 2 pieces 210
in chili gravy *(Old El Paso)*, 3 pieces 320
beef *(Hormel)*, 7.5-oz. can 290
beef, hot-spicy or regular *(Hormel)*, 3 pieces 280
beef, jumbo *(Hormel)*, 2 pieces 270
chicken *(Hormel)*, 3 pieces 210
tortellini:
cheese *(Chef Boyardee)*, 1 cup 230
cheese *(Franco-American)*, 1 cup 240
meat *(Chef Boyardee)*, 1 cup 260
meat *(Franco-American)*, 1 cup 260
ground beef *(Chef Boyardee)*, 7.5 oz. 220
turkey:
gravy and dressing *(Dinty Moore American Classics)*,
10 oz. 290
gravy and dressing *(Libby's Diner)*, 7 oz. 180
stew *(Dinty Moore)*, 1 cup 150
stew *(Dinty Moore Cup)*, 7.5 oz. 130
turkey hash, roast *(Mary Kitchen)*, 1 cup 210
vegetables:
Chinese, mixed *(La Choy)*, 2/3 cup 15

chop suey *(La Choy)*, ²/₃ cup 15
curry *(Patak's)*, ½ cup 180

ENTREES, FREEZE-DRIED
*See also "Entrees, Canned & Packaged," "Entrees, Frozen,"
and "Entrees, Mixes"*

---

calories

beef:
    (AlpineAire), ⅓ cup 106
    with peppers, onions, and rice *(Mountain House)*, 1 cup . . . 230
    stew *(Mountain House)*, 1 cup 150
    Stroganoff, with noodles *(Mountain House)*, 1 cup 240
    teriyaki, with rice *(Mountain House)*, 1 cup 250
chicken, 1 cup:
    à la king, and noodles *(Mountain House)* 290
    honey lime, with rice *(Mountain House)* 240
    noodles and *(Mountain House)* 200
    Polynesian, with rice *(Mountain House)* 200
    rice and *(Mountain House)* 300
    stew *(Mountain House)* 220
chili:
    beef and beans *(Mountain House)*, 1 cup 190
    beef and macaroni *(Mountain House)*, 1 cup 220
    meatless *(AlpineAire Mountain)*, 1½ cups 340
lasagna *(Mountain House)*, 1 cup 240
pasta primavera *(Mountain House)*, 1 cup 220
pasta Roma *(AlpineAire)*, 1⅓ cups 328
pork, sweet and sour, with rice *(Mountain House)*, 1 cup 270
shrimp Alfredo *(AlpineAire)*, 1½ cups 300
shrimp Newburg *(AlpineAire)*, 1½ cups 318
spaghetti with meat and sauce *(Mountain House)*, 1 cup 200
turkey, diced *(AlpineAire)*, ⅓ cup 80
turkey tetrazzini *(Mountain House)*, 1 cup 210
wild rice pilaf, with almonds *(AlpineAire)*, 1⅓ cups 291

ENTREES, FROZEN
See also "Vegetables, Frozen," "Vegetable Dishes, Frozen,"
"Dinners, Frozen," "Entree Mixes, Frozen," "Potpies, Frozen,"
"Meat & Poultry, Frozen or Refrigerated," "Fish & Seafood,
Frozen or Refrigerated," "Pasta, Frozen," "Rice Dishes,
Frozen," "Pasta Side Dishes, Frozen," "Pizza, Frozen," and
"Sandwiches, Frozen or Refrigerated"

---

                                                          calories

angel-hair pasta:
   (Lean Cuisine), 10 oz. 260
   (Smart Ones), 9 oz. 170
   with sausage *(Marie Callender's)*, 1 cup, 8 oz. 370
beans, white, Parisian style *(Weight Watchers International*
   Selections), 9.87 oz. 220
beef:
   casserole *(Schwan's)*, 1 cup 340
   chipped *(Banquet Topper)*, 4-oz. bag 100
   chipped, creamed *(Freezer Queen Cook-In-Pouch)*,
     4-oz. pkg. 100
   chipped, creamed *(Schwan's)*, 1 cup 310
   chipped, creamed *(Stouffer's)*, approx. ½ cup, 4.4 oz. 160
   chopped, BBQ *(Schwan's)*, ½ cup 220
   enchilada, *see "enchilada" below*
   goulash *(Schwan's)*, 1 cup 280
   ground, with rice *(Goya)*, 1 pkg. 860
   macaroni *(Healthy Choice)*, 8.5 oz. 210
   mesquite, with rice *(Lean Cuisine Cafe Classics)*, 9 oz. . . . 280
   Oriental *(The Budget Gourmet Light)*, 9 oz. 250
   Oriental *(Lean Cuisine)*, 9¼ oz. 270
   patty *(Swanson Fun Feast)*, 1 pkg. 470
   patty, charbroiled, gravy and *(Morton)*, 9 oz. 290
   patty, charbroiled, mushroom gravy and *(Freezer Queen*
     Family), ⅙ of 28-oz. pkg. 190
   patty, gravy and *(Banquet Homestyle)*, 9.5 oz. 300
   patty, mushroom or onion gravy and *(Banquet Family)*,
     4.7-oz. patty 180
   patty, onion gravy and *(Freezer Queen Family)*,
     ¼ of 28-oz. pkg. 170
   pepper steak *(The Budget Gourmet)*, 10 oz. 290
   pepper steak *(Stouffer's)*, 10½ oz. 330
   pepper steak *(Weight Watchers)*, 10 oz. 240

pepper steak Oriental *(Healthy Choice)*, 9.5 oz. 250
and peppers, with rice *(Freezer Queen Homestyle)*, 9 oz. . . . 210
pot roast *(Freezer Queen Deluxe Family)*, 1 cup, 8.5 oz. . . . 190
pot roast *(Freezer Queen Homestyle)*, 9 oz. 170
pot roast, with gravy *(Marie Callender's)*, 1 cup, 7.5 oz. . . . 180
pot roast, with potatoes *(Lean Cuisine)*, 9 oz. 210
pot roast, with potatoes *(Stouffer's Homestyle)*, 8⅞ oz. . . . 250
roast *(Healthy Choice Hearty Handfuls)*, 6.1 oz. 310
Salisbury steak *(Banquet Homestyle)*, 9.5 oz. 310
Salisbury steak, grilled *(Weight Watchers)*, 8.5 oz. 260
Salisbury steak and gravy, with potatoes *(Freezer Queen
  Homestyle)*, 9 oz. 300
Salisbury steak, gravy and *(Banquet Family)*, 1 patty,
  4.7 oz. 200
Salisbury steak, gravy and *(Banquet Toppers)*, 5-oz. bag . . . 220
Salisbury steak, gravy and *(Freezer Queen Cook-In-Pouch)*,
  5-oz. pkg. 140
Salisbury steak, gravy and *(Freezer Queen Family)*,
  ⅙ of 28-oz. pkg. 140
Salisbury steak, gravy and *(Morton)*, 9 oz. 210
Salisbury steak, with gravy, mashed potato *(Swanson)*,
  1 pkg. 310
Salisbury steak, sirloin *(The Budget Gourmet Light)*, 9 oz. . 240
Salisbury steak, with macaroni and cheese *(Lean Cuisine)*,
  9.5 oz. 290
Salisbury steak, with macaroni and cheese *(Stouffer's
  Homestyle)*, 9⅝ oz. 350
shepherd's pie *(Schwan's)*, 1 cup 250
shredded, with rice *(Goya)*, 1 pkg. 830
sirloin, cheddar melt *(The Budget Gourmet)*, 9.4 oz. 370
sirloin, in herb sauce *(The Budget Gourmet Light)*, 9.5 oz. . 260
sirloin, peppercorn *(Lean Cuisine Cafe Classics)*, 8¾ oz. . . . 220
sirloin, roast, supreme *(The Budget Gourmet)*, 9 oz. 300
sirloin tips, and noodles *(Swanson)*, 1 pkg. 200
sirloin tips, with vegetables *(The Budget Gourmet)*, 10 oz. . 250
sliced *(Banquet Country)*, 9 oz. 240
sliced, gravy and *(Banquet Family)*, 2 slices, 5.6 oz. 100
sliced, gravy and *(Banquet Topper)*, 4-oz. bag 70
sliced, gravy and *(Freezer Queen Cook-In-Pouch)*,
  4-oz. pkg. 70
sliced, gravy and *(Freezer Queen Family)*, ⅔ cup, 4.9 oz. . . . 80
steak, chicken fried *(Banquet Country)*, 10 oz. 400

Entrees, Frozen, beef *(cont.)*

    steak, Philly *(Healthy Choice Hearty Handfuls)*, 6.1 oz. 290
    steak patty, grilled peppercorn *(Healthy Choice)*, 9 oz. 220
    stew *(Banquet* Family), 1 cup, 8.7 oz. 160
    stew *(Freezer Queen* Family), 1 cup, 8.6 oz. 180
    stew, with rice *(Goya)*, 1 pkg. 770
    Stroganoff *(The Budget Gourmet* Light), 8¾ oz. 290
    Stroganoff *(Stouffer's)*, 9¾ oz. 390
    Stroganoff, and noodles *(Marie Callender's)*, 1 cup, 6.5 oz. . 440
    tips, Français *(Healthy Choice)*, 9.5 oz. 280
    tips, and gravy *(Schwan's)*, 1 cup 220
blintzes, 2 pieces:
    apple *(Empire* Kosher) 220
    blueberry or potato *(Empire* Kosher) 190
    cheese or cherry *(Empire* Kosher) 200
blue hake, breaded *(Schwan's)*, 1 piece, 3 oz. 150
bow-tie pasta and chicken Marsala *(Weight Watchers*
    International Selections), 9.65 oz. 280
bow-ties and chicken *(Lean Cuisine* Cafe Classics), 9.5 oz. 270
burrito:
    bean, black *(Amy's)*, 6 oz. 320
    bean and cheese *(Old El Paso)*, 5 oz. 300
    bean and cheese *(Tina's)*, 5 oz. 340
    bean and rice *(Amy's)*, 6 oz. 250
    bean, rice and cheese *(Amy's)*, 6 oz. 280
    beef *(Hormel Quick Meal)*, 4 oz. 300
    beef *(Tina's* Red Hot), 5 oz. 370
    beef, nacho *(Patio Britos)*, 10 pieces, 6 oz. 410
    beef and bean *(Patio Britos)*, 10 pieces, 6 oz. 420
    beef and bean *(Schwan's)*, 4.3 oz. 260
    beef and bean, all varieties *(Old El Paso)*, 5 oz. 320
    beef steak *(Don Miguel)*, 7 oz. 370
    cheese *(Hormel Quick Meal)*, 4 oz. 250
    chicken *(Don Miguel)*, 7 oz. 360
    chicken and cheese, spicy *(Patio Britos)*, 10 pieces, 6 oz. . 400
    chicken con queso *(Healthy Choice)*, 10.55 oz. 360
    chili, red *(Hormel Quick Meal)*, 4 oz. 280
    pizza, cheese *(Old El Paso)*, 3.5 oz. 240
    pizza, pepperoni *(Old El Paso)*, 3.5 oz. 260
    pizza, sausage *(Old El Paso)*, 3.5 oz. 250
cabbage, stuffed, with potato *(Lean Cuisine)*, 9.5 oz. 180
cannelloni, cheese *(Lean Cuisine)*, 9⅛ oz. 230

catfish fingers, breaded *(Schwan's)*, 4 oz. 170
cavatelli *(Celentano)*, 3.2 oz. 400
chicken:
  à la king *(Banquet* Toppers), 4.5-oz. bag 100
  à la king *(Freezer Queen* Cook-In-Pouch), 4-oz. pkg. 70
  à la king *(Stouffer's)*, 9.5 oz. 350
  au gratin *(The Budget Gourmet* Light), 9.1 oz. 250
  baked, and gravy, whipped potato *(Stouffer's* Homestyle),
    8⅞ oz. 270
  baked, with whipped potato and stuffing *(Lean Cuisine)*,
    8.5 oz. 250
  barbecue *(Tyson)*, 8.9 oz. 270
  barbecue style *(Banquet* Country), 9 oz. 320
  with basil cream sauce *(Lean Cuisine Cafe Classics)*,
    8.5 oz. 260
  biryani *(Curry Classics)*, 10 oz. 460
  and biscuits *(Freezer Queen* Family), 1 cup 210
  blackened, with rice and corn *(Tyson)*, 8.9 oz. 260
  breaded cutlet, pasta marinara *(Celentano)*, 10 oz. 170
  breast, with gravy *(Schwan's)*, 1 cup 260
  breast, in wine sauce *(Lean Cuisine* Cafe Classics), 8⅛ oz. . 220
  breast, skinless, stuffed *(Barber Foods)*, 6-oz. piece 300
  breast, stuffed with asparagus and cheese *(Barber Foods)*,
    6-oz. piece 350
  breast, stuffed with asparagus and cheese *(Schwan's)*,
    6-oz. piece 290
  breast, stuffed with broccoli and cheese *(Barber Foods)*,
    6-oz. piece 330
  breast, stuffed with broccoli and cheese *(Schwan's)*,
    4-oz. piece 220
  breast, stuffed with broccoli, cheese, and ham *(Schwan's)*,
    5-oz. piece 250
  breast, stuffed, Cordon Bleu *(Barber Foods)*, 6-oz. piece . . . 360
  breast, stuffed, Cordon Bleu *(Schwan's)*, 5-oz. piece 260
  breast, stuffed, Kiev *(Schwan's)*, 5-oz. piece 350
  breast strips, breaded *(Schwan's)*, 3 strips, 4 oz. 170
  breast tenderloin, breaded *(Schwan's)*, 2 pieces, 2.86 oz. . . . 190
  breast tenderloin, breaded, Southern *(Schwan's)*, 2 pieces,
    3 oz. 210
  breast tenders *(Tyson)*, 5 pieces, 3 oz. 220
  breast tenders, regular or Southern *(Banquet)*, 3 pieces,
    3 oz. 260

Entrees, Frozen, chicken *(cont.)*

and broccoli *(Healthy Choice Hearty Handfuls)*, 6.1 oz. 320
with broccoli and cheese *(Tyson)*, 8.9 oz. 270
cacciatore *(Tyson)*, 14.9 oz. 560
calypso *(Lean Cuisine* Cafe Classics)*, 8.5 oz. 280
carbonara *(Lean Cuisine* Cafe Classics)*, 9 oz. 280
casserole *(Schwan's)*, 1 cup 360
chow mein *(Banquet)*, 9 oz. 210
chow mein *(Chun King)*, 13 oz. 370
chow mein *(Lean Cuisine)*, 9 oz. 240
chow mein *(Smart Ones)*, 9 oz. 200
chow mein *(Stouffer's)*, 10⅝ oz. 260
chunks, breaded *(Country Skillet)*, 5 pieces, 3.3 oz. 270
chunks, breaded, and cheddar *(Banquet)*, 4 pieces, 2.9 oz. . 280
chunks, breaded, Southern *(Banquet)*, 5 pieces, 3.1 oz. . . . 270
chunks, breaded, Southern *(Country Skillet)*, 5 pieces,
   3.3 oz. 250
Cordon Bleu *(Weight Watchers)*, 9 oz. 230
creamed *(Stouffer's)*, 6.5 oz. 260
creamy, and broccoli *(Stouffer's)*, 8⅞ oz. 320
croquettes *(Goya)*, 3 pieces 280
croquettes *(Tyson)*, 3.5 oz. 290
croquettes, gravy and *(Freezer Queen* Family)*,
   ⅙ of 28-oz. pkg. 140
drumlets *(Swanson Fun Feast)*, 1 pkg. 470
drumsticks, breaded *(Schwan's)*, 2.3-oz. piece 180
and dumplings *(Banquet* Family Size)*, 1 cup, 7 oz. 290
and dumplings *(Banquet* Homestyle)*, 10 oz. 260
enchilada, *see "enchilada," below*
escalloped, and noodles *(Stouffer's)*, 10 oz. 450
escalloped, and noodles *(Stouffer's 76 oz.)*, 8.4 oz. 360
fajita, *see "fajita," below*
fettuccine *(The Budget Gourmet)*, 10 oz. 380
fettuccine *(Lean Cuisine)*, 9¼ oz. 300
fettuccine *(Stouffer's* Homestyle)*, 10.5 oz. 390
fettuccine *(Weight Watchers)*, 10 oz. 290
fettuccine, Alfredo *(Healthy Choice)*, 8.5 oz. 260
fiesta *(Lean Cuisine)*, 8.5 oz. 250
fiesta *(Smart Ones)*, 8.5 oz. 220
fillet, thigh, breaded, Southern style *(Schwan's)*,
   3.5-oz. piece 220
Français *(Tyson)*, 8.9 oz. 260

French recipe *(The Budget Gourmet Light)*, 9 oz. 180
fried *(Banquet Country)*, 9 oz. 470
fried *(Country Skillet)*, 3 oz. 270
fried *(Kid Cuisine High Flying)*, 10.1 oz. 440
fried *(Morton)*, 9 oz. 420
fried *(Swanson Fun Feast Frazzlin')*, 1 pkg. 570
fried, breast *(Banquet)*, 5.5-oz. piece 410
fried, country, original or Southern *(Banquet)*, 3 oz. 270
fried, drums and thighs or hot 'n spicy *(Banquet)*, 3 oz. . . . 260
fried, skinless, original or honey BBQ *(Banquet)*, 3 oz. 210
fried, Southern *(Banquet Country)*, 8¾ oz. 530
fried, with mashed potatoes and gravy *(Tyson)*, 10.9 oz. . . . 360
fried, with whipped potato *(Stouffer's Homestyle)*, 7.5 oz.   . 310
fried, with whipped potatoes *(Swanson)*, 1 pkg. 400
fried, white meat *(Banquet Country)*, 8¾ oz. 470
fried, wing, hot and spicy *(Banquet)*, 4 pieces, 4 oz. 230
garlic *(Healthy Choice Hearty Handfuls)*, 6.1 oz. 330
garlic, Milano *(Healthy Choice)*, 9.5 oz. 240
glazed *(Stouffer's 63 oz.)*, 4.2 oz. 100
glazed, country *(Healthy Choice)*, 8.5 oz. 210
glazed, with rice, broccoli, and carrots *(Tyson)*, 9.1 oz. . . . 240
glazed, with vegetable rice *(Lean Cuisine)*, 8.5 oz. 240
grilled *(Healthy Choice Sonoma)*, 9 oz. 240
grilled, with angel-hair pasta *(Stouffer's)*, 10⅞ oz. 380
grilled, with corn and beans *(Tyson)*, 8.9 oz. 240
grilled, gumbo *(Goya Asopao de Pollo)*, 1 pkg. 190
grilled, Italian, with linguine *(Tyson)*, 8.9 oz. 190
grilled, with mashed potatoes *(Healthy Choice)*, 8 oz. 170
grilled, salsa *(Lean Cuisine Cafe Classics)*, 8⅞ oz. 270
honey mustard *(Healthy Choice)*, 9.5 oz. 260
honey mustard *(Lean Cuisine Cafe Classics)*, 8 oz. 270
honey mustard *(Smart Ones)*, 8.5 oz. 200
honey mustard *(Tyson)*, 11.35 oz. 340
imperial *(Healthy Choice)*, 9 oz. 230
imperial, with rice *(Freezer Queen Homestyle)*, 9 oz. 250
Italian, with fettuccine *(Lean Cuisine)*, 9 oz. 270
Kiev *(Tyson)*, 9.1 oz. 440
lo mein *(Banquet)*, 10.5 oz. 270
mandarin *(The Budget Gourmet Light)*, 10 oz. 270
mandarin *(Healthy Choice)*, 10 oz. 280
mandarin *(Lean Cuisine Lunch Classics)*, 9 oz. 260
marinara rotini *(Lean Cuisine Lunch Classics)*, 9.5 oz. 260

Entrees, Frozen, chicken *(cont.)*

Marsala *(The Budget Gourmet)*, 9 oz. 270
Marsala, with potato and carrots *(Tyson)*, 8.9 oz. 180
Marsala, and vegetables *(Healthy Choice)*, 11.5 oz. 230
Mediterranean *(Lean Cuisine* Cafe Classics), 10.5 oz. 230
mesquite *(Tyson)*, 8.9 oz. 320
Mirabella *(Smart Ones)*, 9.2 oz. 170
Monterey *(Stouffer's* Homestyle), 9⅜ oz. 410
and mushroom *(Healthy Choice Hearty Handfuls)*, 6.1 oz. . 300
with mushroom sauce *(Tyson)*, 8.9 oz. 220
nibbles *(Swanson)*, 1 pkg. 340
noodle casserole *(Swanson)*, 1 pkg. 290
noodle casserole with vegetables *(Swanson)*, 1 pkg. 320
and noodles *(The Budget Gourmet)*, 9 oz. 360
nuggets *(Banquet)*, 6 pieces, 3 oz. 240
nuggets *(Banquet)*, 6 pieces, 4.5 oz. 320
nuggets *(Banquet* Homestyle), 6¾ oz. 410
nuggets *(Country Skillet)*, 10 pieces, 3.3 oz. 280
nuggets *(Freezer Queen* Family), 6 pieces, 3 oz. 240
nuggets *(Kid Cuisine* Cosmic), 9.1 oz. 440
nuggets *(Morton)*, 7 oz. 320
nuggets, breaded *(Schwan's)*, 6 pieces, 3 oz. 230
nuggets, mozzarella *(Banquet)*, 6 pieces, 2.9 oz. 250
nuggets, Southern *(Banquet)*, 6 pieces, 4.5 oz. 340
à l'orange *(Lean Cuisine)*, 9 oz. 250
orange glazed *(The Budget Gourmet* Light), 9 oz. 300
Oriental *(Banquet)*, 9 oz. 260
Oriental *(Lean Cuisine)*, 9 oz. 250
Oriental, and vegetables *(The Budget Gourmet* Light), 9 oz. . 300
Parmesan *(Lean Cuisine* Cafe Classics), 10⅞ oz. 240
parmigiana *(Banquet)*, 9.5 oz. 290
parmigiana *(Banquet* Family), 4.7-oz. piece 240
parmigiana *(Stouffer's* Homestyle), 12 oz. 460
parmigiana *(Tyson)*, 13.8 oz. 430
parmigiana, Italian style *(Banquet)*, 4.6-oz. piece 250
patties, breaded *(Banquet)*, 2.3-oz. piece 180
patties, breaded *(Banquet* Country), 10.2 oz. 380
patties, breaded *(Country Skillet)*, 2.5-oz. piece 190
patties, breaded *(Morton)*, 6¾ oz. 280
patties, breaded strips *(Swanson)*, 1 pkg. 340
patties, breaded, breast *(Schwan's)*, 3-oz. piece 220
patties, breaded, Southern *(Banquet)*, 2.3-oz. piece 170

patties, breaded, Southern *(Country Skillet)*, 3.3-oz. piece . 190
in peanut sauce *(Lean Cuisine)*, 9 oz. 280
penne pollo *(Weight Watchers)*, 10 oz. 290
piccata *(Lean Cuisine Cafe Classics)*, 9 oz. 270
piccata, lemon herb *(Smart Ones)*, 8.5 oz. 200
piccata, with potato and broccoli *(Tyson)*, 8.9 oz. 190
primavera, pasta *(Banquet)*, 10.5 oz. 330
primavera, pasta *(Tyson)*, 11.35 oz. 320
and rice, stir-fry casserole *(Swanson)*, 1 pkg. 240
roasted, herb *(Lean Cuisine Cafe Classics)*, 8 oz. 210
roasted, herb *(Tyson)*, 11.35 oz. 290
roasted, with pasta and vegetables *(Tyson)*, 8.9 oz. 210
sesame *(Healthy Choice)*, 9.75 oz. 240
sliced, gravy and *(Freezer Queen Cook-In-Pouch)*,
    4-oz. pkg. 60
sweet and sour *(The Budget Gourmet)*, 10 oz. 330
sweet and sour, with rice *(Freezer Queen Homestyle)*, 9 oz. . 240
tikka *(Curry Classics Makhanwala)*, 10 oz. 480
and vegetables *(Lean Cuisine)*, 10.5 oz. 250
and vegetables, with linguine *(Freezer Queen Deluxe
    Family)*, 1 cup, 8.6 oz. 250
and vegetables, with noodles *(Freezer Queen Homestyle)*,
    9 oz. 210
walnut, crunchy *(Chun King)*, 13 oz. 470
wings *(Schwan's Hot Wings)*, 6 pieces, 3.3 oz. 210
wings *(Tyson Wings of Fire)*, 4 pieces, 3.4 oz. 220
wings, barbecue *(Schwan's)*, 6 pieces, 3.3 oz. 210
wings, barbecue *(Tyson)*, 4 pieces, 3.4 oz. 210
wings, breaded *(Schwan's Drummies)*, 3 pieces, 2.75 oz. . 240
chili:
    with beans *(Stouffer's)*, 8¾ oz. 270
    three bean *(Lean Cuisine)*, 10 oz. 260
    vegetarian *(Tabatchnik Side Dish)*, 7.5 oz. 210
chimichanga:
    (Banquet), 9.5 oz. 470
    beef *(Old El Paso)*, 4.3-oz. piece 360
    beef steak and bean *(Don Miguel)*, 7 oz. 410
    chicken *(Don Miguel)*, 7 oz. 400
    chicken *(Old El Paso)*, 4.3-oz. piece 340
clams, fried *(Gorton's Crunchy)*, 3 oz. 260
clams, fried *(Mrs. Paul's)*, 3 oz. 280

Entrees, Frozen *(cont.)*
cod:
    battered *(Schwan's Battercrisp)*, 1 fillet, 2 oz. 120
    breaded *(Mrs. Paul's* Premium), 1 fillet 250
    breaded, lightly *(Van de Kamp's)*, 1 fillet 220
    nuggets *(Schwan's)*, 6 pieces, 3 oz. 200
crab cake, deviled *(Mrs. Paul's)*, 1 piece 170
crab cakes, deviled, miniature *(Mrs. Paul's)*, 6 pieces, 3.5 oz. . 230
dumpling, Oriental *(Lean Cuisine)*, 9 oz. 320
egg roll, vegetable *(Lean Cuisine)*, 9 oz. 330
eggplant:
    cutlets *(Celentano)*, 5 oz. 210
    parmigiana *(Celentano)*, 10-oz. pkg. 420
    parmigiana *(Celentano* 14 oz.), ½ pkg. 320
    parmigiana *(Celentano* Value Pack), 1 cup, 8 oz. 360
    parmigiana *(Mrs. Paul's)*, ½ cup 220
    rollettes *(Celentano)*, 10 oz. 350
    rollettes *(Celentano* Great Choice), 10 oz. 330
enchilada:
    beef *(Banquet)*, 11 oz. 380
    beef *(Patio* Family), 2 pieces, 5.7 oz. 200
    beef or beef and cheese *(Patio* Chili 'n Beans Large),
      2 pieces, 7¾ oz. 250
    beef and tamale, chili gravy with *(Morton)*, 10 oz. 260
    black bean *(Amy's* Family Size), 4.38 oz. 120
    black bean and vegetable *(Amy's)*, 4.75 oz. 130
    cheese *(Amy's)*, 4.75 oz. 210
    cheese *(Amy's* Family Size), 4.38 oz. 200
    cheese *(Banquet)*, 11 oz. 340
    cheese *(Patio* Family), 2 pieces, 5.7 oz. 170
    cheese and rice *(Stouffer's)*, 9¾ oz. 370
    chicken *(Banquet)*, 11 oz. 360
    chicken *(Stouffer's* 57 oz.), 4.75 oz. 230
    chicken and rice *(Stouffer's)*, 10 oz. 370
    chicken Suiza *(Healthy Choice)*, 10 oz. 270
    chicken Suiza *(Weight Watchers)*, 9 oz. 270
    chicken Suiza, with rice *(Lean Cuisine)*, 9 oz. 280
fajita, chicken *(Healthy Choice* Fiesta), 7 oz. 260
fajita, chicken *(Schwan's)*, 4-oz. piece 130
fettuccine:
    Alfredo *(Banquet)*, 10.5 oz. 370
    Alfredo *(Healthy Choice)*, 8 oz. 250

Alfredo *(Lean Cuisine)*, 9 oz. 300
Alfredo *(Marie Callender's)*, 1 cup, 6.5 oz. 350
Alfredo *(Stouffer's)*, 10 oz. 520
Alfredo, with broccoli *(Weight Watchers)*, 8.5 oz. 230
Alfredo, with four cheeses *(The Budget Gourmet)*, 11.5 oz. . 480
with broccoli and chicken *(Marie Callender's)*, 1 cup,
    6.5 oz. 420
and meatballs in wine sauce *(The Budget Gourmet)*,
    10¼ oz. 320
primavera *(Lean Cuisine)*, 10 oz. 280
primavera *(Marie Callender's)*, 1 cup, 7 oz. 310
primavera *(Stouffer's)*, 10 oz. 430
primavera in herb sauce with chicken *(The Budget
    Gourmet)*, 10 oz. 270
fish *(see also specific fish listings)*:
    (Van de Kamp's Fish 'n Fries), 6.5 oz. 380
    baked, with shells *(Lean Cuisine)*, 9 oz. 260
    cakes *(Mrs. Paul's)*, 2 pieces 200
    and chips *(Swanson)*, 1 pkg. 310
    fillets, baked, breaded *(Mrs. Paul's Crisp & Healthy)*,
        2 pieces 150
    fillets, baked, garlic and herb *(Mrs. Paul's/Van de Kamp's
        Crunchy)*, 1 piece 150
    fillets, baked, lemon pepper *(Mrs. Paul's/Van de Kamp's
        Crunchy)*, 1 piece 140
    fillets, battered *(Gorton's)*, 2 pieces 280
    fillets, battered *(Mrs. Paul's)*, 1 piece 170
    fillets, battered *(Van de Kamp's)*, 1 piece 180
    fillets, battered, lemon pepper *(Gorton's)*, 2 pieces 250
    fillets, breaded *(Gorton's Crunchy)*, 2 pieces 270
    fillets, breaded *(Mrs. Paul's)*, 2 pieces 240
    fillets, breaded *(Van de Kamp's)*, 2 pieces 280
    fillets, breaded *(Van de Kamp's Crisp & Healthy)*, 2 pieces . 150
    fillets, breaded, cornmeal *(Mrs. Paul's)*, 1 piece 180
    fillets, breaded, cornmeal *(Van de Kamp's Country)*, 1 piece . 180
    fillets, breaded, garlic and herb *(Gorton's Crunchy)*, 1 piece . 180
    fillets, breaded, garlic and herb *(Gorton's Crunchy)*, 2
        pieces 250
    fillets, breaded, hot and spicy *(Gorton's Crunchy)*, 2 pieces . 250
    fillets, breaded, with potato *(Gorton's)*, 2 pieces 290
    fillets, breaded, Southern fried *(Gorton's Crunchy)*, 2 pieces . 270
    fillets, in butter sauce *(Mrs. Paul's)*, 1 piece 120

Entrees, Frozen, fish (cont.)

fillets, grilled, garlic butter, Italian herb, or lemon pepper
  (Mrs. Paul's/Van de Kamp's), 1 piece 130
fillets, grilled, Italian herb (Gorton's), 1 piece 130
fillets, grilled, lemon pepper (Gorton's), 1 piece 120
grilled, with vegetables (Lean Cuisine Cafe Classics),
  8 7/8 oz. 170
with macaroni and cheese (Stouffer's Homestyle), 9 oz. . . . 430
with macaroni and cheese (Swanson), 1 pkg. 350
nuggets (Van de Kamp's), 8 pieces 280
portions, battered (Gorton's), 1 piece 160
portions, battered (Van de Kamp's), 2 pieces 350
portions, breaded (Mrs. Paul's), 2 pieces 190
portions, breaded (Van de Kamp's), 3 pieces 330
sticks (Kid Cuisine Funtastic), 8 1/4 oz. 370
sticks (Swanson Fun Feast Frenzied), 1 pkg. 360
sticks, baked, breaded (Mrs. Paul's Crisp & Healthy),
  6 pieces 180
sticks, battered (Gorton's), 5 pieces 290
sticks, battered (Mrs. Paul's), 6 pieces 240
sticks, battered (Van de Kamp's), 6 pieces 260
sticks, breaded (Gorton's Crunchy), 6 pieces 250
sticks, breaded (Gorton's Value Pack), 6 pieces 220
sticks, breaded (Mrs. Paul's), 6 pieces 200
sticks, breaded (Mrs. Paul's Value Pack), 6 pieces 210
sticks, breaded (Van de Kamp's), 6 pieces 290
sticks, breaded (Van de Kamp's Crisp & Healthy), 6 pieces . 180
sticks, breaded (Van de Kamp's Snack/Value Pack),
  6 pieces 260
sticks, breaded, mini (Van de Kamp's), 13 pieces 250
sticks, breaded, with potato (Gorton's), 6 pieces 220
flounder fillets (Mrs. Paul's Premium), 1 piece 170
flounder fillets, breaded, lightly (Van de Kamp's), 1 piece 230
haddock:
  (Mrs. Paul's Premium), 1 piece 230
  battered (Van de Kamp's), 2 pieces 260
  breaded (Van de Kamp's), 2 pieces 280
  breaded, lightly (Van de Kamp's), 1 piece 220
  breaded, squares (Schwan's), 1 piece, 4 oz. 200
  breaded, sticks (Schwan's), 3 pieces, 3 oz. 160
halibut, battered (Van de Kamp's), 3 pieces 330
ham and asparagus bake (Stouffer's), 9.5 oz. 520

hush puppies *(Schwan's)*, 3 pieces, 2.25 oz. 180
hush puppies *(Stilwell)*, 3 pieces 140
lamb curry *(Curry Classics)*, 10 oz. 480
lasagna:
    (Celentano), 10 oz. 400
    (Celentano 14 oz.), ½ pkg. 280
    (Celentano 25 oz.), 1 cup 360
    (Celentano Great Choice), 10 oz. 260
    (Celentano Value Pack), 1 cup 320
    (Healthy Choice Roma), 13.5 oz. 390
    Alfredo *(Weight Watchers)*, 9 oz. 300
    Alfredo, with broccoli *(The Budget Gourmet)*, 9 oz. 360
    bake *(Stouffer's)*, 10¼ oz. 370
    Bolognese, with meat sauce *(The Budget Gourmet)*, 9 oz. . 340
    Bolognese, with meat sauce *(Weight Watchers)*, 9 oz. 300
    cheese *(Lean Cuisine* Classic), 11.5 oz. 290
    cheese, casserole *(Lean Cuisine Lunch Classics)*, 10 oz. . . . 280
    cheese, with chicken scallopini *(Lean Cuisine* Cafe
      Classics), 10 oz. 290
    cheese, five *(Lean Cuisine* 96 oz.), approx. 1 cup 230
    cheese, five *(Stouffer's)*, 10¾ oz. 360
    cheese, four *(Wolfgang Puck's)*, 12 oz. 480
    cheese, Italian *(Weight Watchers)*, 11 oz. 300
    cheese, three *(The Budget Gourmet)*, 10.5 oz. 390
    extra cheese *(Marie Callender's)*, 1 cup, 7 oz. 330
    chicken *(Lean Cuisine)*, 10 oz. 290
    chicken *(Lean Cuisine* 96 oz.), 8 oz. 230
    Florentine *(Smart Ones)*, 10 oz. 200
    garden *(Weight Watchers)*, 11 oz. 270
    meat sauce *(Banquet)*, 10.5 oz. 290
    meat sauce *(Banquet* Bake at Home), 1 cup, 8 oz. 240
    meat sauce *(Banquet* Family), 1 cup, 7 oz. 230
    meat sauce *(The Budget Gourmet* Light), 9.4 oz. 250
    meat sauce *(Freezer Queen* Deluxe Family), 1 cup, 8.3 oz. . 270
    meat sauce *(Freezer Queen* Homestyle), 10.5 oz. 320
    meat sauce *(Lean Cuisine)*, 10.5 oz. 290
    meat sauce *(Marie Callender's)*, 1 cup, 7 oz. 370
    meat sauce *(Marie Callender's* Multi-Serve), 1 cup, 8.9 oz. . 350
    meat sauce *(Schwan's)*, 1 cup 320
    meat sauce *(Smart Ones)*, 9 oz. 240
    meat sauce *(Stouffer's)*, 10.5 oz. 370
    meat sauce *(Stouffer's* 21 oz.), approx. 1 cup, 7 oz. 260

Entrees, Frozen, lasagna *(cont.)*

meat sauce *(Stouffer's* 40 oz.), approx. 1 cup, 8 oz. 270
meat sauce *(Stouffer's* 96 oz.), approx. 1 cup, 7.4 oz. 290
meat sauce *(Swanson)*, 10 oz. 410
meat sauce *(Weight Watchers)*, 10¼ oz. 270
meat sauce casserole *(Swanson)*, 1 pkg. 330
mozzarella *(The Budget Gourmet)*, 9 oz. 360
primavera *(Celentano* Great Choice), 10 oz. 240
primavera *(Celentano* Selects), 10 oz. 210
sausage, Italian *(The Budget Gourmet)*, 10.5 oz. 450
vegetable *(Amy's* Family Size), 7 oz. 200
vegetable *(Banquet)*, 10.5 oz. 260
vegetable *(Lean Cuisine)*, 10.5 oz. 270
vegetable *(Schwan's)*, 1 cup 280
vegetable *(Stouffer's)*, 10.5 oz. 440
vegetable *(Stouffer's* 96 oz.), approx. 1 cup 340
vegetable, with cheese *(Amy's)*, 9.5 oz. 300
vegetable, cheesy *(Swanson)*, 1 pkg. 350
vegetable, tofu *(Amy's)*, 9.5 oz. 300
zucchini *(Healthy Choice)*, 13.5 oz. 330

linguine:

with bay shrimp and clams, marinara *(The Budget
  Gourmet)*, 9 oz. 270
with shrimp and clams *(The Budget Gourmet* Light),
  9.5 oz. 280
with tomato sauce and sausage *(The Budget Gourmet)*,
  10¼ oz. 380

macaroni:

and beef *(Banquet* Bake at Home), 1 cup, 8 oz. 230
and beef *(Freezer Queen* Homestyle), 9 oz. 220
and beef *(Kid Cuisine* Rip-Roaring), 9.6 oz. 370
and beef *(Lean Cuisine)*, 10 oz. 280
and beef *(Marie Callender's)*, 1 cup, 7 oz. 310
and beef *(Stouffer's)*, 11.5 oz. 420
and beef casserole *(Swanson)*, 1 pkg. 270
broccoli *(Swanson Mac & More)*, 1 pkg. 220
and cheddar, white *(Swanson Mac & More)*, 1 pkg. 200
and cheese *(Amy's)*, 9 oz. 450
and cheese *(Banquet)*, 10.5 oz. 350
and cheese *(Banquet* Bake at Home), 1 cup, 8 oz. 300
and cheese *(Banquet* Family), 1 cup, 7 oz. 210
and cheese *(The Budget Gourmet* Homestyle), 9 oz. 360

and cheese *(Freezer Queen* Family Side Dish), 1 cup,
  8.6 oz. 240
and cheese *(Healthy Choice)*, 9 oz. 290
and cheese *(Kid Cuisine* Magical), 10.6 oz. 420
and cheese *(Lean Cuisine)*, 10 oz. 290
and cheese *(Marie Callender's)*, 1 cup, 6.5 oz. 420
and cheese *(Morton)*, 6.5 oz. 200
and cheese *(Morton* 16/28 oz.), 1 cup 230
and cheese *(Schwan's)*, 1 cup 340
and cheese *(Smart Ones)*, 9 oz. 220
and cheese *(Stouffer's* 12 oz.), approx. 1 cup, 6 oz. 330
and cheese *(Stouffer's* 20 oz.), approx. 1 cup, 8 oz. 340
and cheese *(Stouffer's* 40 oz.), approx. 1 cup, 8 oz. 380
and cheese *(Stouffer's* 76 oz.), approx. 1 cup, 8.4 oz. 360
and cheese *(Swanson* Entree), 1 pkg. 280
and cheese *(Swanson* Entree), 1 cup 260
and cheese *(Swanson Mac & More* Classic), 1 pkg. 240
and cheese *(Tabatchnik* Side Dish), 7.5 oz. 280
and cheese *(Weight Watchers)*, 9 oz. 300
and cheese, with broccoli *(Lean Cuisine Lunch Classics)*,
  9¾ oz. 240
and cheese, with broccoli *(Stouffer's)*, 10.5 oz. 360
and cheese, with cheddar and Romano *(The Budget*
  Gourmet), 9 oz. 310
and cheese, salsa *(Swanson Mac & More)*, 1 pkg. 210
and cheese bake, casserole, three-cheese *(Swanson)*,
  1 pkg. 400
and cheese pie *(Banquet)*, 6.5 oz. 200
Italiano *(Swanson Mac & More)*, 1 pkg. 180
soy cheeze *(Amy's)*, 9 oz. 360
manicotti:
  cheese *(Celentano)*, 10 oz. 450
  cheese *(Celentano* 14 oz.), ½ pkg. 310
  cheese *(Celentano* Great Choice), 10 oz. 250
  cheese *(Celentano* Value Pack), 2 pieces, 8 oz. 320
  cheese *(Stouffer's)*, 9 oz. 380
  cheese *(Weight Watchers)*, 9¼ oz. 260
  cheese, with meat sauce *(The Budget Gourmet)*, 10 oz. . . 420
  cheese, three *(Healthy Choice)*, 11 oz. 260
  Florentine *(Celentano)*, 10 oz. 220
  Florentine *(Celentano* Great Choice), 10 oz. 210

Entrees, Frozen *(cont.)*

meat loaf:

    (Banquet Homestyle), 9.5 oz. 280

    with whipped potato *(Lean Cuisine),* 9⅜ oz. 240

    with whipped potato *(Stouffer's* Homestyle), 9⅞ oz. 330

    tomato sauce and *(Freezer Queen* Family), ⅙ of 28-oz. pkg. . 150

    tomato sauce with *(Morton),* 9 oz. 250

    with sauce and vegetables *(Swanson),* 1 pkg. 260

meatballs:

    Italian *(Schwan's),* 6 pieces, 3 oz. 250

    Italian style, and vegetables in wine *(The Budget Gourmet),*

        10 oz. 280

    spaghetti and, *see "spaghetti," below*

    Swedish *(The Budget Gourmet),* 10 oz. 550

    Swedish *(Healthy Choice),* 9.1 oz. 280

    Swedish *(Stouffer's),* 10¼ oz. 480

    Swedish *(Weight Watchers),* 9 oz. 300

    Swedish, with pasta *(Lean Cuisine),* 9⅛ oz. 280

Mexican *(Banquet),* 11 oz. 400

Mexican combination *(Banquet),* 11 oz. 380

noodles:

    and beef *(Banquet* Family), 1 cup, 7 oz. 140

    with beef *(Freezer Queen* Family), 1 cup, 8.5 oz. 200

    and chicken *(Banquet* Bake at Home), 1 cup, 8 oz. 210

    escalloped, and chicken *(Marie Callender's),* 1 cup, 6.5 oz. . 270

    escalloped, and chicken *(Marie Callender's* Multi-Serve),

        1 cup, 5.7 oz. 270

    and turkey, escalloped *(The Budget Gourmet),* 10¾ oz. . . . 430

    kung pao, and vegetables *(Weight Watchers International*

        Selections), 10 oz. 260

    Romanoff *(Stouffer's),* 12 oz. 490

pasta *(see also specific pasta listings):*

    bow ties, and creamy tomato sauce *(Lean Cuisine Lunch*

        Classics), 9.5 oz. 290

    cheddar bake with *(Lean Cuisine),* 9 oz. 260

    cheddar, with beef and tomatoes *(Stouffer's),* 11 oz. 450

    cheddar and broccoli *(Banquet),* 10.5 oz. 350

    primavera *(Schwan's),* 1 cup 220

    primavera, Alfredo *(Lean Cuisine Lunch Classics),* 10 oz. . . 300

    primavera, with chicken *(Marie Callender's),* 1 cup, 6.5 oz. . 310

    rings *(Swanson Fun Feast* Razzlin'), 1 pkg. 380

    sausage and peppers *(Banquet),* 10.5 oz. 340

shells and cheese *(Stouffer's)*, ½ of 12-oz. pkg. 260
and spicy Italian sausage in cream sauce *(The Budget
   Gourmet)*, 10.5 oz. 440
and spinach Romano *(Weight Watchers International
   Selections)*, 10.4 oz. 240
with tomato basil sauce *(Weight Watchers International
   Selections)*, 9.6 oz. 260
vegetable Italiano *(Healthy Choice)*, 10 oz. 240
wheels and cheese *(Swanson Fun Feast)*, 1 pkg. 390
wide ribbon with ricotta *(The Budget Gourmet)*, 10¼ oz. . . . 430
in wine and mushroom sauce with chicken *(The Budget
   Gourmet)*, 10 oz. 290
penne:
   Bolognese *(Lean Cuisine)*, 9.5 oz. 270
   with chunky tomato sauce and sausage *(The Budget
      Gourmet)*, 9 oz. 290
   spicy, and ricotta *(Weight Watchers International
      Selections)*, 10.2 oz. 280
   with sun-dried tomatoes *(Weight Watchers)*, 10 oz. 290
   with tomato sauce *(Healthy Choice)*, 8 oz. 230
   with tomato basil sauce *(Lean Cuisine Lunch Classics)*,
      10 oz. 290
pepper steak, *see "beef," above*
pepper "steak," vegetarian *(Hain)*, 10 oz. 310
perch, ocean, battered *(Van de Kamp's)*, 2 pieces 300
pizza, deluxe *(Marie Callender's)*, 1 cup, 6.5 oz. 350
pork:
   cutlet *(Banquet Country)*, 10¼ oz. 410
   fritter *(Schwan's)*, 1 piece, 4 oz. 250
   patty *(Tyson)*, 3.8-oz. patty 200
   rib, barbecue *(Schwan's)*, 5.7-oz. piece 420
   ribs, barbecue sauce *(Swanson Fun Feast)*, 1 pkg. 450
   rib-shape patty, barbecue *(Swanson)*, 1 pkg. 460
   sweet and sour *(Chun King)*, 13 oz. 450
potatoes mozzarella with chicken *(The Budget Gourmet)*,
   10.13 oz. 390
radiatore, vegetarian *(Hain Bolognese)*, 10 oz. 290
ravioli:
   cheese *(Amy's)*, 9.5 oz. 350
   cheese *(Kid Cuisine Raptor)*, 9.8 oz. 320
   cheese *(Lean Cuisine)*, 8.5 oz. 240
   cheese *(Stouffer's)*, 10⅝ oz. 380

Entrees, Frozen, ravioli *(cont.)*

cheese *(Swanson Fun Feast* Roaring), 1 pkg. 440
cheese, Florentine *(Smart Ones)*, 8.5 oz. 220
cheese, four *(Wolfgang Puck's)*, 13 oz. 330
cheese, in marinara sauce *(Marie Callender's)*, 1 cup, 8 oz. . 370
cheese, parmigiana *(Healthy Choice)*, 9 oz. 260
mushroom and spinach *(Wolfgang Puck's)*, 13 oz. 260

rice:

and beans, Santa Fe *(Weight Watchers International
  Selections)*, 10 oz. 290
four cheese, pasta and chicken *(The Budget Gourmet)*,
  10.5 oz. 330
fried, with chicken *(Chun King)*, 8 oz. 270
fried, with pork *(Chun King)*, 8 oz. 290
Hunan style, and vegetables *(Weight Watchers International
  Selections)*, 10.34 oz. 250
Italian style, and chicken with mozzarella *(The Budget
  Gourmet)*, 10 oz. 270
paella, and vegetables *(Weight Watchers International
  Selections)*, 10.33 oz. 280
Peking style, and vegetables *(Weight Watchers International
  Selections)*, 10.5 oz. 270
pilaf Florentine *(Weight Watchers International Selections)*,
  10.13 oz. 290
risotto with cheese and mushrooms *(Weight Watchers
  International Selections)*, 10 oz. 290
and vegetables, stir fry *(The Budget Gourmet)*, 8.5 oz. 410
wild, pilaf, with vegetables *(The Budget Gourmet)*, 8.5 oz. . . 400

rigatoni:

cream sauce, with broccoli and chicken *(The Budget
  Gourmet)*, 9 oz. 230
creamy, with broccoli and chicken *(Smart Ones)*, 9 oz. 230
with meat sauce *(Freezer Queen* Family), 1 cup, 8.3 oz. . . . 250
parmigiana *(Marie Callender's)*, 1 cup, 7.5 oz. 300
parmigiana *(Marie Callender's* Multi-Serve), 1 cup, 8 oz. . . . 320

shells, pasta, stuffed:

(Celentano), 10 oz. 400
(Celentano 14 oz.), ½ pkg. 300
(Celentano Great Choice), 10 oz. 250
(Celentano Value Pack), 3 shells, 8 oz. 340
broccoli *(Celentano* Great Choice), 10 oz. 190
cheese *(Lean Cuisine* 80 oz.), 8.9 oz. 210

Florentine *(Celentano)*, 10 oz. 240
shrimp:
  beer batter *(Gorton's)*, 6 pieces 250
  breaded *(Gorton's)*, 6 pieces 230
  breaded *(Schwan's)*, approx. 11 pieces, 4 oz. 230
  breaded *(Van de Kamp's)*, 7 pieces, 4 oz. 240
  breaded, butterfly *(Van de Kamp's)*, 7 pieces 280
  breaded, fantail *(Schwan's)*, 4 pieces, 4 oz. 230
  breaded, oven-ready, *(Schwan's)*, 7 pieces, 3 oz. 200
  breaded, with pasta *(Marie Callender's)*, 1 cup, 7.5 oz. . . . 300
  breaded, scampi *(Gorton's)*, 6 pieces 250
  marinara *(Smart Ones)*, 9 oz. 190
  popcorn, breaded *(Gorton's)*, 1 cup, 3.2 oz. 260
  popcorn, breaded *(Van de Kamp's)*, 20 pieces, 4 oz. 270
  popcorn, breaded, garlic and herb *(Gorton's)*, 1¼ cups,
    3.5 oz. 270
sloppy joe *(Swanson Fun Feast)*, 1 pkg. 290
sole *(Mrs. Paul's Premium)*, 1 fillet 170
sole, breaded, lightly *(Van de Kamp's)*, 1 fillet 220
spaghetti:
  Bolognese *(Banquet)*, 10.5 oz. 370
  with chunky tomato and meat sauce *(The Budget
    Gourmet)*, 10 oz. 320
  marinara *(The Budget Gourmet)*, 9 oz. 290
  marinara *(Marie Callender's)*, 1 cup, 8 oz. 270
  marinara *(Weight Watchers)*, 9 oz. 280
  with meat sauce *(Lean Cuisine)*, 11.5 oz. 300
  with meat sauce *(Marie Callender's)*, 1 cup, 6.8 oz. 260
  with meat sauce *(Morton)*, 8.5 oz. 170
  with meat sauce *(Stouffer's)*, 10 oz. 350
  with meat sauce *(Weight Watchers)*, 10 oz. 290
  with meatballs *(Lean Cuisine)*, 9.5 oz. 280
  with meatballs *(Stouffer's)*, 12⅝ oz. 440
  and sauce, with seasoned beef *(Healthy Choice)*, 10 oz. . . . 260
taco:
  beef *(Schwan's Barquito)*, 1 piece, 5 oz. 350
  beef *(Schwan's Taquito)*, 5 pieces, 5 oz. 350
  chicken *(Schwan's Taquito)*, 5 pieces, 5 oz. 360
  mini, with cheese sauce *(Swanson Fun Feast)*, 1 pkg. 380
  three meat *(Schwan's Barquito)*, 5 oz. 390
tamale *(Goya)*, 1 piece 300
tamale pie, Mexican *(Amy's)*, 8 oz. 220

Entrees, Frozen *(cont.)*

teriyaki *(Lean Cuisine Lunch Classics)*, 10 oz. 270
tortellini, spicy chiken *(Wolfgang Puck's)*, 12 oz. 490
tuna noodle casserole:
    (Stouffer's), 10 oz. 320
    (Swanson), 1 pkg. 320
    (Weight Watchers), 9.5 oz. 270
turkey:
    (Lean Cuisine Homestyle)*, 9³/₈ oz. 240
    breast, with gravy *(Schwan's)*, 4 oz. 140
    breast, stuffed *(Weight Watchers)*, 9 oz. 230
    croquettes, breaded, gravy and *(Freezer Queen* Family),
      ¹/₆ of 28-oz. pkg. 130
    glazed *(The Budget Gourmet* Light), 9 oz. 250
    glazed *(Lean Cuisine* Cafe Classics), 9 oz. 250
    and gravy, with dressing *(Banquet* Homestyle), 9¹/₄ oz. 270
    and gravy, with dressing *(Freezer Queen* Deluxe Family),
      ¹/₄ of 28-oz. pkg. 170
    and gravy, with dressing *(Swanson)*, 1 pkg. 230
    and gravy, with dressing and potatoes *(Freezer Queen*
      Homestyle), 9 oz. 210
    gravy and *(Banquet* Family), 2 slices, 4.8 oz. 120
    gravy and *(Banquet* Toppers), 5-oz. bag 90
    gravy and, with dressing *(Morton)*, 9 oz. 230
    medallions, roast, and mushrooms *(Smart Ones)*, 8.5 oz. . 190
    roast, breast, and stuffing *(Lean Cuisine)*, 9³/₄ oz. 290
    roast, with mushrooms *(Healthy Choice* Country), 8.5 oz. . 220
    roast, and stuffing *(Stouffer's* Homestyle), 9⁵/₈ oz. 320
    sliced, and gravy *(Freezer Queen* Family), 4.5 oz. 60
    sliced, gravy and *(Freezer Queen* Cook-In-Pouch),
      5-oz. pkg. 70
    tetrazzini *(Stouffer's)*, 10 oz. 360
    and vegetables *(Healthy Choice* Hearty Handfuls), 6.1 oz. . . . 310
veal parmigiana:
    (Banquet), 9 oz. 320
    (Morton), 8.75 oz. 280
    (Swanson), 1 pkg. 310
    breaded *(Freezer Queen* Deluxe Family), 1 patty 170
    breaded, with tomato sauce *(Freezer Queen* Cook-In-
      Pouch), 5-oz. pkg. 190
    with spaghetti *(Stouffer's* Homestyle), 11⁷/₈ oz. 430
    patties *(Banquet* Family), 1 patty, 4.7 oz. 230

vegetables:
    Chinese style, and chicken *(The Budget Gourmet)*, 9 oz. . . . 260
    country, and beef *(Lean Cuisine)*, 9 oz. 220
    Italian style, and chicken *(The Budget Gourmet)*, 9 oz. . . . 240
    kofta curry *(Deep)*, 5 oz. 245
    pilaf, Indian *(Deep)*, 1 cup 230
    spicy Szechuan style and chicken *(The Budget Gourmet)*,
      10 oz. 330
    spicy Szechuan style and chicken *(Smart Ones)*, 9 oz. 220
Welsh rarebit *(Stouffer's)*, ¼ cup 120
Western style *(Banquet Country)*, 9.5 oz. 350
ziti mozzarella *(Weight Watchers)*, 9 oz. 280
ziti Parmesano *(The Budget Gourmet)*, 9 oz. 350

POTPIES, FROZEN
See also "Dinners, Frozen," and "Entrees, Frozen"

---

                                                    calories

beef:
    (Banquet), 7-oz. pie 330
    (Stouffer's), 10-oz. pie 450
    (Swanson), 1 pie 400
    (Swanson Hungry Man), 1 pie 710
    Yankee *(Marie Callender's)*, 10-oz. pie 690
    Yankee *(Marie Callender's)*, 1 cup, 7.5 oz. 640
broccoli, with cheddar *(Amy's)*, 7.5-oz. pie 430
chicken:
    (Banquet), 7-oz. pie 350
    (Banquet Family Size), 1 cup, 8 oz. 480
    (Empire Kosher), 1 pie 440
    (Lean Cuisine), 9.5-oz. pie 310
    (Marie Callender's), 10-oz. pie 680
    (Marie Callender's), 1 cup, 8.5 oz. 620
    (Stouffer's), 10-oz. pie 560
    (Stouffer's), approx. 1 cup, ½ of 16-oz. pie 540
    (Swanson), 1 pie 410
    (Swanson Deluxe), 1 pie 470
    (Swanson Hungry Man), 1 pie 650
    (Tyson/Tyson All Meat), 8.9-oz. pie 470
    au gratin *(Marie Callender's)*, 10-oz. pie 720
    au gratin *(Marie Callender's)*, 1 cup, 8.5 oz. 740
    and broccoli *(Marie Callender's)*, 10-oz. pie 780

Potpies, Frozen, chicken *(cont.)*
　　and broccoli *(Marie Callender's)*, 1 cup, 8.5 oz. 800
macaroni and cheese, *see "Entrees, Frozen," page 178*
turkey:
　　(Banquet), 7-oz. pie 370
　　(Empire Kosher), 1 pie 470
　　(Lean Cuisine), 9.5-oz. pie 320
　　(Marie Callender's), 10-oz. pie 710
　　(Marie Callender's), 1 cup, 8½ oz. 740
　　(Stouffer's), 10-oz. pie 530
　　(Swanson), 1 pie 440
　　(Swanson Hungry Man), 1 pie 650
　　(Tyson), 8.9-oz. pie 470
vegetable:
　　(Amy's), 7.5-oz. pie 360
　　(Amy's Nondairy), 7.5-oz. pie 320
　　with beef *(Morton)*, 7-oz. pie 310
　　broccoli and cheese *(Tyson)*, 8.9-oz. pie 210
　　with cheese *(Banquet)*, 7-oz. pie 390
　　with chicken *(Morton)*, 7-oz. pie 320
　　with turkey *(Morton)*, 7-oz. pie 300
　　shepherd's pie, nondairy *(Amy's)*, 8-oz. pie 160

ENTREES, REFRIGERATED
See also "Lunch Combinations, Refrigerated," "Meat & Poultry, Frozen or Refrigerated," and "Fish & Seafood, Frozen or Refrigerated"

　　　　　　　　　　　　　　　　　　　　　　　　　　　calories
beef, corned, hash *(Jones Dairy Farm)*, 2 oz. 120
chicken:
　　cutlet, breaded *(Perdue)*, 3.5-oz. piece 230
　　Italian *(Perdue Short Cuts)*, 3 oz. 110
　　lemon pepper *(Perdue Short Cuts)*, 3 oz. 110
　　mesquite *(Perdue Short Cuts)*, 3 oz. 110
　　nuggets, breaded *(Perdue)*, 5 pieces, 3 oz. 200
　　nuggets, breaded, and cheese *(Perdue)*, 5 pieces, 3 oz. . . . 220
　　oven roasted *(Perdue Short Cuts)*, 3 oz. 110
　　oven roasted, dark meat *(Perdue)*, 3 oz. 170
　　oven roasted, white meat *(Perdue)*, 3 oz. 140
　　tenderloins, breaded *(Perdue)*, 3 oz. 160
　　wings, barbecued *(Perdue)*, 3 oz. 200

wings, hot and spicy *(Perdue)*, 3 oz. 190
chicken breast, seasoned, 4 oz.:
    Cajun, garlic and herb or lemon herb *(Chicken By George)* . 120
    Caribbean grill *(Chicken By George)* 150
    Italian bleu cheese *(Chicken By George)* 130
    lemon oregano or teriyaki *(Chicken By George)* 130
    mesquite barbecue *(Chicken By George)* 120
    mustard dill or tomato herb with basil *(Chicken By George)* . 140
    roasted *(Chicken By George)* 110
turkey:
    nuggets, breaded *(Louis Rich)*, 4 pieces, 3.25 oz. 260
    patty, breaded *(Empire* Kosher), 1 piece 200
    patty, breaded *(Louis Rich)*, 1 piece 220
    sticks, breaded *(Louis Rich)*, 3 pieces 230

ENTREE MIXES, FROZEN, as packaged, except as noted
See also "Dinners, Frozen," "Entrees, Frozen," and "Entrees, Mixes"

---

                                                calories

Alfredo, creamy *(Green Giant Create A Meal!)*, 2 cups 210
Alfredo, creamy *(Green Giant Create A Meal!)*, 1¼ cups* 380
beef, Oriental, with vegetables and rice:
    (Schwan's Meal Kit), 1½ cups 180
    (Schwan's Meal Kit), 1 cup* 180
broccoli stir-fry *(Green Giant Create A Meal!)*, 2⅓ cups 120
broccoli stir-fry *(Green Giant Create A Meal!)*, 1⅓ cups* 290
cacciatore *(Birds Eye Easy Recipe Meal Starter)*, 2 cups 180
cacciatore *(Birds Eye Easy Recipe Meal Starter)*, 2 cups* 280
cheddar, creamy *(Green Giant Create A Meal!)*, 1¾ cups 200
cheddar, creamy *(Green Giant Create A Meal!)*, 1½ cups* 290
cheese and herb primavera *(Green Giant Create A Meal!)*,
    1¾ cups 200
cheese and herb primavera *(Green Giant Create A Meal!)*,
    1¼ cups* 330
chicken breast:
    with fried rice and vegetables *(Schwan's* Meal Kit),
        1½ cups 240
    with fried rice and vegetables *(Schwan's* Meal Kit), 1 cup* . . 240

* *Prepared according to package directions*

Entree Mixes, Frozen, chicken breast *(cont.)*

stir-fry, with rice and vegetables *(Schwan's* Meal Kit),
1½ cups 210

stir-fry, with rice and vegetables *(Schwan's* Meal Kit),
1 cup* . . 210

chicken noodle, creamy *(Green Giant Create A Meal!),*
1½ cups 200

chicken noodle, creamy *(Green Giant Create A Meal!),*
1¼ cups* 350

garlic herb *(Green Giant Create A Meal!),* 2⅓ cups 220

garlic herb *(Green Giant Create A Meal!),* 1¼ cups* 340

hot and spicy Asian stir-fry:

(Birds Eye Easy Recipe Meal Starter), 2¼ cups 230

(Birds Eye Easy Recipe Meal Starter), 2¼ cups* 330

lemon herb *(Green Giant Create A Meal!),* 1½ cups 210

lemon herb *(Green Giant Create A Meal!),* 1½ cups* 380

lo mein *(Green Giant Create A Meal!),* 2⅓ cups 170

lo mein *(Green Giant Create A Meal!),* 1¼ cups* 320

mushroom and wine *(Green Giant Create A Meal!),* 1¾ cups . 210

mushroom and wine *(Green Giant Create A Meal!),* 1¼ cups* . 390

Oriental stir-fry *(Birds Eye Easy Recipe Meal Starter),* 2¼ cups . 210

Oriental stir-fry *(Birds Eye Easy Recipe Meal Starter),*
2¼ cups* 300

primavera *(Birds Eye Easy Recipe Meal Starter),* 1¾ cups 180

primavera *(Birds Eye Easy Recipe Meal Starter),* 1¾ cups* . . . 250

sweet and sour stir-fry *(Green Giant Create A Meal!),* 1¾ cups . 130

sweet and sour stir-fry *(Green Giant Create A Meal!),*
1¼ cups* 290

Szechuan stir-fry *(Green Giant Create A Meal!),* 1¾ cups 170

Szechuan stir-fry *(Green Giant Create A Meal!),* 1¼ cups* 340

teriyaki *(Green Giant Create A Meal!),* 1¾ cups 90

teriyaki *(Green Giant Create A Meal!),* 1¼ cups* 240

vegetable almond stir-fry *(Green Giant Create A Meal!),*
1¾ cups 160

vegetable almond stir-fry *(Green Giant Create A Meal!),*
1⅓ cups* 320

vegetable stew, hearty *(Green Giant Create A Meal!),* 1¼ cups . 130

vegetable stew, hearty *(Green Giant Create A Meal!),*
1¼ cups* 280

* *Prepared according to package directions*

ENTREES, MIXES
See also "Entree Mixes, Frozen," "Pasta & Noodle Dishes, Mixes," and "Rice Dishes, Mixes"

	calories
au gratin *(Tuna Helper)*, ½ cup mix	190
au gratin *(Tuna Helper)*, 1 cup*	310
beef:	
pasta *(Hamburger Helper)*, ⅔ cup mix	120
pasta *(Hamburger Helper)*, 1 cup*	250
Romanoff *(Hamburger Helper)*, ⅔ cup mix	150
Romanoff *(Hamburger Helper)*, 1 cup*	290
stew *(Hamburger Helper Homestyle)*, ½ cup mix	110
stew *(Hamburger Helper Homestyle)*, 1 cup*	250
Stroganoff *(Dinner Sensations)*, 1 cup mix	160
Stroganoff *(Dinner Sensations)*, 1 cup*	320
taco *(Hamburger Helper)*, ½ cup mix	160
taco *(Hamburger Helper)*, 1 cup*	310
teriyaki *(Dinner Sensations)*, ½ cup mix	170
teriyaki *(Dinner Sensations)*, 1 cup*	320
teriyaki *(Hamburger Helper)*, ¼ cup mix	150
teriyaki *(Hamburger Helper)*, 1 cup*	290
broccoli, creamy *(Tuna Helper)*, ⅔ cup mix	190
broccoli, creamy *(Tuna Helper)*, 1 cup*	310
burrito *(Old El Paso)*, 1 piece*	280
cheddar:	
and bacon *(Hamburger Helper)*, ⅔ cup mix	170
and bacon *(Hamburger Helper)*, 1 cup*	350
garden *(Tuna Helper)*, ⅔ cup mix	190
garden *(Tuna Helper)*, 1 cup*	310
melt *(Hamburger Helper)*, ¾ cup mix	150
melt *(Hamburger Helper)*, 1 cup*	310
cheese, three *(Hamburger Helper)*, ½ cup mix	180
cheese, three *(Hamburger Helper)*, 1 cup*	340
chicken:	
Alfredo *(Dinner Sensations)*, 1 cup mix	210
Alfredo *(Dinner Sensations)*, 1 cup*	310
Alfredo, low-fat recipe *(Dinner Sensations)*, 1 cup*	300
stir-fry *(Skillet Chicken Helper)*, ¼ cup mix	140
stir-fry *(Skillet Chicken Helper)*, 1 cup*	270

* Prepared according to package directions

Entrees, Mixes, chicken *(cont.)*
    sweet and sour *(Dinner Sensations)*, ⅔ cup mix 240
    sweet and sour *(Dinner Sensations)*, 1 cup* 330
cheeseburger macaroni *(Hamburger Helper)*, ⅓ cup mix 180
cheeseburger macaroni *(Hamburger Helper)*, 1 cup* 360
chili:
    (Hamburger Mate), ⅕ pkg. mix 160
    all varieties *(Health Valley Chili in a Cup)*, ⅓ cup mix 120
    3 bean *(Spice Islands Quick Meal)*, 1 pkg. mix 180
    4 bean *(Knorr Cup)*, 1 pkg. mix 230
    macaroni *(Hamburger Helper)*, ⅓ cup mix 140
    macaroni *(Hamburger Helper)*, 1 cup* 290
    vegetarian *(Spice Islands Quick Meal)*, 1 pkg. mix 180
fajita *(Old El Paso)*, 2 pieces* 330
fettuccine Alfredo:
    (Hamburger Helper), ½ cup mix 140
    (Hamburger Helper), 1 cup* 300
    (Tuna Helper), ¾ cup mix 170
    (Tuna Helper), 1 cup* 310
hamburger:
    with cheese *(Hamburger Mate)*, ⅕ pkg. mix 160
    with noodles *(Hamburger Mate)*, ⅕ pkg. mix 150
    with pasta and tomato sauce *(Hamburger Mate)*, ⅕ pkg.
       mix 160
Italian:
    cheesy *(Hamburger Helper)*, ½ cup mix 150
    cheesy *(Hamburger Helper)*, 1 cup 330
    rigatoni *(Hamburger Helper Homestyle)*, ⅓ cup mix 140
    rigatoni *(Hamburger Helper Homestyle)*, 1 cup* 180
    zesty *(Hamburger Helper)*, ⅓ cup mix 160
    zesty *(Hamburger Helper)*, 1 cup* 320
lasagna:
    (Hamburger Helper), ⅔ cup mix 140
    (Hamburger Helper), 1 cup* 280
    (Master-A-Meal), ⅕ pkg. mix 150
macaroni and cheese, *see "Pasta & Noodle Dishes, Mixes,"*
    page 223
meat loaf *(Hamburger Helper)*, 1½ tbsp. mix 50
meat loaf *(Hamburger Helper)*, ⅙ loaf* 280
Mexican, zesty *(Hamburger Helper)*, ⅔ cup mix 160

* *Prepared according to package directions*

Mexican, zesty *(Hamburger Helper)*, 1 cup* 300
mushroom and wild rice *(Hamburger Helper)*, ¼ cup mix 150
mushroom and wild rice *(Hamburger Helper)*, 1 cup* 310
nacho cheese *(Hamburger Helper)*, ½ cup mix 160
nacho cheese *(Hamburger Helper)*, 1 cup* 320
pasta:
   cheesy *(Tuna Helper)*, ¾ cup mix 170
   cheesy *(Tuna Helper)*, 1 cup* 280
   creamy *(Tuna Helper)*, ¾ cup mix 190
   creamy *(Tuna Helper)*, 1 cup* 300
   salad *(Tuna Helper)*, ⅓ cup mix 120
   salad *(Tuna Helper)*, ⅔ cup* 380
   salad, low-fat recipe *(Tuna Helper)*, ⅔ cup* 230
pizza:
   (Hamburger Helper Pizzabake), ⅓ cup mix 140
   (Hamburger Helper Pizzabake), ⅙ pan* 270
   pasta *(Hamburger Helper)*, ½ cup mix 150
   pasta *(Hamburger Helper)*, 1 cup* 290
potpie *(Tuna Helper)*, ½ cup mix 340
potpie *(Tuna Helper)*, 1 cup* 440
potato:
   au gratin *(Hamburger Helper)*, ⅔ cup mix 120
   au gratin *(Hamburger Helper)*, 1 cup* 290
   Stroganoff *(Hamburger Helper)*, ⅔ cup mix 120
   Stroganoff *(Hamburger Helper)*, 1 cup* 270
rice, Oriental *(Hamburger Helper)*, ¼ cup mix 160
rice, Oriental *(Hamburger Helper)*, 1 cup 310
Romanoff *(Tuna Helper)*, ⅔ cup mix 210
Romanoff *(Tuna Helper)*, 1 cup* 280
Salisbury *(Hamburger Helper Homestyle)*, ¾ cup mix 130
Salisbury *(Hamburger Helper Homestyle)*, 1 cup* 270
shells, cheesy *(Hamburger Helper)*, ½ cup mix 180
shells, cheesy *(Hamburger Helper)*, 1 cup* 340
shrimp, Creole *(Luzianne)*, ⅕ pkg. mix 150
spaghetti *(Hamburger Helper)*, ½ cup mix 150
spaghetti *(Hamburger Helper)*, 1 cup* 300
stew *(Hamburger Helper)*, ⅔ cup mix 100
stew *(Hamburger Helper)*, 1 cup* 250
Stroganoff:
   (Hamburger Helper), ⅔ cup mix 170

---

* *Prepared according to package directions*

Entrees, Mixes, Stroganoff *(cont.)*

(Hamburger Helper), 1 cup* 350

vegetarian *(Natural Touch)*, 4 tbsp. mix 90

Swedish meatball *(Hamburger Helper Homestyle)*, ⅔ cup mix . 160

Swedish meatball *(Hamburger Helper Homestyle)*, 1 cup* 300

sweet and sour *(La Choy)*, ¼ pkg. mix 90

taco:

    (Lawry's), ⅕ pkg. mix 150

    (Old El Paso), 2 tacos* 270

    (Pancho Villa), 2 tacos* 270

    with rice *(Old El Paso One Skillet Mexican)*, 2 pieces* 440

    with rice, cheese flavor *(Old El Paso One Skillet*

       Mexican), 2 pieces* 490

    with rice, salsa flavor *(Old El Paso One Skillet Mexican)*,

       2 pieces* 460

    soft *(Old El Paso)*, 2 pieces* 380

tetrazzini *(Tuna Helper)*, ⅔ cup mix 180

tetrazzini *(Tuna Helper)*, 1 cup* 310

tofu:

    burger *(Fantastic* Classics), ⅛ cup mix 70

    chow mein, Mandarin *(Fantastic* Classics), ⅝ cup 170

    shells 'n curry *(Fantastic* Classics), ½ cup mix 200

    Stroganoff, creamy *(Fantastic* Classics), ½ cup mix 190

vegetable stew *(Knorr)*, 1 pkg. mix 160

LUNCH COMBINATIONS, REFRIGERATED, one package
See also "Entrees, Refrigerated"

---

	calories
bologna/American *(Lunchables)*	470
bologna/wild cherry *(Lunchables)*	530
chicken/turkey deluxe *(Lunchables)*	390
ham/cheddar *(Lunchables)*	360
ham/Swiss *(Lunchables)*	340
ham/fruit punch *(Lunchables)*	440
ham/fruit punch, low-fat *(Lunchables)*	350
ham/*Surfer Cooler* *(Lunchables)*	390
pizza, mozzarella/fruit punch *(Lunchables)*	450

pizza/pepperoni:

    mozzarella *(Lunchables)* 330

---

* *Prepared according to package directions*

orange *(Lunchables)* 450
pizza, two cheese *(Lunchables)* 300
salami/American *(Lunchables)* 430
turkey/cheddar *(Lunchables)* 350
turkey/ham *(Lunchables)* 370
turkey/Monterey Jack *(Lunchables)* 350
turkey/*Pacific Cooler (Lunchables)* 450
turkey/*Pacific Cooler,* low-fat *(Lunchables)* 360
turkey/*Surfer Cooler (Lunchables)* 430

Chapter 11

MEAT, FISH, AND POULTRY

MEAT & POULTRY, CANNED OR IN JARS
See also "Appetizers & Snacks, Canned or in Jars," "Entrees,
Canned or Packaged," "Meat, Fish, & Poultry Spreads," and
"Luncheon Meat & Poultry"

---

calories

beef:

corned *(Goya)*, 2 oz.	120
corned *(Libby's)*, 2 oz.	120
corned *(Hormel)*, 2 oz.	120
cubed *(Hormel)*, ½ cup	130

chicken, chunk, 2 oz. or ¼ cup, except as noted:

(Hormel)	70
breast *(Hormel/Hormel No Salt)*	60
in broth *(Swanson Mixin')*	110
in water *(Swanson Premium)*	70
in water *(Swanson Premium)*, 3 oz.	100
white *(Swanson)*, 3 oz.	80
white, in water *(Swanson Premium)*	60

ham, refrigerated or canned, 3 oz., except as noted:

(Black Label Refrigerated)	100
(Black Label Shelf)	110
(Curemaster Half)	80
(Hormel Light & Lean)	90
(John Morrell Boneless)	140
(Jones Dairy Farm Country Club)	100
(Jones Dairy Farm Homestead)	140
(Jones Dairy Farm Old Fashioned)	220
(Jones Dairy Farm Country Carved Family/Dainty)	100
(Schwan's Haugin's Farm), 2 oz.	60
(Swift Premium Water Added)	100
baked *(Louis Rich Dinner)*, 3.3-oz. slice	80
Black Forest *(Boar's Head Baby)*	90
chunk *(Hormel)*, 2 oz.	90
fully cooked *(Jones Dairy Farm)*	240

honey *(Jones Dairy Farm Country Carved* Family) 100
honey *(Patrick Cudahy ReaLean)* 90
maple *(Boar's Head Baby Honey Coat)* 90
maple *(Jones Dairy Farm Country Carved* Family) 100
semi-boneless *(Jones Dairy Farm)* 180
skinless, shankless *(Jones Dairy Farm)* 160
slice *(Oscar Mayer)* 80
slice, smoked or maple glaze *(Boar's Head Sweet Slice)* . . . 110
smoke flavor *(Patrick Cudahy ReaLean)* 80
smoked, semi-boneless *(Boar's Head)* 130
spiral, sliced *(Jones Dairy Farm)* 180
spiral, sliced *(Spiral Cure 81* Half) 150
steak *(Jones Dairy Farm Lean Choice/Rock River)* 100
steak *(Oscar Mayer),* 2 oz. 60
steak, honey *(Patrick Cudahy)* 100
steak, smoke flavor *(Patrick Cudahy)* 90
Virginia *(Boar's Head* Ready-to-Eat) 100
Virginia, smoked *(Boar's Head* Baby Gourmet) 90
meat, potted, *see "Meat, Fish, & Poultry Spreads," page 211*
(Spam/Spam Less Salt), 2 oz. 170
(Spam Lite), 2 oz. 110
turkey, chunk, 2 oz., ¼ cup:
   (Hormel) 70
   (Swanson Premium) 100
   white *(Hormel)* 60
   white *(Swanson* Premium) 90

MEAT & POULTRY, FROZEN OR REFRIGERATED
*See also "Dinners, Frozen," "Entrees, Frozen," "Entrees,
Refrigerated," and "Luncheon Meat & Poultry"*

calories

beef:
   ribeye, salted *(Hebrew National),* 4 oz. 400
   sirloin tips *(Schwan's),* 4 oz. 150
   steak *(Schwan's Big Sam),* 6 oz. 210
   steak, chopped *(Schwan's),* 5.3 oz. 390
   steak, cubed, breaded *(Schwan's),* 4 oz. 290
   steak, sirloin ball tip *(Schwan's),* 6 oz. 250
   steak, sirloin fillet *(Schwan's),* 4 oz. 150
   steak, sirloin, top *(Schwan's),* 9.3 oz. 640
   steak, sirloin, tri tip *(Schwan's),* 5 oz. 240

Meat & Poultry, Frozen or Refrigerated *(cont.)*
beef, ground:
    80% lean *(Schwan's)*, 4-oz. patty 290
    90% lean *(Schwan's)*, 3.75-oz. patty 180
    melt *(Schwan's)*, 4-oz. patty 340
    pizza *(Schwan's)*, 3.3-oz. patty 300
chicken:
    whole, barbecued *(Empire* Kosher), 5 oz. edible 280
    whole, cooked, dark meat *(Perdue)*, 3 oz. 210
    whole, cooked, dark meat *(Perdue Oven Stuffer)*, 3 oz. 200
    whole, cooked, white meat *(Perdue/Perdue Oven Stuffer)*,
      3 oz. 160
    half, roasted, skinless *(Tyson)*, 3 oz. 140
    cutlet, battered, breaded *(Empire* Kosher), 3.3-oz. piece . . . 200
    diced, *(Tyson)*, 3 oz. 130
    diced, cooked *(Schwan's)*, 3 oz. 130
    frying parts, raw *(Tyson)*, 4 oz. 250
    gizzards, raw *(Tyson)*, 4 oz. 90
    ground, raw *(Perdue/Perdue* Burger), 4 oz. 180
    ground, cooked *(Perdue/Perdue* Burger), 3 oz. 170
    necks, raw *(Tyson)*, 4 oz. 330
chicken breast, raw, 4 oz.:
    halves *(Tyson)* 190
    halves, skinless *(Tyson)* 140
    quarters *(Tyson)* 210
chicken breast, raw, boneless, 4 oz., except as noted:
    (Perdue/Perdue Oven Stuffer/Perdue Family Pack) 130
    (Tyson) 110
    fillet *(Schwan's)* 110
    fillet, breaded *(Schwan's)*, 5-oz. piece 260
    tenderloins *(Perdue)* 110
    tenderloins *(Tyson)* 110
    thin sliced *(Perdue)*, 3 oz. .80
    seasoned, barbecue *(Perdue)* 130
    seasoned, lemon pepper *(Schwan's)*, 4.5-oz. piece 180
    seasoned, lemon pepper or Italian *(Perdue)* 110
    seasoned, Oriental *(Perdue)* 120
    seasoned, teriyaki *(Schwan's)* 120
chicken breast, cooked, 3 oz., except as noted:
    whole *(Perdue)* 160
    whole *(Perdue Oven Stuffer)* 150
    boneless *(Perdue/Perdue Oven Stuffer)* 120

quartered *(Perdue)* 180
roundelet *(Tyson)*, 2.6-oz. piece 170
tenderloins *(Perdue)* 100
thin sliced *(Perdue)*, 2 oz. 80
fried, battered & breaded *(Empire* Kosher), 3 oz. edible 170
roasted *(Perdue)*, 6.7-oz. half 370
roasted *(Tyson)*, ½ breast 250
roasted, boneless *(Perdue)*, 3.6-oz. half 140
roasted, boneless *(Perdue Fit 'n Easy)*, 3.6-oz. half 150
roasted, skinless *(Perdue)*, 5.9-oz. half 250
seasoned, boneless, barbecue *(Perdue)* 110
seasoned, boneless, lemon pepper *(Perdue)* 90
seasoned, boneless, Italian or Oriental *(Perdue)* 100
seasoned, strips, fajita *(Schwan's)* 110
chicken leg:
   whole, roasted *(Perdue)*, 5.5 oz. 370
   whole, roasted *(Perdue Jumbo Family/Value)*, 5.5 oz. 360
   drum and thigh, fried *(Empire* Kosher), 3 oz. edible 240
   drumstick, roasted *(Perdue)*, 2.2-oz. piece 110
   drumstick, roasted *(Perdue Oven Stuffer)*, 3.6-oz. piece . . . 190
   drumstick, roasted *(Tyson)*, 3 pieces 330
   drumstick, roasted, skinless *(Perdue Pick)*, 2 pieces,
      3.5 oz. 150
   drumsticks, thighs, and wings, raw *(Tyson* Multipak), 4 oz. . 230
   quarters, raw *(Tyson)*, 4 oz. 290
   quarters, cooked *(Perdue)*, 3 oz. 210
   thigh, raw *(Tyson)*, 4 oz. 250
   thigh, raw, boneless, skinless *(Tyson/Tyson* Jumbo), 4 oz. . 160
   thigh, roasted, *(Perdue)*, 3.2-oz. piece 240
   thigh, roasted, boneless *(Perdue)*, 2 thighs, 3.6 oz. 200
   thigh, roasted, boneless *(Perdue Fit 'n Easy)*, 2 pieces 190
   thigh, roasted, boneless *(Perdue Oven Stuffer)*, 3.3 oz. 170
   thigh, roasted, skinless *(Perdue)*, 2.7 oz. 160
   thigh, roasted, skinless *(Tyson)*, 3.6-oz. piece 270
chicken liver, raw *(Tyson)*, 4 oz. 140
chicken wing:
   raw, whole *(Tyson)*, 4 oz. 250
   roasted *(Perdue)*, 2 pieces 210
   roasted *(Perdue* Wingettes), 3 pieces 200
   roasted *(Perdue Oven Stuffer* Drummettes), 2 pieces 170
   roasted *(Perdue Oven Stuffer* Wingettes), 3 pieces 220
chicken nuggets *(Empire* Kosher), 5 pieces, 3 oz. 180

Meat & Poultry, Frozen or Refrigerated *(cont.)*

chicken sticks *(Empire* Kosher Stix), 4 pieces, 3.1 oz. 180
Cornish hen:
   cooked, dark meat *(Perdue)*, 3 oz. 200
   cooked, white meat *(Perdue)*, 3 oz. 170
   roasted, half, dark meat *(Perdue)*, 6.5 oz. 210
   roasted, half, white meat *(Perdue)*, 6.5 oz. 200
ham, refrigerated, *see "Meat & Poultry, Canned or in Jars,"*
   page 194
ham patty *(Hormel)*, 2-oz. patty 180
ham patty, and cheese *(Hormel)*, 2-oz. patty 190
pork, raw:
   chop, center cut *(Schwan's)*, 5.3-oz. chop 270
   loin, center *(John Morrell Table Trim)*, 4 oz. 190
   smoked shoulder butt *(Oscar Mayer Sweet Morsel)*, 3 oz. . 180
   tenderloin *(John Morrell Table Trim)*, 4 oz. 120
pork, cooked:
   shredded, barbecued *(Lloyd's)*, ¼ cup 90
   spareribs *(Lloyd's)*, 3 ribs with sauce 380
   spareribs, baby back *(Lloyd's)*, 3 ribs with sauce 330
turkey, 4 oz., except as noted:
   whole, raw, young *(Norbest* Family Tradition, 8–16 lb.) 190
   whole, raw, young *(Norbest* Family Tradition, 16–24 lb.) . . . 170
   whole, raw, young, basted *(Norbest,* 8–16 lb.) 180
   whole, raw, young, basted *(Norbest,* 16–24 lb.) 165
   whole, cooked, dark meat *(Perdue)*, 3 oz. 200
   whole, cooked, white meat *(Perdue)*, 3 oz. 170
   whole, barbecued *(Empire* Kosher), 5 oz. 250
   ground, *see "turkey, ground" below*
   breast, *see "turkey breast" below*
   maple glaze *(Boar's Head Honey Coat)*, 3 oz. 100
   roast, boneless *(Norbest)* 135
   smoked, hickory *(Norbest* Young), 3 oz. 145
   steak, cubed, raw *(Perdue)* 110
   thigh, cooked *(Perdue)*, 3 oz. 180
   wing, cooked *(Perdue* Tom), 3 oz. 160
   wing portion, cooked *(Perdue)*, 3 oz. 170
   wing, roasted *(Perdue)*, 3-oz. wing 180
   wing, roasted *(Perdue* Drummettes), 3½-oz. piece 180
turkey breast, raw, 4 oz., except as noted:
   basted *(Norbest)* 170
   boneless *(Perdue)* 130

cutlets, thin sliced *(Perdue)*, 3½ oz. 100
fillet, boneless and skinless *(Schwan's)*, 3 oz. 70
fillets or tenderloins *(Perdue)* 120
roast, boneless *(Norbest)* 135
turkey breast, cooked:
    (Perdue Whole/Half), 3 oz. 170
    boneless, fillets or tenderloins *(Perdue)*, 3 oz. 110
    cutlets, thin sliced *(Perdue)*, 2.5 oz. 90
    oven roasted *(Hebrew National)*, 2 oz. 60
    oven roasted, skinless *(Hebrew National)*, 2 oz. 50
turkey breast, smoked:
    (Hebrew National), 2 oz. 60
    (Hormel Light & Lean 97), 3 oz. 80
    (Perdue), 3 oz. 150
turkey, ground, 4 oz., except as noted:
    raw *(Louis Rich)* 190
    raw *(Norbest)* 170
    raw *(Perdue)* 160
    raw *(Shady Brook Farms)* 170
    raw, breast *(Perdue)* 120
    raw, breast *(Shady Brook Farms)* 120
    raw, patty, white *(Louis Rich)* 150
    cooked, breast *(Perdue)*, 3 oz. 110
    cooked, regular or burger *(Perdue)*, 3 oz. 170
turkey nuggets, breaded *(Louis Rich)*, 4 pieces 260
turkey patty, breaded *(Louis Rich)*, 3-oz. piece 220
turkey sticks, breaded *(Louis Rich)*, 3 pieces 230

FRANKFURTERS, one link, except as noted
See also "Sausages"

                                     calories

(Boar's Head) 150
(Hormel 10), 1.6-oz. link 140
(Hormel 8), 2-oz. link 180
(Hormel Big 8), 2-oz. link 180
(Hormel Light & Lean 97), 1.6-oz. link 45
(Hormel Light & Lean 97 Jumbo), 2-oz. link 60
(John Morrell Fat Free), 1.4-oz. link 45
(John Morrell Lite) 90
(Louis Rich Wieners) 70
(Oscar Mayer Wieners) 150

Frankfurters *(cont.)*
(Oscar Mayer Wieners Light) 110
(Oscar Mayer Wieners, Little), 6 links, 2 oz. 180
(Oscar Mayer Wieners, Little Hot & Spicy), 6 links, 2 oz. 170
(Oscar Mayer Big & Juicy Wieners) 240
(Oscar Mayer Bun-Length Wieners) 190
(Schwan's Old Fashioned Wieners) 170
(Schwan's Skinless) 140
beef:
    (Boar's Head Giant) 160
    (Boar's Head Lite) 90
    (Boar's Head Skinless) 120
    (Hebrew National), 1.7-oz. link 150
    (Hebrew National 8 oz.) 140
    (Hebrew National Bulk), 2.7-oz. link 240
    (Hebrew National Family Pack), 2-oz. link 180
    (Hebrew National Picnic Pack), 1.6-oz. link 140
    (Hebrew National Quarter Pound/Jumbo) 350
    (Hebrew National Reduced Fat), 1.7-oz. link 120
    (Hebrew National Reduced Fat 3 lb.), 2.7-oz. link 180
    (Hormel 8) 170
    (Hormel Light & Lean 97) 45
    (Louis Rich) 70
    (Oscar Mayer) 140
    (Oscar Mayer Fat Free) .35
    (Oscar Mayer Light) 110
    (Oscar Mayer Big & Juicy), 2.7-oz. link 240
    (Oscar Mayer Big & Juicy ¼ lb.) 350
    (Oscar Mayer Big & Juicy Deli), 2.7-oz. link 230
    (Oscar Mayer Bun-Length) 190
    (Wranglers) 170
cheese *(Oscar Mayer)* 140
cheese *(Wranglers)* 170
chicken *(Empire* Kosher), 2-oz. link 100
cocktail:
    (Hormel), 5 links 160
    beef *(Boar's Head),* 5 links 170
    beef *(Hebrew National),* 4 links 180
    beef *(Hebrew National* 32 oz.), 6 links 160
    smoked *(Hormel* Smokies), 5 links 180
hot and spicy *(Oscar Mayer Big & Juicy)* 220
smoked *(Oscar Mayer Big & Juicy* Smokie) 220

smoked *(Wranglers)* 170
turkey:
    (Empire Kosher) 90
    and beef *(Oscar Mayer Fat Free)* 40
    and chicken *(Louis Rich* 8 links, 12 oz.), 1.5-oz. link 80
    and chicken *(Louis Rich* 10 links, 16 oz.), 1.6-oz. link 90
    and chicken *(Louis Rich Bun-Length)* 110
    and chicken, cheese *(Louis Rich)* 90

LUNCHEON MEAT & POULTRY, two ounces, except as noted
*See also "Meat & Poultry, Canned or in Jars," "Meat &
Poultry, Frozen or Refrigerated," "Sausages," and "Meat, Fish,
& Poultry Spreads"*

---

                                                calories

abruzzese *(Boar's Head Cinghiale),* 1 oz. 100
beef:
    corned *(Hebrew National)* 80
    corned, brisket *(Boar's Head)* 80
    corned, round *(Healthy Deli)* 80
    corned, round *(Hebrew National)* 60
    cut *(Boar's Head* Deluxe Low Sodium) 90
    dried, sliced *(Hormel),* 1 oz. 50
    dried, sliced *(Hormel 2.5-oz. pkg.),* 1 oz. 45
    roast *(Hormel)* 60
    roast *(Hormel* Chuck) 110
    roast *(Hormel* Top Round) 50
    roast *(Hormel Light & Lean 97)* 60
    roast *(Oscar Mayer Deli-Thin),* 4 slices, 1.8 oz. 60
    roast, Cajun *(Boar's Head)* 80
    roast, Italian or seasoned *(Healthy Deli)* 70
    roast, top round *(Boar's Head* No Salt) 90
    round *(Boar's Head* No Salt) 90
    round, eye, pepper seasoned *(Boar's Head)* 90
    round, top *(Boar's Head* Low Sodium) 90
bologna:
    (Boar's Head) 150
    (Boar's Head 28% Lower Sodium) 150
    (Healthy Deli Regular/German 95% Fat Free) 70
    (John Morrell) 180
    (Oscar Mayer), 1-oz. slice 90
    (Oscar Mayer Fat Free), 1-oz. slice 20

Luncheon Meat & Poultry, bologna *(cont.)*
  (Oscar Mayer Light), 1-oz. slice 60
  (Oscar Mayer Wisconsin Ring) 180
  beef *(Boar's Head)* 150
  beef *(Hebrew National)* 180
  beef *(Hebrew National* Lean) 90
  beef *(Hebrew National* Reduced Fat) 130
  beef *(Oscar Mayer)*, 1-oz. slice 90
  beef *(Oscar Mayer* Light), 1-oz. slice 60
  garlic *(Boar's Head)* 150
  garlic *(Oscar Mayer)*, 1.5-oz. slice 130
  ham *(Boar's Head)* 80
braunschweiger:
  (Jones Dairy Farm Chub) 150
  (Jones Dairy Farm Chunk) 180
  (Oscar Mayer), 1-oz. slice 100
  with bacon or onion *(Jones Dairy Farm* Chub) 150
  light *(Boar's Head)* 120
  light *(Jones Dairy Farm* Chub/Chunk) 100
  sliced *(Jones Dairy Farm)*, 1.2-oz. slice 110
  sliced *(Jones Dairy Farm)*, 2 slices, 1.6 oz. 150
  tube *(Oscar Mayer)* 190
capocolla, *see "ham," below*
chicken:
  breast, all varieties *(Tyson)*, 2 slices, 1.5 oz. 35
  breast, baked, grilled or honey glazed *(Louis Rich Carving*
    Board), 2 slices, 1.6 oz. 45
  breast, honey glazed *(Oscar Mayer Deli-Thin)*, 4 slices,
    1.8 oz. 60
  breast, oven roasted *(Boar's Head* Golden) 50
  breast, oven roasted *(Hebrew National)* 45
  breast, oven roasted *(Hebrew National)*, 5 slices, 1.8 oz. 45
  breast, oven roasted *(Louis Rich* Deluxe), 1-oz. slice 30
  breast, oven roasted *(Louis Rich Deli-Thin)*, 4 slices,
    1.8 oz. 50
  breast, oven roasted *(Oscar Mayer* Fat Free), 4 slices,
    1.8 oz. 45
  breast, smoked *(Boar's Head* Hickory) 60
  white, sliced, oven roasted *(Louis Rich)*, 1-oz. slice 40
  white meat roll *(Tyson)*, 2 slices, 1.3 oz. 60
ham *(see also "prosciutto, below")*:
  (Boar's Head Deluxe) 60

(Boar's Head Lower Sodium Extra Lean) 50
(Healthy Deli Cinnamon Apple Grove) 70
(Healthy Deli Deluxe/Less Sodium/Old Tyme Taverne) 60
(Hormel Light & Lean 97), 1 oz. 25
(Hormel Light & Lean 97 Deli) 50
(Jones Dairy Farm Lean Choice), 2 slices, 2 oz. 50
(Menumaster) 30
(Old Tyme) 35
(Oscar Mayer Lower Sodium), 3 slices, 2.2 oz. 70
baked *(Louis Rich Carving Board),* 2 slices, 1.6 oz. 50
baked *(Oscar Mayer),* 3 slices, 2.2 oz. 70
baked *(Oscar Mayer* Fat Free), 3 slices, 1.7 oz. 35
baked, Virginia *(Healthy Deli)* 60
baked, Virginia *(Healthy Deli* Less Sodium) 70
Black Forest *(Boar's Head)* .60
Black Forest *(Healthy Deli)* .60
boiled *(Oscar Mayer),* 3 slices, 2.2 oz. 60
boiled *(Oscar Mayer Deli-Thin),* 4 slices, 1.8 oz. 50
boiled *(Patrick Cudahy),* 1 oz. 30
capocolla *(Boar's Head* Cappy) 60
capocolla *(Healthy Deli* Cappi) 60
chopped *(Black Label)* 140
chopped *(Oscar Mayer),* 1-oz. slice 50
cooked *(Alpine Lace)* 60
cooked *(Hormel* Deli/Low Salt) 60
cooked *(Patrick Cudahy* Less Sodium), 1 oz. 30
honey *(Healthy Deli* Honey Valley Farms) 60
honey *(Louis Rich Carving Board* Thin), 6 slices, 2.1 oz. 70
honey *(Louis Rich Carving Board* Traditional), 2 slices,
    1.6 oz. 50
honey *(Oscar Mayer),* 3 slices, 2.2 oz. 70
honey *(Oscar Mayer Deli-Thin),* 4 slices, 1.8 oz. 60
honey *(Oscar Mayer* Fat Free), 3 slices, 1.7 oz. 35
honey *(Patrick Cudahy),* 1 oz. 35
honey or smoked *(Louis Rich* Fat Free), 2 slices, 1.7 oz. 35
hot *(Healthy Deli* Rodeo) 60
jalapeño *(Healthy Deli)* 60
maple *(Boar's Head* Honey Coat) 60
maple *(Healthy Deli* Vermont) 60
maple *(Patrick Cudahy),* 1 oz. 35
pepper *(Boar's Head)* 70
pepper *(Healthy Deli)* 60

Luncheon Meat & Poultry, ham *(cont.)*

smoked *(Boar's Head Gourmet)* 60
smoked *(Hormel Light & Lean 97 Deli)* 50
smoked *(Louis Rich Carving Board)*, 2 slices, 1.6 oz. 45
smoked *(Oscar Mayer)*, 3 slices, 2.2 oz. 60
smoked *(Oscar Mayer Deli-Thin)*, 4 slices, 1.8 oz. 50
smoked, double *(Healthy Deli)* 60
spiced *(Boar's Head)* 120
Virginia *(Boar's Head)* 60
Virginia *(Healthy Deli)* 60
ham and cheese loaf *(Oscar Mayer)*, 1-oz. slice 70
head cheese *(Oscar Mayer)*, 1-oz. slice 50
honey loaf *(Oscar Mayer)*, 1-oz. slice 35
liver cheese *(Oscar Mayer)*, 1.3-oz. slice 120
liverwurst, 2 oz. or ¼ cup:
    (Boar's Head Strassburger/Smoked) 170
    (Spam) 100
    (Underwood) 160
mortadella *(Boar's Head Cinghiale)* 160
mortadella, with pistachios *(Boar's Head Cinghiale)* 170
old-fashioned loaf *(Oscar Mayer)*, 1-oz. slice 70
olive loaf *(Boar's Head)* 130
olive loaf *(Oscar Mayer)*, 1-oz. slice 70
pastrami:
    (Healthy Deli) .80
    (Hebrew National) 80
    brisket or Romanian *(Boar's Head)* 90
    round *(Boar's Head)* 70
    round *(Hebrew National)* 70
pepperoni:
    (Boar's Head), 1 oz. 140
    (Hormel/Leoni/Rosa Grande), 1 oz. 140
    (Oscar Mayer), 15 slices, 1.1 oz. 140
    (Patrick Cudahy 3 oz.), 16 slices, 1.1 oz. 150
    (Patrick Cudahy 6 oz.), 15 slices, 1.1 oz. 170
    (Patrick Cudahy Stick), 1 oz. 150
pickle and pepper loaf *(Boar's Head)* 150
pickle and pimiento loaf *(Oscar Mayer)*, 1-oz. slice 80
pork *(Hormel Deli Pork Roast)* 70
pork, seasoned *(Boar's Head)* 80
prosciutto *(Primissimo)* 210

salami:
    beef *(Boar's Head* Chub) 120
    beef *(Hebrew National)* 170
    beef *(Hebrew National* Lean) 90
    beef *(Hebrew National* Reduced Fat) 110
    beer *(Oscar Mayer)*, 2 slices, 1.6 oz. 110
    beef *(Oscar Mayer* Machiach), 2 slices, 1.6 oz. 120
    cooked *(Boar's Head)* 130
    cotto *(Oscar Mayer)*, 2 slices, 1.6 oz. 110
    cotto, beef *(Oscar Mayer)*, 2 slices, 1.6 oz. 90
    dry or hard *(Boar's Head)*, 1 oz. 110
    dry or hard *(Hormel Homeland/Sandwich Maker)*, 1 oz. 110
    Genoa *(Boar's Head)* 180
    Genoa *(Di Lusso)*, 1 oz. 120
    Genoa *(Hormel Pillow Pack/Hormel Sandwich Maker)*, 1 oz. . .120
    Genoa *(San Remo Brand)*, 1 oz. 120
    Genoa or hard *(Oscar Mayer)*, 3 slices, 1 oz. 100
scrapple *(Jones Dairy Farm)* 120
sopressata *(Boar's Head Cinghiale* Mini), 1 oz. 100
spiced loaf *(Oscar Mayer)*, 1-oz. slice 70
summer sausage *(Old Smokehouse)* 110
summer sausage, regular or beef *(Oscar Mayer)*, 2 slices,
    1.6 oz. 140
turkey bologna:
    (Empire), 3 slices 90
    (Louis Rich), 1-oz. slice 50
    (Norbest) 130
turkey breast:
    (Boar's Head Premium Lower Sodium) 60
    (Boar's Head Premium Lower Sodium Skinless) 60
    (Boar's Head Ovengold/Boar's Head Ovengold Skinless) 60
    (Boar's Head Salsalito) 60
    (Hormel Deli No Salt) 60
    (Hormel Deli Premium/*Hormel Light & Lean 97)* 50
    (Hormel Light & Lean 97), 1-oz. slice 30
    (Hormel Sandwich Maker) 45
    (Norbest Bronze Label/Gold Label Golden Browned) 60
    (Norbest Gold Label/Silver Label) 55
    barbecued or honey roasted *(Louis Rich)* 60
    Black Forest or honey roasted *(Healthy Deli)* 60
    cured *(Norbest* Gourmet) 70
    honey roasted *(Hormel Light & Lean 97)* 50

Luncheon Meat & Poultry, turkey breast *(cont.)*

honey roasted *(Louis Rich)* 60
honey roasted, and white *(Louis Rich)*, 1-oz. slice 30
lemon garlic *(Hebrew National)*, 5 thin slices 50
maple honey *(Boar's Head)* 70
oven roasted *(Alpine Lace)* 50
oven roasted *(Boar's Head* Golden/Golden Skinless) 60
oven roasted *(Empire)*, 3 slices 50
oven roasted *(Healthy Deli* Gourmet/Gourmet Brick Oven) . .60
oven roasted *(Healthy Deli* Less Sodium/Natural Shape) 60
oven roasted *(Hebrew National)*, 5 thin slices 50
oven roasted *(Louis Rich)* 50
oven roasted *(Louis Rich* Fat Free), 1-oz. slice 25
oven roasted *(Louis Rich Carving Board* Thin Sliced),
    6 slices, 2.1 oz. 60
oven roasted *(Louis Rich Carving Board* Traditional
    Sliced), 2 slices, 1.6 oz. 40
oven roasted *(Louis Rich Deli-Thin* Fat Free), 4 slices,
    1.8 oz. 45
oven roasted *(Oscar Mayer)*, 1-oz. slice 30
oven roasted *(Oscar Mayer* Fat Free), 4 slices, 1.8 oz. 40
oven roasted, glazed *(Healthy Deli* Gourmet) 60
oven roasted, Italian *(Healthy Deli)* 70
oven roasted, white *(Oscar Mayer)*, 1-oz. slice 30
oven roasted, and white *(Louis Rich* Chunk) 60
oven roasted, and white *(Louis Rich)*, 1-oz. slice 30
roast, and white *(Oscar Mayer Deli-Thin)*, 4 slices, 1.8 oz. . .50
rotisserie flavor *(Louis Rich)* 50
rotisserie flavor *(Louis Rich Carving Board)*, 2 slices,
    1.6 oz. 45
skinless *(Hormel/Hormel* Deli) 50
smoked *(Boar's Head* Hickory) 70
smoked *(Boar's Head Cracked Pepper Mill)* 60
smoked *(Empire)*, 3 slices 40
smoked *(Healthy Deli* Mesquite) 60
smoked *(Hebrew National)*, 5 thin slices 60
smoked *(Hebrew National* Hickory) 60
smoked *(Hormel* Mesquite) 60
smoked *(Hormel Light & Lean 97* Mesquite), 1 oz. 30
smoked *(Louis Rich* Hickory) 50
smoked *(Louis Rich* Hickory Fat Free), 1-oz. slice 25
smoked *(Louis Rich Carving Board)*, 2 slices, 1.6 oz. 40

smoked *(Louis Rich Deli-Thin* Hickory), 4 slices, 1.8 oz. 50
smoked *(Norbest* Gold Label) 60
smoked *(Oscar Mayer* Fat Free), 4 slices, 1.8 oz. 40
smoked, honey roasted *(Oscar Mayer Deli-Thin)*, 4 slices,
   1.8 oz. 50
smoked, and white *(Louis Rich)*, 1-oz. slice 30
smoked, white *(Oscar Mayer)*, 1-oz. slice 30
turkey ham:
   (Healthy Deli) 70
   (Louis Rich/Louis Rich Honey Cured), 1-oz. slice 30
   (Louis Rich Chunk) 70
   (Louis Rich Deli-Thin), 4 slices, 1.8 oz. 60
   canned *(Hormel)* 70
   chopped *(Louis Rich)*, 1-oz. slice 45
turkey pastrami:
   (Boar's Head) 60
   (Empire), 3 slices 60
   (Louis Rich), 1-oz. slice 30
   (Louis Rich Chunk) 60
   (Healthy Deli) 70
   (Hebrew National) 60
   (Norbest) 70
turkey salami:
   (Empire), 3 slices 70
   (Louis Rich Salami) 100
   (Norbest) 85
   cooked or cotto *(Louis Rich)*, 1-oz. slice 40

SAUSAGES, cooked or ready-to-serve, except as noted
See also "Appetizers & Snacks, Canned or in Jars,"
"Frankfurters," and "Luncheon Meat & Poultry"

---

                                                  calories

(Hormel Special Recipe), 1 link 111
(Hormel Special Recipe), 1 patty 178
beef:
   (Jones Dairy Farm Golden Brown), 2 links 170
   roll *(Jones Dairy Farm* All Natural), 2 oz. 170
   smoked *(Oscar Mayer* Smokies), 1 link 120
bratwurst:
   (Boar's Head), 4 oz. 300
   (Jones Dairy Farm Dinner), 1 link 230

Sausages, bratwurst *(cont.)*

uncooked *(Schwan's)*, 3-oz. link 270
brown and serve:
    (Little Sizzlers), 3 links 230
    (Little Sizzlers), 2 patties 190
    beef, smoked *(Jones Dairy Farm)*, 2 links 180
    light *(Jones Dairy Farm)*, 2 links 110
    pork *(Jones Dairy Farm)*, 2 links 190
    pork and bacon *(Jones Dairy Farm)*, 2 links 180
canned *(Diana Salchichas)*, 3 links 130
cheese, smoked *(Oscar Mayer* Little Smokies), 6 links 180
cheese, smoked *(Oscar Mayer* Smokies), 1 link 130
chicken:
    apple *(Gerhard's Sausage)*, 2.5 oz. 110
    and apricot *(Bilinski)*, 3.3-oz. link 120
    and broccoli *(Bilinski)*, 3.3-oz. link 110
    with chilies and tequila *(Gerhard's Sausage)*, 2.5 oz. 110
    Italian, with pepper and onion *(Bilinski)*, 3.3-oz. link 120
    and jalapeño *(Bilinski)*, 3.3-oz. link 130
    and pesto *(Bilinski)*, 3.3-oz. link 110
    smoked, and chardonnay *(Gerhard's Sausage)*, 2.5 oz. 110
    and spinach *(Bilinski)*, 3.3-oz. link 100
    and sun-dried tomato with basil *(Bilinski)*, 3.3-oz. link . . . 120
    Thai *(Gerhard's Sausage)*, 2.5 oz. 110
chorizo *(Goya)*, 1.6-oz. link 160
dinner, 1 link or patty:
    (Jones Dairy Farm) 210
    (Jones Dairy Farm All Natural) 130
    Italian *(Jones Dairy Farm)* 140
    sandwich patty *(Jones Dairy Farm)* 140
kielbasa *(Boar's Head)*, 2 oz. 120
kielbasa *(Jones Dairy Farm* Dinner), 1 link 190
knockwurst, beef *(Boar's Head)*, 4 oz. 310
knockwurst, beef *(Hebrew National)*, 3-oz. link 260
New England *(Oscar Mayer)*, 1.6 oz. 60
pickled, smoked or hot *(Hormel)*, 6 links 140
Polish:
    (Schwan's), 2.7-oz. link 270
    beef *(Hebrew National)*, 3-oz. link 240
    beef *(Hebrew National)*, 4-oz. link 330
    skinless *(John Morrell)*, 2 oz. 180

pork *(see also specific sausage listings):*
    (Jones Dairy Farm All Natural Light), 2 links 130
    (Jones Dairy Farm All Natural Little Links), 3 links 190
    (Little Sizzlers), 3 links 180
    (Oscar Mayer), 2 links 180
    hot and spicy *(Little Sizzlers),* 3 links 180
    Italian, hot or sweet, uncooked *(Perri),* 2.7-oz. link 230
    light *(Jones Dairy Farm Golden Brown),* 2 links 110
    maple or milk *(Jones Dairy Farm Golden Brown),* 2 links . . . 190
    mild or spicy *(Jones Dairy Farm Golden Brown),* 2 links . . . 190
    uncooked *(Schwan's),* 3 links 340
pork, patty:
    (Jones Dairy Farm All Natural), 1 patty 130
    (Jones Dairy Farm Golden Brown), 1 patty 150
    (Little Sizzlers), 2 patties 210
    uncooked *(Schwan's),* 2-oz. patty 230
pork roll, regular or hot *(Jones Dairy Farm All Natural),* 2 oz. . 230
smoked:
    (Boar's Head), 4.5 oz. 400
    (John Morrell Bun Size), 1 link 270
    (John Morrell Bun Size Less Fat), 1 link 180
    (Light & Lean 97 Dinner Link), 1 link 60
    (Oscar Mayer Little Smokies), 6 links 170
    (Oscar Mayer Smokie Links), 1 link 130
    hot *(Boar's Head),* 3.2 oz. 280
sticks:
    (Tombstone Snappy Sticks), .75-oz. piece 110
    beef *(Boar's Head),* .6-oz. piece 100
    beef *(Old Dutch),* 1 oz. 110
    beef *(Rustlers Roundup Jerky),* 1 piece 30
    beef *(Tombstone Jerky),* .45-oz. piece 35
    beef *(Tombstone Stick),* .75-oz. piece 110
    hot *(Rustlers Roundup),* 1 piece 40
    smoked *(Rustlers Roundup Steak Stick),* 1 piece 60
    smoked, mild or spicy *(Slim Jim),* 1.4-oz. box 210
    spicy *(Rustlers Roundup),* 1 piece 50
    summer sausage *(Old Dutch),* 1 oz. 110
turkey:
    (Shady Brook Farms Old World), 4 oz. 190
    breakfast, raw *(Shady Brook Farms),* 4 oz. 160
    breakfast, raw or cooked *(Perdue),* 2 links 100
    Italian, hot or sweet *(Louis Rich),* 2.5 oz. 120

Sausages, turkey *(cont.)*
    Italian, hot or sweet *(Shady Brook Farms)*, 4 oz. 170
    Italian, hot or sweet, raw or cooked *(Perdue)*, 1 link 110
    smoked *(Louis Rich/Louis Rich Polska)*, 2 oz. 90
turkey and duck, smoked *(Gerhard's Sausage)*, 2.5 oz. 100
Vienna, canned:
    (Goya), 4 links 170
    (Hormel), 2 oz. 140
    (Libby's), 3 links 130
    chicken *(Hormel)*, 2 oz. 110
    chicken *(Libby's)*, 3 links 100
    with barbecue sauce *(Libby's BBQ)*, 3 links 130
    with hot sauce *(Goya)*, 3 links 130

BACON, cooked, two slices, except as noted

---

                                                    calories

(Agar Prestige) 80
(Black Label/Black Label Low Salt) 80
(Black Label Center Cut), 3 slices 60
(Black Label Thin/Thin Low Salt) 60
(Boar's Head) 60
(Hormel Microwave) 70
(Hormel Layout Pack/Hormel Layout Pack Low Salt) 80
(John Morrell Hardwood Smoked) 100
(Jones Dairy Farm) 90
(Jones Dairy Farm Thick), 1 slice 70
(Old Smokehouse) 80
(Oscar Mayer/Oscar Mayer Center Cut/Lower) 60
(Oscar Mayer Thick), 1 slice 60
(Patrick Cudahy) 80
(Patrick Cudahy Rind) 100
(Range Brand Thick) 100
(Red Label) 80
(Rock River/Sinnissippi) 80
(Schwan's), 1 slice 70
(Sweet Applewood Farms) 80
precooked *(Fast'N Easy)* 80
Canadian-style:
    (Boar's Head), 2 oz. 70
    (Hormel), 2 oz. 70
    (Jones Dairy Farm Lean Choice), 3 slices 70

(Oscar Mayer), 2 slices 50
turkey bacon *(Louis Rich)*, .5-oz. slice 30

MEAT, FISH, & POULTRY SPREADS
See also "Appetizers & Snacks, Canned or in Jars," "Meat & Poultry, Canned or in Jars," "Luncheon Meat & Poultry," and "Fish & Seafood, Canned or in Jars"

---

                                calories

anchovy paste *(Reese)*, 1 tbsp. 30
caviar spread *(Krinos* Taramosalata), 1 tbsp. 90
chicken:
    chunky *(Underwood)*, ¼ cup 120
    chunky, with crackers *(Red Devil* Snackers), 1 pkg. 280
    chunky, salad *(Libby's Spreadables)*, ⅓ cup 140
    salad *(Swanson* Lunch Kit), 1 pkg. 300
ham:
    deviled *(Cure 81)*, 2 oz. 150
    deviled *(Underwood)*, ¼ cup 160
    deviled, with crackers *(Red Devil* Snackers), 1 pkg. 310
    honey *(Underwood)*, ¼ cup 190
    honey, with crackers *(Red Devil* Snackers), 1 pkg. 340
    salad *(Libby's Spreadables)*, ⅓ cup 110
liverwurst, 2 oz. or ¼ cup:
    (Hormel) 130
    (Underwood) 190
    pâté *(Boar's Head)* 150
potted meat:
    (Goya), ¼ cup 60
    (Hormel), 2 oz. 100
    or deviled *(Libby's)*, 3 oz. 160
roast beef spread *(Underwood)*, ¼ cup 140
salmon, smoked, spread *(Vita)*, ¼ cup, 2 oz. 180
sandwich spread *(Oscar Mayer)*, 2 oz. 130
tuna spread:
    (Underwood), ¼ cup 50
    salad *(Bumble Bee)*, 2.75-oz. can 70
    salad *(Libby's Spreadables)*, ⅓ cup 130
    salad, with 6 crackers *(Bumble Bee)*, 2.75-oz. pkg. 150
    salad, with 6 crackers *(StarKist* Tuna Salad), 1 pkg. 190
turkey spread, chunky *(Underwood)*, ¼ cup 110
turkey spread, salad *(Libby's Spreadables)*, ⅓ cup 150

FISH & SEAFOOD, CANNED OR IN JARS
See also "Appetizers & Snacks, Canned or in Jars" and "Meat, Fish, & Poultry Spreads"

calories

clam juice:
   (Bookbinder's), 10.5 oz. .10
   (Doxsee), 1 tbsp. 0
   (S&W), 9.6 fl. oz. 20
clams, 2 oz. or ¼ cup:
   baby, whole *(S&W)* .50
   chopped *(S&W)* 20
   chopped or minced *(Doxsee)* 25
   minced *(Progresso)* 60
   minced *(S&W)* 20
   smoked *(S&W)* 130
crab, Dungeness *(S&W)*, ⅓ cup, 3 oz. 80
cuttlefish, in ink *(Goya)*, ¼ cup 120
gefilte fish, drained:
   (Manischewitz Gold/Jelled Broth), 1 ball with jell 110
   (Manischewitz Gold Vegetable Medley), 1 ball, ⅙ carrot 80
   (Manischewitz Gold with Olives/Carrots), 1 ball, ¼ carrot 60
   zesty *(Manischewitz* Gold/Brine), 1 ball 70
herring, drained:
   (Vita Homestyle), 2 oz. 130
   (Vita Party Snacks), 2 oz. 120
   lunch, sliced *(Vita)*, 2 oz. 130
   in sour cream *(Vita)*, ¼ cup, 2¼ oz. 120
   roll mops *(Vita)*, approx. 1 piece, 2½ oz. 140
herring salad *(Vita)*, ¼ cup 110
mackerel, boneless, skinless, drained *(Reese)*, 4.375-oz. can . . . 240
octopus:
   (Goya), ¼ cup 140
   in garlic sauce *(Goya)*, ¼ cup 160
   à la marinara *(Goya)*, ¼ cup 180
   in olive oil *(Goya)*, ¼ cup 150
   spiced, in red sauce *(Reese)*, 2 oz. 120
oysters:
   whole *(S&W)*, 2 oz. 70
   smoked *(Reese* Petite), 2 oz. 110
   smoked *(S&W)*, 2 oz. 100

salmon, ¼ cup, except as noted:
   chum *(Peter Pan)* 90
   coho *(Peter Pan)* 90
   king *(Peter Pan)* 140
   Norwegian fillet *(Abelvaer)*, 3 oz. 170
   pink, skinless fillet *(Bumble Bee)* 70
   pink, skinless fillet *(Chicken of the Sea)*, 2 oz. 60
   pink, skinless fillet *(Libby's)*, 2 oz. 90
   pink, skinless fillet *(Libby's)*, ⅓ cup 70
   pink, skinless fillet *(Peter Pan)* 90
   red *(Libby's)* 110
   red *(Peter Pan)* 110
   red, blueback *(Rubinstein's)* 110
   red, sockeye *(S&W)* 110
   red, sockeye *(S&W)*, 3¾-oz. can 190
sardines:
   in lemon *(Goya)*, ¼ cup 120
   in mustard sauce *(Underwood)*, 3¾-oz. can 180
   in olive oil, drained *(Goya)*, ¼ cup 130
   in olive oil, drained, Norway brisling, *(S&W)*, 3¾-oz. can . . 160
   in olive oil, drained, skinless, boneless *(Granadaisa)*, ¼ cup . 120
   in olive oil, drained, skinless, boneless *(S&W)*, 3¾-oz. can . 100
   in olive oil, drained, small *(Goya Sardinilla)*, ¼ cup 120
   in soy oil, drained *(Underwood)*, 3 oz. 220
   in soy oil, drained, skinless, boneless *(King Oscar)*,
     3 pieces 120
   spiced *(Goya)*, ¼ cup 120
   in tomato sauce *(Del Monte)*, ½ fish with sauce, 2 oz. 80
   in tomato sauce *(Goya)*, ¼ cup 130
   in tomato sauce *(Goya Oval)*, ¼ cup 80
   in tomato sauce *(Goya Tinapa)*, 2 pieces 50
   in tomato sauce *(Underwood)*, 3¾-oz. can 180
shrimp, all sizes *(Goya)*, 2 oz. 44
shrimp, deveined, small/medium *(S&W)*, ¼ cup 45
squid *(Goya)*, ⅓ can .45
squid, in juice *(Goya)*, ¼ cup 120
tuna, drained, 2 oz. or ¼ cup, except as noted:
   chunk light, in oil *(Bumble Bee)* 110
   chunk light, in oil *(Chicken of the Sea)* 110
   chunk light, in oil *(S&W)* 110
   chunk light, in oil *(StarKist)* 110
   chunk light, in oil *(StarKist)*, 2.7 oz. 140

Fish & Seafood, Canned or in Jar, tuna *(cont.)*

chunk light, in water *(Bumble Bee)* 60
chunk light, in water *(StarKist Low Fat/Sodium)*, 2.7 oz. 70
chunk light, in water *(S&W)* 70
chunk light or white, in water *(StarKist/StarKist Low Fat/ Sodium)* 60
chunk white, in water *(StarKist/StarKist Low Fat/Sodium)*, 2.7 oz. 80
fillet, in water *(StarKist Prime Light)* 60
fillet, in water *(StarKist Prime Light)*, 2.7 oz. 80
solid, in olive oil *(Progresso)* 160
solid white, in oil *(Bumble Bee)* 90
solid white, in oil *(Chicken of the Sea)* 90
solid white, in oil *(S&W)* .80
solid white, in oil *(StarKist)* 90
solid white, in oil *(StarKist)*, 3-oz. can 130
solid white, in water *(Bumble Bee)* 70
solid white, in water *(StarKist)* 70
solid white, in water *(StarKist)*, 3-oz. can 100

FISH & SEAFOOD, FROZEN OR REFRIGERATED, uncooked, except as noted
See also "Dinners, Frozen," "Entrees, Frozen," and "Entrees, Refrigerated"

---

                                             calories

catfish, 4 oz.:
fillets *(Delta Pride)* 90
nuggets *(Delta Pride)* 170
steaks *(Delta Pride)* 170
whole *(Delta Pride)* 130
cod:
fillet *(Schwan's)*, 4 oz. .90
Pacific, loins *(Peter Pan)*, 4 oz. 90
crab, chunks, cooked *(Tyson Delight)*, 3 oz. 70
crab, imitation:
(Captain Jac Easy Shreds), ½ cup, 3 oz. 80
(Peter Pan), 3 oz. 70
flaked *(Captain Jac Crab Tasties)*, ½ cup, 3 oz. 100
flaked *(Louis Kemp Crab Delights)*, ½ cup, 3 oz. 80
flaked *(Pacific Mate Fat Free)*, ½ cup, 3 oz. 90
flaked *(Seafest)*, ½ cup, 3 oz. 100

flaked or chunk *(Louis Kemp Crab Delights)*, ½ cup, 3 oz. . .80
leg style *(Louis Kemp Crab Delights)*, 3 legs, 3 oz. 80
leg style, with crab *(Captain Jac Crab Tasties)*, 3 legs,
   3 oz. 100
crab, legs and claws *(Pride of Alaska)*, ¾ cup edible 100
flounder *(Van de Kamp's)*, 4 oz. 110
haddock, fillet *(Schwan's)*, 4 oz. 100
hake, blue, loins *(Schwan's)*, 4 oz. 70
halibut *(Peter Pan)*, 4 oz. 110
lobster, chunks *(Tyson Delight)*, 3 oz. 80
lobster, imitation:
   chunks *(Captain Jac Lobster Tasties)*, ½ cup, 3 oz. 90
   chunks *(Louis Kemp Lobster Delights)*, ½ cup, 3 oz. 80
   salad style *(Louis Kemp Lobster Delights)*, ½ cup, 3 oz. 80
   tail style *(Captain Jac Lobster Tasties)*, 4-oz. tail 120
mackerel, meat only, smoked *(Spence & Co.)*, 2 oz. 180
mahi mahi, fillet *(Peter Pan)*, 4 oz. 100
ocean perch *(Schwan's)*, 4 oz. 90
orange roughy *(Schwan's)*, 4 oz. 80
salmon, boneless, skinless:
   burger *(Salmon Chef)*, 3-oz. burger 80
   chum, fillet or steak *(Peter Pan)*, 4 oz. 130
   coho, fillet *(Peter Pan)*, 4 oz. 160
   cuts *(Salmon Chef)*, 5-oz. piece 110
   cuts, in dill-sorrel-chive marinade *(Salmon Chef)*,
      5-oz. piece 140
   kabob *(Salmon Chef)*, 3.3 oz. 100
   kabob, in teriyaki sesame marinade *(Salmon Chef)*, 3.3 oz. . 110
   loin *(Salmon Chef)*, 2 pieces, 4 oz. 110
   loin, in chili-cilantro marinade *(Salmon Chef)*, 2 pieces,
      4 oz. 130
   tenderloin *(Salmon Chef)*, 6-oz. piece 110
   tenderloin, in sweet pepper-sage marinade *(Salmon Chef)*,
      6-oz. piece 160
salmon, smoked, lox or Nova *(Vita)*, 3-oz. pkg. 80
scallop, fried *(Mrs. Paul's)*, 12 pieces 200
shrimp:
   jumbo *(Schwan's)*, 6 pieces 100
   medium *(Schwan's)*, 4 oz. 60
   regular or tail on, cooked *(Contessa)*, about 1 cup, 3 oz. 60
shrimp, imitation, jumbo *(Captain Jac Shrimp Tasties)*,
   3 pieces, 3 oz. 90

Fish & Seafood, Frozen or Refrigerated *(cont.)*
sole *(Van de Kamp's* Natural), 4 oz. 110
swordfish, steaks *(Peter Pan)*, 4 oz. 160
trout, rainbow, fillet, smoked, peppered *(Spence & Co.)*, 2 oz. . 100
tuna, yellowtail *(Peter Pan)*, 4 oz. 110

Chapter 12

PASTA, NOODLES, RICE, AND GRAIN DISHES

PASTA, REFRIGERATED, uncooked
See also "Entrees, Frozen," "Pasta & Noodles, Dry, Plain," "Pasta, Frozen," and "Pasta Side Dishes, Frozen"

	calories
angel-hair *(Contadina)*, 1¼ cups	240
angel-hair *(Di Giorno)*, 2 oz.	160
fettuccine:	
(Contadina), 1¼ cups	240
artichoke *(Tutta Pasta)*, 2 oz.	190
black squid *(Tutta Pasta)*, 2 oz.	180
plain or spinach *(Di Giorno)*, 2.5 oz.	190
spinach *(Contadina)*, 1¼ cups	260
linguine *(Contadina)*, 1¼ cups	250
linguine, plain or herb *(Di Giorno)*, 2.5 oz.	190
penne, fusilli, or rigatoni *(Tutta Pasta)*, 1 cup	290
ravioli:	
(Monterey Pasta Company Mediterranean), 3 oz.	250
beef and garlic *(Contadina)*, 1¼ cups	350
cheddar roasted garlic *(Monterey Pasta Company)*, 3 oz.	240
cheese *(Contadina Family Pack)*, 1 cup	290
cheese, four *(Contadina)*, 1 cup	290
cheese, four *(Contadina Light)*, 1 cup	240
cheese and garlic *(Di Giorno Light)*, 1 cup	270
chicken, rosemary *(Contadina)*, 1¼ cups	330
chicken and rosemary *(Real Torino)*, 1 cup	300
crab, snow *(Monterey Pasta Company)*, 3 oz.	230
garden vegetable *(Contadina Light)*, 1 cup	250
garlic basil cheese *(Monterey Pasta Company)*, 3 oz.	240
Gorgonzola *(Contadina)*, 1¼ cups	360
Gorgonzola roasted walnut *(Monterey Pasta Company)*, 3 oz.	240
herb and cheese *(Di Giorno)*, 1 cup	350

Pasta, Refrigerated, ravioli *(cont.)*

    Monterey Jack, smoked *(Monterey Pasta Company)*, 3 oz. . 240

    with Italian sausage *(Di Giorno)*, ¾ cup 340

    spinach and ricotta *(Real Torino)*, 1 cup 310

    tomato and cheese *(Di Giorno Light)*, 1 cup 280

shells *(Tutta Pasta)*, ⅞ cup 300

tortellini:

    cheese *(Di Giorno)*, ¾ cup 260

    cheese or herb chicken *(Contadina)*, ¾ cup 260

    cheese, herb and garlic *(Real Torino)*, 1 cup 320

    cheese, three *(Contadina)*, ¾ cup 250

    with meat *(Di Giorno)*, ¾ cup 290

    spinach *(Contadina)*, ¾ cup 270

tortelloni:

    cheese, four *(Real Torino)*, 1 cup 310

    cheese and basil *(Contadina)*, 1 cup 360

    cheese and garlic *(Contadina)*, 1 cup 280

    chicken *(Real Torino)*, 1 cup 300

    with chicken and herbs *(Di Giorno)*, 1 cup 260

    chicken and prosciutto *(Contadina)*, 1 cup 350

    hot red pepper and cheese *(Di Giorno)*, 1 cup 310

    mozzarella garlic *(Di Giorno)*, 1 cup 300

    mushroom *(Contadina)*, 1 cup 310

    mushroom *(Di Giorno)*, 1 cup 290

    pumpkin *(Real Torino)*, 11 pieces, 3.2 oz. 210

    sausage *(Contadina)*, 1 cup 320

PASTA & NOODLES, DRY, PLAIN, uncooked, two ounces,
except as noted
See also "Pasta, Refrigerated"

---

                                     calories

all varieties:

    (Creamette/Prince) 210

    (Delverde) 200

    (Goya Estrellas*)* 210

    (Mueller's) 210

    (San Giorgio Cholesterol Free*)* 200

    with egg *(Herb's)* 220

    except angel hair and garlic herb fettuccine *(San Giorgio)* . 210

alphabets, vegetable *(Eden* Organic*)*, ½ cup or 2 oz. 200

angel-hair *(San Giorgio)* 200

elbows:
    (Creamette Macaroni) 210
    (Goya Coditos) 210
    regular or hot pepper *(Eden* Organic), ½ cup or 2 oz. 210
extra fine *(Eden* Organic), ½ cup or 2 oz. 210
fettuccine *(Prince)* 220
fettuccine, garlic herb *(San Giorgio)* 200
finbows, parsley-garlic *(Eden* Organic), ½ cup or 2 oz. 210
kamut and quinoa *(Eden* Organic Twisted Pair), ½ cup or 2 oz. . 210
kuzu and sweet potato or kuzu kiri *(Eden)* 190
linguine, tomato-basil *(Prince)* 200
macaroni, *see "elbows," above*
mung bean *(Eden* Harusame) 190
noodles, chow mein, *see "Appetizers & Snacks, Canned or in*
    Jars," page 152
noodles, egg:
    (Creamette/Penn Dutch) 210
    (Kluski) 220
    (Manischewitz) 210
    all varieties *(Creamette/Goodman's)* 220
    all varieties *(Eden* Organic) 220
    bow ties *(Mueller's)* 220
    and spinach *(Prince* Paglia E Fieno) 220
    yolk free *(Borden)* 210
    yolk free *(Mueller's)* 210
noodles, Japanese:
    (Nasoya), 1 cup, 2¾ oz. 210
    soba, buckwheat *(Eden* 100%) 200
    soba, buckwheat *(Eden* Traditional 40%) 190
    soba, lotus root, mugwort, or wild yam *(Eden)* 190
    somen *(Eden* Organic Traditional) 200
    spinach *(Nasoya)*, 1 cup, 2¾ oz. 210
    udon *(Eden)* 190
    udon, regular or brown rice *(Eden* Organic Traditional) . . . 200
penne, tomato-pepper-basil *(Prince)* 210
ribbons, bell pepper–basil, parsley-basil, pesto, saffron,
    or vegetable *(Eden* Organic) 210
ribbons, regular or spinach, whole wheat *(Eden* Organic) 200
rice *(Eden* Bifun) 200
shells *(Goya* Conchas) 210
shells, vegetable *(Eden* Organic) 200

Pasta & Noodles, Dry, Plain *(cont.)*
spaghetti:
    (Eden Organic) 200
    (Prince Square/Thin) 200
    parsley-garlic or whole wheat *(Eden* Organic) 210
spaghetti or spirals, kamut *(Eden* Organic) 190
spirals, sesame-rice or vegetable *(Eden* Organic) 200
spirals, spinach *(Eden* Organic) 210
tri-color *(Mueller's)* 210
tubes, endless *(Eden* Organic), ½ cup or 2 oz. 210
twists, pesto *(Eden* Organic) 200
vegetable rotini, spirals, shells *(Eden/Herb's)* 210
vegetable spirals, whole wheat *(Eden)* 210

PASTA, FROZEN
*See also "Dinners, Frozen," "Entrees, Frozen," "Pasta,
Refrigerated," and "Pasta Side Dishes, Frozen,"*

---

                             calories

manicotti *(Celentano)*, 2 pieces, 7 oz. 410
manicotti, mini *(Celentano)*, 2 pieces, 4.8 oz. 110
ravioli:
    cheese *(Amy's)*, 9.5 oz. 340
    cheese *(Celentano)*, ½ of 13-oz. pkg. 400
    cheese *(Celentano* Great Choice), ½ of 13-oz. pkg. 360
    cheese mini or round mini *(Celentano)*, 4 oz. 270
    cheese *(Schwan's)*, 5 pieces 320
    parsley *(Putney)*, 1 cup 250
    tofu *(Tofutti)*, 1 cup 320
shells, stuffed, without sauce:
    (Celentano), 4 shells 330
    (Celentano Value Pack), 3 shells 240
    (Schwan's), 3 shells 330
tortellini:
    cheese *(Schwan's)*, 1 cup 240
    chicken *(Schwan's)*, 1 cup 230
    spinach *(Putney)*, 1 cup 290
    tofu *(Soy-Boy)*, ⅞ cup 190
    tofu *(Tofutti)*, 1 cup 320

PASTA SIDE DISHES, FROZEN
See also "Dinners, Frozen," "Entrees, Frozen," "Pasta, Refrigerated," and "Pasta, Frozen"

---

calories

Alfredo *(Green Giant Pasta Accents)*, 2 cups 210
cheddar, creamy *(Green Giant Pasta Accents)*, 2⅓ cups 250
cheddar, white *(Green Giant Pasta Accents)*, 1¾ cups 300
Florentine *(Green Giant Pasta Accents)*, 2 cups 310
garden blend, early *(Schwan's)*, ½ cup 45
garden blend, summer *(Schwan's)*, 1 cup 90
garden herb *(Green Giant Pasta Accents)*, 2 cups 230
garlic *(Green Giant Pasta Accents)*, 2 cups 260
Italian blend *(Schwan's)*, 1 cup 60
primavera *(Green Giant Pasta Accents)*, 2¼ cups 320
primavera *(Schwan's)*, 1 cup 220
rotini, with vegetables *(Schwan's)*, 1 cup 130

PASTA & NOODLE DISHES, MIXES, dry, except as noted
See also "Vegetable Dishes, Mixes" and "Entrees, Mixes"

---

calories

angel-hair:
    chicken broccoli *(Lipton Pasta & Sauce)*, ½ pkg. 210
    chicken broccoli *(Lipton Pasta & Sauce)*, 1 cup* 260
    with herbs *(Pasta Roni)*, approx. 1 cup* 320
    lemon and butter *(Pasta Roni)*, approx. 1 cup* 360
    Parmesan *(Lipton Pasta & Sauce)*, ½ pkg. 240
    Parmesan *(Lipton Pasta & Sauce)*, 1 cup* 280
    Parmesan *(Pasta Roni)*, approx. 1 cup* 320
bow ties:
    and beans with herb sauce *(Knorr)*, ⅔ cup 260
    chicken primavera *(Lipton Pasta & Sauce)*, ½ pkg. 210
    chicken primavera *(Lipton Pasta & Sauce)*, 1 cup* 290
    Italian cheese *(Lipton Pasta & Sauce)*, ½ pkg. 220
    Italian cheese *(Lipton Pasta & Sauce)*, 1 cup* 300
butter and herb *(Lipton Pasta & Sauce)*, ½ pkg. 220
butter and herb *(Lipton Pasta & Sauce)*, 1 cup* 270
cheese *(see also "macaroni and cheese," below)*:
    cheddar, mild *(Lipton Pasta & Sauce)*, ½ pkg. 210

---

* *Prepared according to package directions*

Pasta & Noodle Dishes, Mixes, cheese *(cont.)*

cheddar, mild *(Lipton* Pasta & Sauce), 1 cup* 290
cheddar broccoli *(Lipton* Pasta & Sauce), ½ pkg. 260
cheddar broccoli *(Lipton* Pasta & Sauce), 1 cup* 340
four, corkscrews *(Pasta Roni),* approx. 1 cup* 410
three *(Lipton* Pasta & Sauce), ½ pkg. 240
chicken:
herb Parmesan *(Lipton* Pasta & Sauce), ½ pkg. 230
herb Parmesan *(Lipton* Pasta & Sauce), 1 cup* 280
primavera *(Lipton* Pasta & Sauce), ½ pkg. 220
roasted garlic *(Lipton* Pasta & Sauce), ½ pkg. 210
roasted garlic *(Lipton* Pasta & Sauce), 1 cup* 290
stir-fry *(Lipton* Pasta & Sauce), ½ pkg. 220
stir-fry *(Lipton* Pasta & Sauce), 1 cup* 270
fagioli, with white beans *(Fantastic* One Pot Meals), ½ pkg. . . . 150
fettuccine:
with Alfredo sauce *(Pasta Roni),* approx. 1 cup* 470
broccoli, au gratin *(Pasta Roni),* approx. 1 cup* 280
cheddar, mild *(Pasta Roni),* approx. 1 cup* 290
chicken sauce *(Pasta Roni),* approx. 1 cup* 320
with creamy basil sauce *(Knorr* Cup), 1 pkg. 220
Romanoff *(Pasta Roni),* approx. 1 cup* 400
fusilli, with creamy pesto *(Knorr),* ⅔ cup 250
garlic:
butter *(Golden Saute),* ½ pkg. 210
creamy *(Lipton* Pasta & Sauce), ½ pkg. 270
creamy *(Lipton* Pasta & Sauce), 1 cup* 350
creamy, corkscrews *(Pasta Roni),* approx. 1 cup* 420
and herb *(Spice Islands* Quick Meal), 1 pkg. 160
roasted, and olive oil, tomatoes *(Lipton* Pasta & Sauce),
    ½ pkg. 220
roasted, and olive oil, tomatoes *(Lipton* Pasta & Sauce),
    1 cup* 270
gemelli and red lentils, Mediterranean *(Fantastic* One Pot
Meals), ⅜ cup 150
herb, savory, with garlic *(Lipton* Pasta & Sauce), ½ pkg. 230
herb, savory, with garlic *(Lipton* Pasta & Sauce), 1 cup* 280
lasagna, tomato and vegetable *(Pasta Roni),* approx. 1 cup* . . . 230
linguine:
chicken and broccoli *(Pasta Roni),* approx. 1 cup* 370

* Prepared according to package directions

chicken Parmesan, creamy *(Pasta Roni)*, approx. 1 cup* . . . 410
garlic and butter *(Lipton* Pasta & Sauce), ½ pkg. 210
garlic and butter *(Lipton* Pasta & Sauce), 1 cup* 260
macaroni and cheese:
   (Creamette), ⅓ pkg. 250
   (Kraft Original Deluxe Dinner), 3½ oz. 320
   (Kraft Original Dinner), 2½ oz. 260
   (Kraft Thick'n Creamy), 2½ oz. 260
   (Land O' Lakes Deluxe Plus Dinner), approx. 1 cup* 340
   (Land O' Lakes Original Dinner), approx. 1 cup* 400
   Alfredo *(Annie's)*, ½ cup 200
   all varieties, except original and white cheddar *(Kraft*
     Dinner), 2½ oz. 260
   cheddar *(Golden Grain)*, 1 cup* 340
   cheddar, white, mild *(Kraft* Dinner), 2½ oz. 260
   cheddar or Parmesan *(Fantastic)*, ⅜ cup 200
   rotini, with broccoli *(Velveeta)*, 4½ oz. 400
   shells *(Velveeta* Original), 4 oz. 360
   shells, with bacon *(Velveeta)*, 4 oz. 360
   shells, creamy *(Land O' Lakes* Dinner), approx. 1 cup* 330
   shells, with salsa *(Velveeta* Original), 4 oz. 380
   three cheese *(Knorr* Cup), 1 pkg. 240
mushroom, creamy *(Lipton* Pasta & Sauce), ½ pkg. 240
mushroom, creamy *(Lipton* Pasta & Sauce), 1 cup* 320
noodles:
   Alfredo *(Lipton* Noodles & Sauce), ½ pkg. 250
   Alfredo *(Lipton* Noodles & Sauce), 1 cup* 330
   Alfredo broccoli *(Lipton* Noodles & Sauce), ½ pkg. 260
   Alfredo broccoli *(Lipton* Noodles & Sauce), 1 cup* 340
   beef *(Lipton* Noodles & Sauce), ½ pkg. 230
   beef *(Lipton* Noodles & Sauce), 1 cup* 280
   butter *(Lipton* Noodles & Sauce), ½ pkg. 260
   butter *(Lipton* Noodles & Sauce), 1 cup* 310
   butter and herb *(Lipton* Noodles & Sauce), ½ pkg. 250
   butter and herb *(Lipton* Noodles & Sauce), 1 cup* 300
   cheddar *(Kraft* Dinner), 2.5 oz. 270
   cheddar *(Master-A-Meal)*, ⅕ 180
   cheddar *(Nissin* Noodles & Sauce), 2.5 oz. 330
   Oriental *(Knorr* Cup), 1 pkg. 210
   Oriental *(Pasta Roni)*, approx. 1 cup* 290

* *Prepared according to package directions*

Pasta & Noodle Dishes, Mixes, noodles *(cont.)*
    Parmesan *(Lipton* Noodles & Sauce), ½ pkg. 250
    Parmesan *(Lipton* Noodles & Sauce), 1 cup* 330
    sour cream and chives *(Lipton* Noodles & Sauce), ½ pkg. . 260
    sour cream and chives *(Lipton* Noodles & Sauce), 1 cup* . 310
    Stroganoff *(Lipton* Noodles & Sauce), ½ pkg. 220
    Stroganoff *(Lipton* Noodles & Sauce), 1 cup* 300
    tomato, Italian *(Nissin* Noodles and Sauce), 2.4 oz. 320
noodles, with chicken or chicken flavor:
    (Kraft Dinner), 2.5 oz. 270
    (Lipton Noodles & Sauce), ½ pkg. 240
    (Lipton Noodles & Sauce), 1 cup* 290
    (Nissin Noodles & Sauce), 2.4 oz. 330
    broccoli *(Lipton* Noodles & Sauce), ½ pkg. 230
    broccoli *(Lipton* Noodles & Sauce), 1 cup* 310
    creamy *(Lipton* Noodles & Sauce), ½ pkg. 240
    creamy *(Lipton* Noodles & Sauce), 1 cup* 320
    tetrazzini *(Lipton* Noodles & Sauce), ½ pkg. 220
    tetrazzini *(Lipton* Noodles & Sauce), 1 cup* 300
pasta:
    broccoli, and mushroom *(Pasta Roni),* approx. 1 cup* 450
    garlic and olive oil *(Pasta Roni),* approx. 1 cup* 360
    mixed *(Buckeye* Oceans of Pasta), 2 oz. 210
    Parmesan *(Pasta Roni* Parmesano), approx. 1 cup* 390
penne:
    Alfredo *(Knorr),* ¾ cup 280
    herb and butter *(Pasta Roni),* approx. 1 cup* 430
    with sun-dried tomato Parmesan *(Knorr),* ½ pkg. 270
primavera:
    (Knorr Cup), 1 pkg. 210
    (Lipton Pasta & Sauce), ½ pkg. 240
    (Spice Islands Quick Meal), 1 pkg. 170
rigatoni, cheddar and broccoli *(Pasta Roni),* approx. 1 cup* . . . 400
rigatoni, tomato basil *(Pasta Roni),* approx. 1 cup* 240
rotini:
    with mushroom sauce *(Knorr),* frs2/3] cup 250
    primavera or three cheese *(Lipton* Pasta & Sauce), ½ pkg. . 240
    primavera or three cheese *(Lipton* Pasta & Sauce), 1 cup* . 320
salad:
    (Buckeye Sunny Day), ¹⁄₁₀ pkg. 130

* Prepared according to package directions

Caesar *(Kraft)*, 2.5 oz. . . . . , ... 350
garden primavera *(Kraft)*, 2.5 oz. 280
hearty *(Buckeye)*, 1/8 pkg. 140
Italian, light *(Kraft)*, 2.5 oz. 190
Italian herb *(Fantastic)*, 2/3 cup 170
Parmesan peppercorn *(Kraft)*, 2.5 oz. 360
ranch, classic, with bacon *(Kraft)*, 2.5 oz. 360
seasoned *(Buckeye* Sunny), 1/9 pkg. 140
spicy Oriental *(Fantastic)*, 2/3 cup 200
shells, white cheddar *(Pasta Roni)*, approx. 1 cup* 390
spaghetti:
    with meat sauce *(Kraft* Dinner), 5.5 oz. 330
    mild *(Kraft* American Dinner), 2 oz. 200
    tangy *(Kraft* Italian Dinner), 2 oz. 200
spinach and mushroom *(Spice Islands* Quick Meal), 1 pkg. . . . 160
tomato, creamy, basil *(Spice Islands* Quick Meal), 1 pkg. 190
tomato, creamy, twists *(Knorr* Cup), 1 pkg. 230

POLENTA, REFRIGERATED, unheated

calories

plain *(Frieda's)*, 4 oz. 100
plain *(San Gennaro)*, 2 slices, 1/2" 70
basil and garlic *(San Gennaro)*, 2 slices, 1/2" 71
sun-dried tomato *(San Gennaro)*, 2 slices, 1/2" 74

RICE, PLAIN, dry, 1/4 cup, except as noted
See also "Rice Dishes, Mixes"

calories

Arborio:
    (Colavita), 2 oz. 200
    (Fantastic Foods) 210
    (Frieda's) 210
basmati, brown:
    (Arrowhead Mills) 150
    (Fantastic Foods) 170
    (Lundberg Organic) 160
    (Lundberg Nutra-Farmed/Lundberg Royal) 170

* Prepared according to package directions

Rice, Plain *(cont.)*
basmati, white:
    (Casbah) 158
    (Fantastic Foods) 180
    (Lundberg Nutra-Farmed/Lundberg Organic) 180
blends *(Lundberg Countrywild/Lundberg Wild Blend)* 150
blends *(Lundberg Jubilee/Black Japonica)* 170
brown:
    (Carolina/Mahatma/River) 150
    (Lundberg Wehani) 170
    (Success), ½ cup 150
brown, long grain:
    (Arrowhead Mills) 150
    (S&W) 150
    (Uncle Ben's Instant), ½ cup 190
    (Uncle Ben's Whole Grain) 170
brown, long or short grain *(Lundberg Nutra-Farmed/Lundberg*
    Organic) 170
brown, medium grain:
    (Arrowhead Mills) 160
    (Arrowhead Mills Quick) 150
    (Lundberg) 160
brown, precooked *(S&W* Quick), ½ cup 150
brown, quick *(Lundberg)* 150
brown, short grain *(Arrowhead Mills)* 170
brown, sweet *(Lundberg* Organic/*Lundberg* Premium) 150
glutinous or sweet *(Goya* Fancy Blue Rose/Valencia) 170
jasmine *(Fantastic Foods)* 170
white, long grain:
    (Canilla) 160
    (Carolina) 150
    (Mahatma) 150
    (Martha White) 170
    (River/Water Maid) 160
    (Success), ½ cup 190
    extra *(Goya)* 160
    instant *(Carolina)* 160
    instant *(Mahatma)* 160
    instant *(Minute)*, ½ cup 170
    instant *(Minute* Boil in Bag), ½ cup 190
    instant *(Minute* Premium), ½ cup 170
    instant *(Uncle Ben's)*, ½ cup 190

parboiled *(Uncle Ben's Converted)* 170
wild, raw *(Fantastic Foods)*, ¼ cup 140

RICE DISHES, CANNED
See also "Entrees, Canned or Packaged"

calories

Chinese fried *(La Choy)*, 1 cup 240
Mexican *(Old El Paso)*, ½ cup 410
Spanish *(Old El Paso)*, 1 cup 130
Spanish *(Van Camp's)*, 1 cup 180

RICE DISHES, FROZEN, one package, except as noted
See also "Vegetable Dishes, Frozen" and "Entrees, Frozen"

calories

and broccoli *(Green Giant)* 320
and broccoli au gratin *(Freezer Queen* Family Side Dish), 1 cup . 180
and vegetables:
    (Green Giant Medley) 240
    Oriental *(Green Giant* International) 180
    pilaf *(Green Giant)* 230
    white and wild *(Green Giant)* 250

RICE DISHES, MIXES, 2 oz. dry*, except as noted
See also "Vegetable Dishes, Mixes," "Entrees, Mixes," and "Rice, Plain"

calories

and beans:
    black *(Carolina/Mahatma)* 200
    black or red *(Goya)* 160
    black, Mediterranean, pilaf *(Near East)*, approx. 1 cup** . . 270
    black, savory *(Good Harvest)*, ⅓ cup 160
    black, spicy *(Spice Islands* Quick Meal), 1 pkg. 180
    Cajun *(Fantastic Foods)*, ⅔ oz. 240
    Cajun style *(Lipton* Rice & Sauce), ½ pkg. 260
    Cajun style *(Lipton* Rice & Sauce), 1 cup** 310
    Caribbean *(Fantastic Foods)*, 2.1 oz. 230

---

* *Yield is approximately 1 cup prepared*
** *Prepared according to package directions*

Rice Dishes, Mixes, and beans *(cont.)*
    curry *(Fantastic Foods),* 2.3 oz. 260
    Italian *(Fantastic Foods),* 2.2 oz. 240
    pinto *(Mahatma)* 190
    red *(Carolina/Mahatma)* 190
    red *(Rice-A-Roni),* approx. 1 cup* 280
    red, pilaf *(Near East),* approx. 1 cup* 220
    red, spicy *(Good Harvest),* ⅓ cup 160
    red, spicy *(Spice Islands* Quick Meal), 1 pkg. 180
    Spanish *(Fantastic Only A Pinch* Cup), 2.2 oz. 210
    Szechuan *(Fantastic Foods),* 1.9 oz. 210
    Tex-Mex *(Fantastic Foods),* 2.4 oz. 270
    tomato herb, pilaf *(Near East),* approx. 1 cup* 270
    vegetables, garden, pilaf *(Near East),* approx. 1 cup* 270
beef/beef flavor:
    (Country Inn) 200
    (Lipton Rice & Sauce), ½ pkg. 220
    (Lipton Rice & Sauce), 1 cup* 270
    (Rice-A-Roni), approx. 1 cup* 320
    (Rice-A-Roni Less Salt), approx. 1 cup* 280
    (Success) 190
    and mushroom *(Rice-A-Roni),* approx. 1 cup* 290
    pilaf *(Near East),* approx. 1 cup* 220
broccoli:
    Alfredo *(Lipton* Rice & Sauce), ½ pkg. 240
    Alfredo *(Lipton* Rice & Sauce), 1 cup* 320
    au gratin *(Country Inn)* 200
    au gratin *(Rice-A-Roni),* approx. 1 cup* 370
    au gratin *(Rice-A-Roni* Less Salt), approx. 1 cup* 320
    au gratin *(Savory Classics),* 1 cup* 390
    cheese *(Mahatma)* 200
    cheese *(Success)* 210
brown and wild *(Success)* 190
brown and wild, herb *(Arrowhead* Quick), ¼ pkg. 140
Cajun style *(Lipton* Rice & Sauce), ½ pkg. 220
Cajun style *(Lipton* Rice & Sauce), 1 cup* 270
cheddar, white, with herbs *(Rice-A-Roni),* approx. 1 cup* 340
cheddar broccoli *(Lipton* Rice & Sauce), ½ pkg. 230
cheddar broccoli *(Lipton* Rice & Sauce), 1 cup* 280
cheese *(Country Inn)* 210

---

* *Prepared according to package directions*

chicken/chicken flavor:
   (Country Inn) 200
   (Lipton Rice & Sauce), ½ pkg. 230
   (Lipton Rice & Sauce), 1 cup* 280
   (Rice-A-Roni), approx. 1 cup* 310
   (Rice-A-Roni Less Salt), approx. 1 cup* 280
   (Savory Classics), 1 cup* 300
   (Success Classic) 150
   creamy *(Lipton* Rice & Sauce), ½ pkg. 240
   creamy *(Lipton* Rice & Sauce), 1 cup* 290
   pilaf *(Eastern Traditions)* 200
   pilaf *(Knorr)*, ⅓ cup 210
   pilaf *(Lundberg* Quick Country) 220
   pilaf *(Near East)*, approx. 1 cup* 220
   pilaf *(Spice Islands* Quick Meal), 1 pkg. 180
   pilaf, with wild rice, Mediterranean *(Near East)*, approx.
     1 cup* 220
   roasted or Southwestern *(Lipton* Side Dish), ½ pkg. 210
   roasted or Southwestern *(Lipton* Side Dish), 1 cup* 260
chicken and broccoli:
   (Country Inn) 200
   (Lipton Rice & Sauce), ½ pkg.* 230
   (Lipton Rice & Sauce), 1 cup* 280
   (Rice-A-Roni), approx. 1 cup* 290
chicken and mushrooms *(Rice-A-Roni)*, approx. 1 cup* 360
chicken with vegetables *(Country Inn)* 200
chicken with vegetables *(Rice-A-Roni)*, approx. 1 cup* 290
chicken and wild rice *(Country Inn)* 190
chicken and wild rice, almond *(Savory Classics)*, 1 cup* 310
chili *(Lundberg One Step)* 180
curry:
   (Lundberg One Step) 160
   basmati, with lentils *(Fantastic* One Pot Meals), ⅜ cup 160
   pilaf *(Near East)*, approx. 1 cup* 220
fried rice *(Rice-A-Roni)*, approx. 1 cup* 320
fried rice *(Rice-A-Roni Less Salt)*, approx. 1 cup* 260
garlic basil *(Lundberg One Step)* 160
gumbo *(Mahatma)* 160
herb and butter:
   (Lipton Rice & Sauce), ½ pkg. 230

* *Prepared according to package directions*

Rice Dishes, Mixes, herb and butter *(cont.)*
   (Lipton Rice & Sauce), 1 cup* 280
   (Rice-A-Roni), approx. 1 cup* 310
jambalaya *(Mahatma)* 190
long grain and wild:
   (Lipton Rice & Sauce Original), ½ pkg. 230
   (Lipton Rice & Sauce Original), 1 cup* 280
   (Mahatma) 190
   (Rice-A-Roni), approx. 1 cup* 240
   (Uncle Ben's Fast/Original) 190
   butter and herb *(Uncle Ben's)* 200
   chicken with almonds *(Rice-A-Roni),* approx. 1 cup* 290
   chicken and herb *(Uncle Ben's)* 200
   mushroom and herb *(Lipton* Rice & Sauce), ½ pkg. 250
   pilaf *(Near East),* approx. 1 cup* 220
   pilaf *(Rice-A-Roni),* approx. 1 cup* 240
   vegetable herb *(Uncle Ben's)* 200
medley *(Lipton* Rice & Sauce), ½ pkg. 220
medley *(Lipton* Rice & Sauce), 1 cup* 270
Mexican:
   (Goya) 160
   (Pritikin) 200
   (Savory Classics Fiesta), 1 cup* 310
   cheesy *(Old El Paso),* ½ pkg. 420
mushroom:
   (Lipton Rice & Sauce), ½ pkg. 220
   (Lipton Rice & Sauce), 1 cup* 270
   brown *(Uncle Ben's)* 190
   and herb *(Lipton* Rice & Sauce), ½ pkg. 240
   and herb *(Lipton* Rice & Sauce), 1 cup* 290
Oriental:
   (Pritikin) 190
   (Rice-A-Roni), approx. 1 cup* 290
   (Savory Classics), 1 cup* 290
   stir-fry *(Lipton* Side Dish), ½ pkg. 220
   stir-fry *(Lipton* Side Dish), 1 cup* 270
   and vegetables *(Spice Islands* Quick Meal), 1 pkg. 180
pilaf:
   (Casbah), 1 oz. 100
   (Country Inn) 200

* *Prepared according to package directions*

(Eastern Traditions/Eastern Traditions Harvest) 190
(Knorr Original), 1/3 cup 220
(Lipton Rice & Sauce), 1/2 pkg. 210
(Lipton Rice & Sauce), 1 cup* 260
(Mahatma) 190
(Near East), approx. 1 cup* 220
(Rice-A-Roni), approx. 1 cup* 310
(Success) 200
almond, toasted *(Near East)*, approx. 1 cup* 230
brown rice *(Near East)*, approx. 1 cup* 220
brown rice, with miso *(Fantastic Foods)*, 1/2 cup 250
four grain with wild rice *(Fantastic* Healthy Complements),
    1/2 cup 160
garden *(Savory Classics)*, 1 cup* 240
garlic herb *(Lundberg* Quick) 210
lemon herb, with jasmine rice *(Knorr)*, 1/3 cup 270
Mediterranean *(Good Harvest)*, 1/3 cup 160
nutted *(Casbah)*, 1 oz. 110
primavera *(Goya)* 160
Spanish fiesta or savory mushroom *(Lundberg* Quick) 190
three grain with herbs *(Fantastic Foods)*, 1/3 cup 240
risotto:
    all varieties *(Lundberg)*, 1/4 pkg. 140
    broccoli au gratin *(Knorr)*, 1/3 cup 260
    chicken and Parmesan *(Lipton* Rice & Sauce), 1/2 pkg. . . 220
    chicken and Parmesan *(Lipton* Rice & Sauce), 1 cup* . . . 270
    classico *(Fantastic* Healthy Complements), 1/4 cup . . . 140
    Milanese *(Knorr)*, 1/3 cup 280
    mushroom *(Fantastic* Healthy Complements), 1/4 cup . . . 140
    mushroom *(Knorr)*, 1/3 cup 300
    onion herb *(Knorr)*, 1/3 cup 310
    primavera *(Knorr)*, 1/3 cup 290
    tomato–wild mushroom *(Good Harvest)*, 1/3 cup 160
salsa style *(Lipton* Side Dish), 1/3 pkg. 170
salsa style *(Lipton* Side Dish), 1 cup* 220
scampi style *(Lipton* Rice & Sauce), 1/2 pkg. 220
scampi style *(Lipton* Rice & Sauce), 1 cup* 270
Spanish:
    (Country Inn) 200
    (Fantastic Healthy Complements), 3/8 cup 160

* Prepared according to package directions

Rice Dishes, Mixes, Spanish (cont.)

(Good Harvest), ⅓ cup 160
(Lipton Rice & Sauce), ½ pkg. 220
(Lipton Rice & Sauce), 1 cup* 270
(Old El Paso), ½ pkg. 410
(Mahatma) 180
(Rice-A-Roni), approx. 1 cup* 270
(Success) 190
brown *(Arrowhead Mills* Quick), ¼ pkg. 150
brown rice pilaf *(Fantastic Foods),* ½ cup 240
pilaf *(Casbah),* 1 oz. 100
pilaf *(Knorr),* ⅓ cup 230
pilaf *(Near East),* approx. 1 cup* 230
pilaf, brown *(Lundberg* Quick Fiesta) 190
sticky, with coconut milk *(Thai Kitchen),* ½ cup* 240
Stroganoff *(Rice-A-Roni),* approx. 1 cup* 360
teriyaki *(Lipton* Rice & Sauce), ½ pkg. 220
teriyaki *(Lipton* Rice & Sauce), 1 cup* 270
vegetable, country *(Spice Islands* Quick Meal), 1 pkg. 180
vegetable herb *(Arrowhead Mills* Quick Meal), ¼ pkg. 150
wild, and bean *(Good Harvest),* ⅓ cup 160
wild, and vegetables *(Spice Islands* Quick Meal), 1 pkg. 170
yellow *(Goya)* 170
yellow, saffron *(Carolina/Mahatma)* 190

GRAIN DISHES, MIXES
See also "Cereal & Grain Products"

---

calories

barley pilaf *(Near East),* approx. 1 cup* 220
bulgur pilaf *(Casbah),* 1 oz. 100
couscous:
  almond chicken, vegetarian *(Casbah),* 1 pkg. 160
  asparagus au gratin *(Casbah),* 1 pkg. 150
  black bean salsa *(Fantastic Cup),* 1 pkg. 240
  cheddar, broccoli, creamy *(Casbah),* 1 pkg. 130
  cheddar, nacho *(Fantastic Cup),* 1 pkg. 200
  corn, sweet *(Fantastic Cup),* 1 pkg. 180
  garlic with red pepper *(Fantastic* Healthy Complements),
    ⅓ cup 200

* *Prepared according to package directions*

with lentils *(Fantastic Only A Pinch* Cup), 1 pkg. 220
pilaf *(Casbah)*, 1 oz. 100
royal Thai *(Fantastic* Healthy Complements), ⅓ cup 200
savory pilaf *(Fantastic Foods)*, ⅓ cup 240
tomato Parmesan *(Casbah)*, 1 pkg. 170
vegetable, Creole *(Fantastic* Cup), 1 pkg. 220
falafel *(Casbah)*, ⅛ pkg. 130
falafel *(Fantastic Falafil)*, ½ cup 250
hush puppy *(Martha White)*, ¼ cup 120
lentil:
  burgoo, spicy *(Buckeye Beans)*, 1 cup* 200
  honey baked *(Buckeye Beans)*, 1 cup* 250
  sausage cassoulet *(Buckeye Beans)*, 1 cup* 170
polenta *(Fantastic Foods)*, 1 cup* 260
tabbouleh *(Casbah* Tabouli), 1 oz. 90
tabbouleh *(Fantastic* Tabouli), ¼ cup 120
wheat pilaf *(Near East)*, approx. 1 cup* 220

Chapter 13

PIZZA AND SANDWICHES

PIZZA, FROZEN
*See also, "Appetizers & Snacks, Frozen or Refrigerated,"
"Pizza, Bread & Roll, Frozen," "Sandwiches, Frozen or
Refrigerated," and "Food Chains & Restaurants"*

	calories
artichoke heart *(Wolfgang Puck's 10")*, ½ pie	340
bacon burger *(Totino's Party)*, ½ pie, 5.25 oz.	380
Canadian bacon:	
(Jeno's Crisp 'n Tasty), 6.9-oz. pie	430
(Schwan's Special Recipe), ⅓ pie, 5.6-oz.	430
(Tombstone Original 12"), ¼ pie	360
(Totino's Party), ½ pie, 5.2 oz.	320
cheese:	
(Amy's), 1 serving	310
(Celentano Thick Crust), ½ pie	390
(Celeste Large), ¼ pie	320
(Celeste Pizza for One), 1 pie	540
(Empire Kosher 3 Pack), 3-oz. pie	210
(Empire Kosher 10 oz.), ½ pie	340
(Jeno's Microwave For One), 3.7-oz. pie	240
(Jeno's Crisp 'n Tasty), 6.9-oz. pie	450
(Kid Cuisine Pirate), 8-oz. pie	430
(Schwan's Deep Dish Single), 6-oz. pie	500
(Schwan's Special Recipe), ⅓ pie, 5.3 oz.	440
(Swanson Fun Feast), 1 pie	350
(Tombstone For One ½ Less Fat), 6.5-oz. pie	360
(Totino's Microwave for One), 3.7-oz. pie	240
(Totino's Party), ½ pie, 4.9 oz.	320
(Totino's Party Family Size), ⅓ pie, 5.6 oz.	360
cheese, extra:	
(Marie Callender's), ½ pie, 4.5 oz.	410
(Tombstone Original 9"), ½ pie	420
(Tombstone Original 12"), ¼ pie	370
(Tombstone For One), 1 pie	540

(Weight Watchers), 5.74 oz. 390
cheese, four:
   (Celeste Pizza for One), 1 pie 540
   (Schwan's Deep Dish 10½"), ¼ pie 310
   (Tombstone Special Order 12"), ⅕ pie 400
   (Wolfgang Puck's), ½ pie 360
   hot and zesty *(Celeste* Pizza for One), 1 pie 530
   zesty *(Celeste* Large), ¼ pie 330
cheese, three:
   (Pappalo's Deep Dish), ¼ pie, 5.3 oz. 370
   (Pappalo's Deep Dish for One), 7.2-oz. pie 540
   (Pappalo's for One), 7.7-oz. pie 500
   (Pappalo's Pizzeria Style 9"), ½ pie 400
   (Pappalo's Pizzeria Style 12"), ¼ pie 340
   (Totino's Select), ⅓ pie, 4.4 oz. 300
   Italian *(Tombstone* ThinCrust), ¼ pie, 4.9 oz. 380
cheese, two:
   with Canadian bacon *(Totino's* Select), ⅓ pie, 4.9 oz. 310
   with pepperoni *(Totino's* Select), ⅓ pie, 4.8 oz. 360
   with sausage *(Totino's* Select), ⅓ pie, 5 oz. 360
chicken, spicy *(Wolfgang Puck's* 10¾"), ½ pie 360
chicken and broccoli *(Marie Callender's)*, ½ pie, 4.5 oz. 350
combination:
   (Jeno's Microwave for One), 4.2-oz. pie 310
   (Jeno's Crisp 'n Tasty), 7-oz. pie 520
   (Totino's Microwave for One), 4.2-oz. pie 310
   (Totino's Party), ½ pie, 3.4 oz. 390
   (Totino's Party Family), ¼ pie, 4.4 oz. 300
   (Weight Watchers Deluxe), 6.57 oz. 380
deluxe:
   (Celeste Large), ¼ pie 350
   (Celeste Pizza for One), 1 pie 540
   (Marie Callender's), ½ pie, 4.5 oz. 380
   (Tombstone Original 9"), ⅓ pie 320
   (Tombstone Original 12"), ¼ pie 320
hamburger:
   (Jeno's Crisp 'n Tasty), 7.3-oz. pie 500
   (Kid Cuisine Big League), 8.3 oz. 400
   (Tombstone Original 9"), ⅓ pie 310
   (Tombstone Original 12"), ⅕ pie 320
   (Totino's Party), ½ pie, 5.5 oz. 370
Italiano, zesty *(Totino's* Party), ½ pie, 5.4 oz. 390

Pizza, Frozen *(cont.)*

with meat *(Celeste* Suprema for One), 1 pie 580
with meat *(Celeste* Suprema Large), 1/5 pie 290
meat, five *(Marie Callender's),* 1/2 pie, 4.5 oz. 330
meat, four:

    (Pappalo's Deep Dish), 1/5 pie, 4.5 oz. 330
    (Pappalo's Pizzeria Style 12"), 1/4 pie 380
    (Tombstone Special Order 9"), 1/3 pie 400
    (Tombstone Special Order 12"), 1/6 pie 350
    combo, Italian *(Tombstone* ThinCrust), 1/4 pie, 5.1 oz. 410
meat, three:

    (Jeno's Crisp 'n Tasty), 7-oz. pie 500
    (Schwan's Deep Dish 10 1/2"), 1/4 pie 340
    (Totino's Party), 1/2 pie, 5.25 oz. 360
Mexican style:

    (Schwan's Deep Dish Single), 5.4-oz. pie 440
    supreme taco *(Tombstone* ThinCrust), 1/4 pie, 5.1 oz. 380
    zesty *(Totino's* Microwave for One), 4.2-oz. pie 280
    zesty *(Totino's Party),* 1/2 pie, 5.5 oz. 370
pepperoni:

    (Celeste Large), 1/4 pie 350
    (Celeste Pizza for One), 1 pie 520
    (Hormel Quick Meal), 5.9-oz. pie 380
    (Jeno's Microwave For One), 4-oz. pie 280
    (Jeno's Crisp 'n Tasty), 6.8-oz. pie 500
    (Marie Callender's), 1/2 pie, 4.5 oz. 440
    (Pappalo's Deep Dish), 1/5 pie, 4.4 oz. 340
    (Pappalo's Deep Dish For One), 7-oz. pie 540
    (Pappalo's for One), 7-oz. pie 520
    (Pappalo's Pizzeria Style 9"), 1/2 pie 440
    (Pappalo's Pizzeria Style 12"), 1/4 pie 390
    (Schwan's Deep Dish Single), 6-oz. pie 530
    (Schwan's Special Recipe), 1/3 pie, 5.4 oz. 480
    (Tombstone Original 9"), 1/3 pie 340
    (Tombstone Original 12"), 1/5 pie 340
    (Tombstone For One), 7-oz. pie 580
    (Tombstone For One 1/2 Less Fat), 6.8-oz. pie 400
    (Tombstone Special Order 9"), 1/3 pie 400
    (Tombstone Special Order 12"), 1/6 pie 360
    (Totino's Microwave for One), 4 oz. 280
    (Totino's Party), 1/2 pie, 5.1 oz. 380
    (Totino's Party Family), 1/3 pie, 5.6 oz. 410

(Weight Watchers), 5.56 oz. 390
double cheese *(Tombstone Double Top)*, ¹/₆ pie, 4.6 oz. 350
Italian *(Tombstone ThinCrust)*, ¹/₄ pie, 5 oz. 420
super *(Schwan's Deep Dish 10½")*, ¹/₄ pie 350
sausage:
   (Celeste Pizza for One), 1 pie 530
   (Jeno's Microwave for One), 4.1-oz. pie 280
   (Jeno's Crisp 'n Tasty), 7-oz. pie 510
   (Pappalo's Deep Dish), ¹/₅ pie, 4.6 oz. 330
   (Pappalo's Pizzeria Style 9"), ¹/₂ pie 440
   (Pappalo's Pizzeria Style 12"), ¹/₄ pie 380
   (Schwan's Deep Dish Single), 6-oz. pie 520
   (Schwan's Special Recipe), ¹/₄ pie, 4.5 oz. 380
   (Tombstone Original 9"), ¹/₃ pie 310
   (Tombstone Original 12"), ¹/₅ pie 320
   (Totino's Microwave for One), 4.1-oz. pie 280
   (Totino's Party), ¹/₂ pie, 5.4 oz. 380
   (Totino's Party Family), ¹/₄ pie, 4.5 oz. 300
   double cheese *(Tombstone Double Top)*, ¹/₆ pie, 4.8 oz. 350
   Italian *(Tombstone ThinCrust)*, ¹/₄ pie, 5.1 oz. 400
   Italian *(Tombstone For One)*, 7-oz. pie 560
   three *(Tombstone Special Order 9")*, ¹/₃ pie 390
   three *(Tombstone Special Order 12")*, ¹/₆ pie 340
sausage and herb *(Wolfgang Puck's 10¾")*, ¹/₂ pie 380
sausage and mushroom *(Tombstone Original 12")*, ¹/₅ pie 320
sausage and pepperoni:
   (Marie Callender's), ¹/₂ pie, 4.5 oz. 430
   (Pappalo's Deep Dish), ¹/₅ pie, 4.6 oz. 530
   (Pappalo's Deep Dish for One), 7.26-oz. pie 550
   (Pappalo's for One), 7.2-oz. pie 570
   (Pappalo's Pizzeria Style 9"), ¹/₂ pie 440
   (Pappalo's Pizzeria Style 12"), ¹/₄ pie 390
   (Schwan's Special Recipe), ¹/₄ pie, 4.4 oz. 390
   (Tombstone Original 9"), ¹/₃ pie 360
   (Tombstone Original 12"), ¹/₅ pie 340
   (Tombstone For One), 7-oz. pie 590
   (Totino's Select), ¹/₃ pie, 5 oz. 360
   double cheese *(Tombstone Double Top)*, ¹/₆ pie, 4.8 oz. 360
spinach and feta *(Amy's)*, 1 serving 320
supreme:
   (Jeno's Crisp 'n Tasty), 7.2-oz. pie 520
   (Pappalo's Deep Dish), ¹/₅ pie, 4.9 oz. 350

Pizza, Frozen, supreme *(cont.)*

(Pappalo's Deep Dish for One), 7.6-oz. pie 540
(Pappalo's for One), 7.6-oz. pie 520
(Pappalo's Pizzeria Style 9"), ½ pie 300
(Pappalo's Pizzeria Style 12"), ¼ pie 390
(Schwan's Deep Dish 10½"), ¼ pie 350
(Schwan's Deep Dish Single), 6-oz. pie 490
(Schwan's Special Recipe), ¼ pie, 5.1 oz. 410
(Tombstone Light), ⅕ pie, 4.9 oz. 270
(Tombstone Original 12"), ⅕ pie 330
(Tombstone For One), 7.6-oz. pie 570
(Tombstone For One ½ Less Fat), 7.7-oz. pie 400
(Totino's Microwave For One), 4.3-oz. pie 290
(Totino's Select), ⅓ pie, 5.5 oz. 360
(Totino's Party), ½ pie, 5.5 oz. 380
Italian *(Tombstone* ThinCrust), ¼ pie, 5.3 oz. 400
super *(Tombstone* Special Order 9"), ⅓ pie 400
super *(Tombstone* Special Order 12"), ⅙ pie 350
tomato and mozzarella *(Marie Callender's),* ½ pie, 4.5 oz. 350
vegetable:
(Celeste Pizza for One), 1 pie 480
(Tombstone Light), ⅕ pie, 4.6 oz. 240
(Tombstone For One ½ Less Fat), 7.3-oz. pie 360
grilled, cheeseless *(Wolfgang Puck's* 10¾"), ½ pie 200
primavera *(Marie Callender's),* ½ pie, 4.5 oz. 350
roasted *(Amy's),* 1 serving 270

PIZZA, BREAD & ROLL, FROZEN
*See also "Pizza, Frozen" and "Sandwiches, Frozen or
Refrigerated"*

---

                                                          calories
bagel *(Empire* Kosher), 2-oz. piece 150
croissant *(Pepperidge Farm),* 1 piece:
    cheese 390
    deluxe 450
    pepperoni 420
English muffin *(Empire* Kosher), 2-oz. piece 130
French bread, 1 piece:
    bacon cheddar *(Stouffer's)* 430
    cheese *(Healthy Choice)* 320
    cheese *(Lean Cuisine)* 320

cheese *(Stouffer's)* 360
cheeseburger *(Stouffer's)* 420
deluxe *(Lean Cuisine)* 320
deluxe *(Stouffer's)* 430
double cheese *(Stouffer's)* 420
meat, three *(Stouffer's)* 460
pepperoni *(Healthy Choice)* 340
pepperoni *(Lean Cuisine)* 310
pepperoni *(Stouffer's)* 440
pepperoni and mushroom *(Stouffer's)* 440
sausage *(Healthy Choice)* 300
sausage *(Stouffer's)* 430
sausage and pepperoni *(Stouffer's)* 450
supreme *(Healthy Choice)* 310
vegetable *(Healthy Choice)* 270
vegetable deluxe *(Stouffer's)* 380
white *(Stouffer's)* 460
Italian bread, 1 piece:
  cheese, four *(Celeste)* 300
  chicken, zesty *(Celeste)* 260
  deluxe *(Celeste)* 290
  pepperoni *(Celeste)* 320

SANDWICHES, FROZEN OR REFRIGERATED
See also "Breakfast Sandwiches," "Entrees, Frozen," and "Pizza, Bread & Roll, Frozen"

calories

beef:
  barbecue *(Hormel Quick Meal)*, 1 pkg. 360
  barbecue *(Hot Pockets)*, 4.5-oz. piece 340
  broccoli *(Lean Pockets)*, 4.5-oz. piece 250
  cheddar *(Hot Pockets)*, 4.5-oz. piece 360
  cheeseburger *(Hormel Quick Meal)*, 1 pkg. 400
  cheeseburger *(White Castle)*, 2 pieces, 3.6 oz. 310
  cheeseburger, bacon *(Hormel Quick Meal)*, 1 pkg. 440
  cheeseburger, chili *(Hormel Quick Meal)*, 1 pkg. 450
  fajita *(Hot Pockets)*, 4.5-oz. piece 360
  hamburger *(Hormel Quick Meal)*, 1 pkg. 350
  hamburger *(White Castle)*, 2 pieces, 3.2 oz. 270
  patty, with cheese *(Kid Cuisine Buckaroo)*, 8.5-oz. pkg. 410
  steak, biscuit *(Hormel Quick Meal)*, 1 pkg. 320
  steak, cheese *(Deli Stuffs)*, 4.5-oz. piece 370

Sandwiches, Frozen or Refrigerated, beef *(cont.)*
    steak, mushroom *(Mrs. Paterson's Aussie Pie)*, 1 pkg. 420
    steak, Philly, and cheese *(Croissant Pockets)*, 4.5-oz. piece . 370
broccoli and cheddar pocket *(Ken & Robert's Veggie Pockets)*,
    1 piece 250
broccoli and cheese *(Stuffed Breads)*, 6-oz. piece 450
broccoli-cheese, in pastry *(Pepperidge Farm)*, 1 piece 240
calzone:
    cheese *(Stefano's)*, 6-oz. piece 510
    pepperoni *(Stefano's)*, 6-oz. piece 520
    spinach *(Stefano's)*, 6-oz. piece 440
cheese, grilled *(Swanson Fun Feast)* 1 pkg. 460
chicken:
    (Hormel Quick Meal), 1 pkg. 340
    (Kid Cuisine Super Charging), 9.4-oz. pkg. 480
    (Schwan's), 3.3-oz. piece 200
    broccoli supreme *(Lean Pockets)*, 4.5-oz. piece 240
    broccoli and cheddar *(Croissant Pockets)*, 4.5-oz. piece . . . 300
    broccoli and cheddar *(Schwan's)*, 4.4-oz. piece 300
    and cheddar with broccoli *(Hot Pockets)*, 4.5-oz. piece 300
    fajita *(Lean Pockets)*, 4.5-oz. piece 260
    fajita *(Totino's* Big & Hearty), 4.8-oz. piece 270
    grilled *(Hormel Quick Meal)*, 1 pkg. 300
    grilled *(Tyson* Microwave), 3.45 oz. 210
    Parmesan *(Lean Pockets)*, 4.5-oz. piece 260
    pastry *(Mrs. Paterson's Aussie Pie)*, 1 piece 460
empanadilla, *see "Appetizers & Snacks, Frozen or*
    Refrigerated," page 153
fish fillet *(Hormel Quick Meal)*, 1 pkg. 400
fish fillet, with cheese *(Mrs. Paul's)*, 1 piece 330
frankfurter, 1 piece:
    (Hormel Quick Meal Jumbo Dog) 350
    bagel wrapped *(Boar's Head* Bagel Dog) 310
    bagel wrapped *(Hebrew National* Bagel Dog) 400
    bagel wrapped, with cheese *(Schwan's)*, 4.5-oz. piece 350
    on bun *(Swanson Fun Feast)* 350
    with cheese *(Hormel Quick Meal* Cheesey Dog) 310
    chili with cheese *(Hormel Quick Meal)* 350
    corn dog *(Hormel/Hormel Quick Meal)* 220
    corn dog *(Schwan's)*, 2.3-oz. piece 190
ham and cheese:
    (Croissant Pockets), 4.5-oz. piece 360
    (Deli Stuffs), 4.5-oz. piece 350

(Hormel Quick Meal), 1 pkg. 330
(Hot Pockets), 4.5-oz. piece 340
(Schwan's), 4.4-oz. piece 290
(Totino's Big & Hearty)*, 4.8-oz. piece 310
bologna and salami *(Schwan's Ranchero)*, 5.5-oz. piece . . . 400
croissant *(Sara Lee)*, 1 piece 300
and turkey *(Schwan's* Croissant)*, 4-oz. piece 310
pepperoni:
    (Schwan's), 4.4-oz. piece 330
    bagel *(Hormel Quick Meal)*, 1 pkg. 350
    and cheese *(Stuffed Breads)*, 6-oz. piece 610
pizza:
    (Amy's Pocketfuls), 4.5-oz. piece 290
    (Deli Stuffs), 4.5-oz. piece 370
    meat, mega *(Totino's* Big & Hearty)*, 4.8-oz. piece . . . 330
    pepperoni *(Croissant Pockets)*, 4.5-oz. piece 350
    pepperoni *(Hot Pockets)*, 4.5-oz. piece 350
    pepperoni *(Totino's* Big & Hearty)*, 4.8-oz. piece 350
    pepperoni, deluxe *(Lean Pockets)*, 4.5-oz. piece 280
    pepperoni and sausage or sausage *(Hot Pockets)*,
        4.5-oz. piece 340
    vegetable *(Ken & Robert's Veggie Pockets)*, 1 piece . . . 270
    vegetable, pepperoni style *(Amy's Pocketfuls)*, 4.5-oz. piece . 220
pork, barbecued *(Hormel Quick Meal)*, 1 piece 350
potato and cheddar *(Ken & Robert's Veggie Pockets)*, 1 piece . 260
spinach and feta cheese *(Amy's Pocketfuls)*, 4.5-oz. piece 200
turkey:
    with broccoli *(Mrs. Paterson's Aussie Pie)*, 1 piece 470
    with broccoli and cheese *(Lean Pockets)*, 4.5-oz. piece 260
    and ham with cheese *(Hot Pockets)*, 4.5-oz. piece 320
    and ham and cheese *(Lean Pockets)*, 4.5-oz. piece 270
    and Swiss *(Croissant Pockets)*, 4.5-oz. piece 300
vegetable, 1 piece:
    barbecue *(Veggie Pockets* Bar-B-Q)* 290
    broccoli & cheddar, Greek, Oriental, potpie, or Santa Fe
        (Veggie Pockets) 250
    Indian or potato and cheddar *(Veggie Pockets)* 260
    pizza *(Veggie Pockets)* 270
    potpie *(Amy's Pocketfuls)*, 5-oz. piece 230
    Tex-Mex *(Veggie Pockets)* 280

Chapter 14

FATS, OILS, AND SALAD DRESSINGS

FATS & OILS, one tablespoon, except as noted

	calories
butter:	
(Land O' Lakes Light)	50
(Land O' Lakes Salted/Unsalted)	100
clarified *(Parity Farms* Ghee), 1 tsp.	45
chicken fat, rendered *(Empire* Kosher)	120
fat, imitation *(Rokeach Nyafat)*	130
lard *(Goya)*	130
margarine:	
(Mazola/Mazola Unsalted)	100
(Mazola Light)	50
(Nucoa)	100
(Smart Beat Nonfat)	10
(Smart Beat Super Light/Trans Fat Free)	20
(Smart Beat Unsalted)	25
(Weight Watchers Light/Light Sodium Free)	45
soft *(Chiffon* Tub)	100
soft *(Parkay* Tub)	100
soft *(Parkay* Diet Tub)	50
spread *(I Can't Believe It's Not Butter* Light)	50
spread *(I Can't Believe It's Not Butter* Salted/Unsalted)	90
spread *(Kraft Touch of Butter* Stick)	90
spread *(Kraft Touch of Butter* Tub)	60
spread *(Land O' Lakes Country Morning* Light)	50
spread *(Land O' Lakes Country Morning* Salted/Unsalted)	100
spread *(Mazola* Light)	50
spread *(Parkay* Stick 53%)	70
spread *(Parkay* Stick 70%)	90
spread *(Parkay* Tub 50%)	60
spread *(Parkay Light* Tub 40%)	50
spread *(Shedd's Spread)*	70
spread, with sweet cream *(Land O' Lakes)*	90
squeeze *(Kraft Touch of Butter)*	80

squeeze *(Parkay)* 80
squeeze *(Smart Beat Smart Squeeze)* 5
whipped *(Chiffon Tub)* 70
whipped *(Parkay Tub)* .70
oil:
    all varieties and blends *(Crisco)* 120
    all varieties and blends *(Wesson)* 122
    corn, all varieties *(Goya)* 120
    corn or canola/corn *(Mazola)* 120
    olive, all varieties *(Progresso)* 120
    Oriental cooking *(House of Tsang Mongolian*
      Fire/Saigon Sizzle), 1 tsp. 45
    peanut or popcorn *(Planters)* 120
    popcorn, popping and topping *(Orville Redenbacher)* 120
    sesame, toasted or hot pepper *(Eden)* 130
    sesame, regular or hot chili *(House of Tsang)*, 1 tsp. 45
    wok *(House of Tsang)* 130
oil substitute *(Baking Healthy)* 30
shortening:
    (Pillsbury Jewel/Snowdrift/Swiftening) 110
    vegetable, regular/butter flavor *(Crisco)* 110

SALAD DRESSINGS, two tablespoons, except as noted
See also "Salad Dressings, Mixes" and "Condiments & Sauces"

                                              calories

bacon and tomato *(Kraft)* 140
bacon and tomato *(Kraft Deliciously Right)* 60
balsamic vinegar *(S&W Vintage)* 35
berry vinaigrette *(Knott's Berry Farm)* 40
blue cheese:
    (Bernstein's Dressing/Dip) 180
    (Bernstein's Dressing/Dip Lite) 80
    (Kraft Free) 50
    (Kraft Roka) 90
    (Marie's Salad Bar Reduced Calorie) 100
    chunky *(Hellmann's)* 140
    chunky *(Marie's)* 180
    chunky *(Marie's Reduced Calorie)* 100
    chunky *(Seven Seas)* .90
    chunky *(Wish-Bone)* 170

Salad Dressings, blue cheese *(cont.)*
chunky *(Wish-Bone* Fat Free) 35
chunky *(Wish-Bone* Lite) .70
creamy *(Bernstein's)* 120
creamy *(Marie's* Low Fat) 30
vinaigrette *(Herb Magic)* 160
Caesar:
(*Bernstein's*) 100
(*Bernstein's* Extra Rich) 110
(*Cardini's* Original) 160
(*Hidden Valley Ranch* Fat Free) 30
(*Kraft*) 130
(*Kraft* Classic) 110
(*Kraft Deliciously Right*) 60
(*Salad Celebrations* Fat Free) 10
(*Wish-Bone*) 110
(*Wish-Bone* Fat Free) .25
creamy *(Hellmann's)* 170
creamy *(Seven Seas)* 140
creamy *(Seven Seas Viva)* 120
creamy *(Wish-Bone)* 180
creamy, with cracked pepper *(Lawry's)* 130
garlic, roasted *(Knott's Berry Farm)* 140
ranch *(Kraft)* 140
three cheese *(Salad Celebrations* Fat Free) 40
cheese *(Bernstein's* Fantastico!) 110
cheese *(Bernstein's Light Fantastic* Fantastico!) 30
chicken salad, Oriental *(Knott's Berry Farm)* 130
citrus vinaigrette *(Knott's Berry Farm)* 40
coleslaw *(Kraft)* 150
coleslaw *(Marie's)* 150
cucumber, creamy *(Herb Magic)* 15
Dijon *(see also "honey Dijon," below)*:
creamy *(Bernstein's Light Fantastic)* 50
vinaigrette, balsamic *(Pritikin)* 30
dill, creamy *(Bernstein's Light Fantastic)* 45
dill, creamy *(Nasoya Vegi-Dressing)* 60
French:
(*Hellmann's* Fat Free) .45
(*Kraft*) 120
(*Kraft Catalina*) 140
(*Kraft Deliciously Right*) 50

(Kraft Deliciously Right Catalina) 80
(Kraft Free) 50
(Kraft Free Catalina) .45
(Nalley) 110
(Salad Celebrations Fat Free) 40
(Wish-Bone Deluxe) 120
(Wish-Bone Lite) 50
herbal, creamy *(Bernstein's)* 130
with honey *(Kraft Catalina)* 140
honey *(Pritikin)* 40
honey and bacon *(Hidden Valley Ranch)* 150
style *(Pritikin)* 35
style *(Wish-Bone Fat Free Deluxe)* 30
sweet 'n spicy *(Wish-Bone)* 140
sweet 'n spicy *(Wish-Bone Fat Free)* 30
tangy *(Marie's)* 130
vinaigrette, true *(Herb Magic)* 170
fruit salad *(Knott's Berry Farm)* 70
fruit vinaigrette *(Knott's Berry Farm)* 45
garden, zesty *(Kraft Salsa)* 70
garlic:
    creamy *(Kraft)* 110
    creamy *(Wish-Bone Fat Free)* 40
    roasted, creamy *(Wish-Bone)* 110
    zesty *(Cardini's)* 120
green goddess *(Seven Seas)* 120
herb, garden *(Nasoya Vegi-Dressing)* 60
herb, Italian, and cheese *(Hidden Valley Ranch Fat Free)* 30
herb vinaigrette, zesty *(Marie's Fat Free)* 30
herbs and spices *(Seven Seas)* 120
honey Dijon:
    (Hellmann's Fat Free) 50
    (Hidden Valley Ranch Fat Free) 35
    (Kraft) 150
    (Kraft Free) 50
    (Pritikin) 45
    (Salad Celebrations Fat Free) 45
    (Wish-Bone Fat Free) 45
    vinaigrette, zesty *(Marie's Fat Free)* 50
honey mustard:
    (Bernstein's Dressing/Dip) 130
    (Knott's Berry Farm) 130

Salad Dressings, honey mustard *(cont.)*
  (Marie's) 160
  (Nalley) 130
Italian:
  (Bernstein's) 140
  (Bernstein's Reduced Calorie) 25
  (Bernstein's Restaurant) 80
  (Bernstein's Wine Country) 110
  (Bernstein's Light Fantastic) 40
  (Hellmann's) 110
  (Herb Magic) 10
  (Kraft House) 120
  (Kraft Oil/Fat Free) 5
  (Kraft Presto) 140
  (Kraft Deliciously Right) 70
  (Kraft Free) 10
  (Ott's Zesty) 90
  (Pritikin) 20
  (Salad Celebrations Fat Free) 10
  (Seven Seas Free) 10
  (Seven Seas Viva) 110
  (Seven Seas Viva Reduced Calorie) 45
  (Wish-Bone) 80
  (Wish-Bone Classic House) 140
  (Wish-Bone Fat Free) 10
  (Wish-Bone Lite) 15
  (Wish-Bone Robusto) 90
  with cheese *(Bernstein's* Reduced Calorie) . . .25
  cheese, 2 *(Seven Seas)* 70
  cheese and garlic *(Bernstein's)* 110
  creamy *(Hellmann's)* 160
  creamy *(Kraft)* 110
  creamy *(Kraft Deliciously Right)* 50
  creamy *(Nasoya Vegi-Dressing)* 60
  creamy *(Salad Celebrations* Fat Free) 30
  creamy *(Seven Seas)* 110
  creamy *(Seven Seas* Reduced Calorie) 60
  creamy *(Wish-Bone)* 110
  creamy *(Wish-Bone* Fat Free) 35
  garlic, creamy *(Marie's)* 180
  garlic, creamy *(Marie's* Reduced Calorie) 90
  herb, creamy *(Marie's* Low Fat) 30

herb and garlic, creamy *(Bernstein's)* 130
olive oil *(Seven Seas* Reduced Calorie) 50
vinaigrette, zesty *(Marie's* Fat Free) 35
zesty *(Kraft)* 110
Italian Parmesan *(Hidden Valley Ranch* Fat Free) 20
mango–key lime vinegar *(S&W* Vintage Lite) 30
mayonnaise, 1 tbsp.:
    (Best Foods Real) 100
    (Blue Plate) 100
    (Hellmann's Real) 100
    (Hellmann's/Best Foods Light) 50
    (Hellmann's/Best Foods Low Fat) 25
    (Kraft Real) 100
    (Master Choice) 100
    (Nalley Real) 100
    (Nalley Light) 50
    (Nalley Cholesterol Free) 40
    (Smart Beat Super Light Reduced Fat) 35
    (Weight Watchers Light/Light Low Sodium) 25
    canola *(Smart Beat* Reduced Fat) 35
    tofu *(Nayonaise)* .35
mayonnaise-type dressing, 1 tbsp.:
    (Kraft Free) 10
    (Kraft Light) 50
    (Miracle Whip Salad) 70
    (Miracle Whip Free) 15
    (Miracle Whip Light) 40
    (Nalley Whip) 60
    (Nayonaise Vegi-Dressing & Spread Fat Free) 10
    (Smart Beat Nonfat) 10
    (Spin Blend) 60
    (Spin Blend Nonfat) 15
    (Weight Watchers Fat Free) 10
    whipped *(Weight Watchers* Fat Free) 15
olive oil vinaigrette *(Wish-Bone)* 60
Oriental *(Bernstein's Light Fantastic)* 60
Oriental rice wine vinegar *(S&W* Vintage Lite) 30
(Ott's Famous Original) .80
(Ott's Famous Fat Free) .35
(Ott's Famous Reduced Calorie) 60
pesto *(Cardini's* Pata) 140
Parmesan, creamy *(Marie's* Low Fat) 35

Salad Dressings *(cont.)*
Parmesan and onion *(Wish-Bone)* 110
Parmesan and onion *(Wish-Bone* Fat Free) 45
peppercorn, ground *(Knott's Berry Farm)* 160
poppy seed:
    (Herb Magic) 170
    (Knott's Berry Farm) 120
    (Marie's) 150
    (Ott's Fat Free) 45
    (Ott's Reduced Calorie) 90
potato salad *(Best Foods/Hellmann's One Step)* 160
potato salad *(Best Foods/Hellmann's One Step* ⅓ Less Fat) . . . 110
ranch:
    (Bernstein's Dressing/Dip) 110
    (Bernstein's Dressing/Dip Lite) 70
    (Bernstein's Light Fantastic) 35
    (Hellmann's Fat Free) .45
    (Herb Magic) 15
    (Hidden Valley Ranch Original) 140
    (Kraft) 170
    (Kraft Deliciously Right) 110
    (Kraft Free) 50
    (Kraft Salsa) 130
    (Marie's Salad Bar Reduced Calorie) 90
    (Nalley) 100
    (Nalley Fat Free) 40
    (Ott's Buttermilk) 140
    (Salad Celebrations Fat Free) 35
    (Seven Seas) 150
    (Seven Seas Reduced Calorie) 100
    (Seven Seas Free) 50
    (Wish-Bone) 160
    (Wish-Bone Fat Free) .40
    (Wish-Bone Lite) 100
    with bacon *(Hidden Valley Ranch* Original) 150
    buttermilk *(Kraft)* 150
    buttermilk *(Marie's)* 180
    cucumber *(Kraft)* 150
    cucumber *(Kraft Deliciously Right)* 60
    creamy *(Hellmann's)* 140
    creamy *(Marie's* Reduced Calorie) 100
    Italian *(Bernstein's)* 150

Parmesan *(Marie's)* 180
Parmesan garlic *(Bernstein's)* 110
Parmesan garlic *(Bernstein's Light Fantastic)* 45
peppercorn *(Kraft)* 170
peppercorn *(Kraft Free)* 50
sour cream and onion *(Kraft)* 170
zesty *(Marie's Low Fat)* 30
raspberry blush vinegar *(S&W Vintage Lite)* 40
raspberry vinaigrette:
  (Knott's Berry Farm Low Fat) 50
  (Pritikin) 45
  zesty *(Marie's Fat Free)* 35
red wine vinaigrette:
  (Wish-Bone) 80
  (Wish-Bone Fat Free) 35
  zesty *(Marie's Fat Free)* 40
red wine vinegar:
  (Kraft Free) 15
  (Seven Seas Free) 15
  with herbs *(S&W Vintage Lite)* 40
  and oil *(Seven Seas)* 110
  and oil *(Seven Seas Reduced Calorie)* 60
Roquefort *(Bernstein's Dressing/Dip)* 140
Russian:
  (Kraft) 130
  (Salad Celebrations Fat Free) 45
  (Seven Seas Viva) 150
  (Wish-Bone) 110
salsa and sour cream *(Bernstein's Dressing/Dip)* 90
sesame garlic *(Nasoya Vegi-Dressing)* 60
sour cream and dill *(Marie's)* 190
sweet and sour *(Herb Magic)* 35
sweet and sour *(Old Dutch)* 50
Thousand Island:
  (Bernstein's Dressing/Dip) 120
  (Herb Magic) 15
  (Kraft) 110
  (Kraft Deliciously Right) 70
  (Kraft Free) 45
  (Marie's) 240
  (Marie's Salad Bar) 170
  (Nalley) 120

Salad Dressings, Thousand Island *(cont.)*
  (Nalley Fat Free) 30
  (Nasoya Vegi-Dressing) 60
  (Salad Celebrations Fat Free) 45
  (Wish-Bone) 140
  (Wish-Bone Fat Free) 35
  (Wish-Bone Lite) 80
  with bacon *(Kraft)* 120
tomato, sun-dried, vinaigrette *(Knott's Berry Farm)* 100
tuna salad *(Best Foods/Hellmann's One Step)* 140
vinaigrette *(Herb Magic)* 10
white wine vinaigrette, zesty *(Marie's* Fat Free) 40
white wine vinegar with herbs *(S&W* Vintage Lite) 40

SALAD DRESSINGS, MIXES, two tablespoons*
See also "Salad Dressings"

	calories
buttermilk, farm *(Good Seasons)*	120
Caesar, gourmet *(Good Seasons)*	150
cheese garlic or garlic and herbs *(Good Seasons)*	140
herb, zesty *(Good Seasons* Free)	.10
honey mustard *(Good Seasons)*	150
honey mustard *(Good Seasons* Free)	.20

Italian:
  (Good Seasons) 140
  (Good Seasons Free) 10
  (Good Seasons Reduced Calorie) 50
  creamy *(Good Seasons* Free) 20
  mild *(Good Seasons)* 150
  zesty *(Good Seasons)* 140
  zesty *(Good Seasons* Reduced Calorie) 50
Mexican spice *(Good Seasons)* 140
Oriental sesame *(Good Seasons)* 150
ranch *(Good Seasons)* 120
ranch *(Good Seasons* Reduced Calorie) 60

---

* Prepared according to package directions

Chapter 15

CONDIMENTS, SAUCES, GRAVIES, AND SEASONINGS

> **CONDIMENTS & SAUCES**
> *See also "Tomato Paste, Puree, & Sauce," "Pickles, Cucumber," "Pickle Relish, Cucumber," "Soups, Mixes," "Dips," "Salsa," "Appetizers & Snacks, Canned or in Jars," "Salad Dressings," "Barbecue Sauces," "Pasta Sauces," "Sauces, Mixes," "Gravies, Canned or in Jars," and "Seasonings, Dry & Mixes"*

calories

bacon bits, 1 tbsp., except as noted:
(Hormel)	.30
(Hormel Pieces)	.25
(Oscar Mayer/Oscar Mayer Pieces)	.25
imitation (Bac'n Pieces), 1½ tbsp.	.30
imitation (Bac-Os)	.30
imitation (Durkee)	0
imitation chips (Durkee)	0
bean sauce, brown, spicy (House of Tsang), 1 tsp.	.15
biryani paste (Patak's), 2 tbsp.	160
black bean garlic sauce (Lee Kum Kee), 1 tbsp.	.25
broth concentrate, beef or vegetable flavor (Knorr), 2 tsp.	5
brown gravy sauce (La Choy), ¼ cup	275
browning sauce (Gravy Master), ¼ tsp.	.10
burrito sauce (Hunt's Manwich), ¼ cup	.25

capers:
(B&G), 1 tbsp.	5
(Crosse & Blackwell), 1 tbsp.	5
(Krinos), 1 tsp.	0
(Progresso), 1 tsp.	0
with pimientos (Goya), ¼ cup	.25

cheese sauce:
(Cheez Whiz Squeezable), 2 tbsp.	100
(Cheez Whiz Zap-A-Pack), 2 tbsp.	.90

Condiments & Sauces, cheese sauce *(cont.)*
   (Franco-American), ¼ cup 40
   all varieties *(Kaukauna Micro Melt)*, 2 tbsp. 80
   Mexican cheddar, mild *(Gracias Cheese Fantastico!)*, ¼ cup . 100
   nacho *(Kaukauna)*, 2 tbsp. .80
   nacho, medium *(Gracias Cheese Fantastico!)*, ¼ cup 90
   nacho jalapeño, hot *(Gracias Cheese Fantastico!)*, ¼ cup 90
   salsa *(Cheez Whiz Zap-A-Pack)*, 2 tbsp. 90
chicken sauce:
   barbecue flavor *(Hunt's Chicken Sensations)*, 1 tbsp. 35
   Caesar *(Lawry's)*, 2 tbsp. .30
   Dijon, country *(Lawry's Chicken Saute)*, 2 tbsp. 40
   garlic Italian *(Lawry's Chicken Saute)*, 2 tbsp. 30
   Italian garlic *(Hunt's Chicken Sensations)*, 1 tbsp. 30
   lemon herb *(Hunt's Chicken Sensations)*, 1 tbsp. 30
   lemon herb *(Lawry's Chicken Saute)*, 2 tbsp. 25
   sherried *(Lawry's)*, 1 tbsp. .20
   Southwestern *(Hunt's Chicken Sensations)*, 1 tbsp. 30
   teriyaki *(Lawry's Chicken Saute)*, 2 tbsp. 40
   Thai, satay *(Lawry's)*, 1 tbsp. 35
   wing *(Stubb's Legendary Original/Inferno)*, 1 tbsp. 10
   wing, Buffalo style *(World Harbors Hot Zings)*, 2 tbsp. 30
   wing, hot *(Nance's)*, 2 tbsp. 15
   wing, mild *(Nance's)*, 2 tbsp. 20
chicken simmer sauce, ½ cup:
   cacciatore or herbed, with wine *(Ragú Chicken Tonight)* . . .80
   country French *(Ragú Chicken Tonight)* 130
   creamy, with mushrooms *(Ragú Chicken Tonight)* 110
   creamy, primavera *(Ragú Chicken Tonight)* 90
   sweet and sour *(Ragú Chicken Tonight)* 120
chili pepper pickle relish *(Patak's)*, 1 tbsp. 45
chili sauce:
   (Del Monte), 1 tbsp. 20
   (Heinz), 1 tbsp. 15
   (Las Palmas), ¼ cup 15
   (Nance's), 2 tbsp. 25
   (S&W Steakhouse), 1 tbsp. 15
   hot dog *(Gebhardt)*, ¼ cup .60
   hot dog *(Just Rite)*, 2 oz. 50
   hot dog *(Wolf)*, 1 tbsp. 15
   hot dog, with beef *(Stenger)*, ¼ cup 70
chowchow pickle *(Crosse & Blackwell)*, 1 tbsp. 10

chowchow pickle *(Stubb's Legendary* Original/Spicy), ½ cup . . .70
chutney:
    mango *(Patak's* Major Grey's), 1 tbsp. 50
    tomato, dried *(Sonoma)*, 1 tbsp. 35
    tropical fruit and nut *(Patak's)*, 1 tbsp. 60
cocktail sauce, *see "seafood sauce, cocktail," below*
coconut cream, canned:
    (Coco Casa), 3 tbsp. 170
    (Coco Goya), 1 tbsp. 140
    (Coco Lopez), 3 tbsp. 170
coconut milk, canned, ¼ cup, except as noted:
    (Goya), 1 tbsp. 50
    (Taste of Thai) 110
    light *(Taste of Thai)* 36
corn relish:
    (Green Giant), 1 tbsp. 20
    (Nance's), 2 tbsp. 25
    (Pickle Eater's), 1 tbsp. .20
cranberry-orange relish *(New England)*, ¼ cup 120
cucumber pickle, *see "Pickles, Cucumber," page 121*
cucumber relish, *see "Pickle Relish, Cucumber," page 122*
curry paste *(Patak's)*, 2 tbsp. 170
curry sauce:
    (Kylin Thai), ¼ cup 25
    hot, Madras *(Patak's)*, ½ cup 300
    hot, tikka masala *(Patak's)*, ½ cup 240
    hot, vindaloo *(Patak's)*, ½ cup 320
    jalfrezzi *(Patak's)*, ½ cup 160
    masala *(Shahi* Cream), ¼ cup 50
    masala *(Shahi* Curry), ¼ cup 50
    rogan josh *(Patak's)*, ½ cup 190
diable sauce *(Escoffier)*, 1 tbsp. 20
duck sauce, *see "sweet and sour sauce," below*
eggplant pickle relish *(Patak's* Brinjal), 1 tbsp. 60
enchilada sauce, ¼ cup:
    (Chi-Chi's) 30
    (La Victoria) 20
    (Rosarita) 25
    all varieties *(Old El Paso)* 30
    green chili *(Las Palmas)* .25
    green chili *(Old El Paso)* .30
    original or hot *(Las Palmas)* 15

Condiments & Sauces *(cont.)*
fajita sauce:
    (S&W Southwestern), 1 tbsp. .10
    and marinade *(World Harbors* Guadalupe), 2 tbsp. 50
    skillet *(Lawry's),* 2 tbsp. 15
garlic dressing *(Christopher Ranch),* 1 tbsp. 53
garlic pickle relish *(Patak's),* 1 tbsp. 45
garlic spread *(Lawry's* Concentrate), 2 tsp. 50
garlic spread *(Lawry's* Ready-to-Spread), 1 tbsp. 100
garlic-basil, chopped *(Paesana),* 1 tsp. 6
ginger, pickled *(Eden),* 1 tbsp. 15
grilling sauce:
    Chardonnay or Tuscan herb *(Knorr),* 2 tbsp. 35
    mandarin ginger *(Knorr* Microwave), 2 tbsp. 45
    Parmesano *(Knorr* Microwave), 3 tbsp. 50
    plum, spicy *(Knorr),* 2 tbsp. .50
    tequila lime *(Knorr),* 2 tbsp. .40
ham glaze *(Crosse & Blackwell),* 1 tbsp. 30
ham glaze *(Marzetti),* 2 tbsp. 35
hoisin sauce *(House of Tsang),* 1 tsp. 15
hoisin sauce *(Lee Kum Kee),* 2 tbsp. 100
hollandaise grilling sauce *(Knorr* Microwave), 2 tbsp. 45
honey hickory sauce *(World Harbors* Ember Wisp), 2 tbsp. . . .45
honey mustard *(Grey Poupon),* 1 tsp. 10
honey mustard, California style *(Rice Road),* 1 tbsp. 20
horseradish, prepared, 1 tsp., except as noted:
    (Boar's Head) 0
    (Heluva Good) 0
    (Kraft) 0
    cream style *(Kraft)* 0
    red *(Gold's)* 0
    red *(Hebrew National),* ½ cup 25
    red *(Rosoff),* 1 tbsp. 8
    white *(Rosoff),* 1 tbsp. 7
horseradish sauce:
    (Heinz), 1 tsp. 25
    (Reese), 2 tbsp. 100
    (Sauceworks), 2 tbsp. 20
jalapeño relish *(Old El Paso),* 1 tbsp. 5
jerk sauce *(World Harbors* Blue Mountain), 2 tbsp. 80
ketchup, 1 tbsp.:
    (Del Monte) 15

(Healthy Choice)	.10
(Heinz)	.15
(Heinz Hot)	.20
(Hunt's/Hunt's No Salt)	.15
(Smucker's)	.25
lemon sauce *(House of Tsang)*, 2 tbsp.	.70
lemon pepper garlic sauce *(World Harbors)*, 2 tbsp.	.35
marinade:	
(House of Tsang Classic), ½ tbsp.	.15
(House of Tsang Mandarin), 1 tbsp.	.25
(Stubb's Legendary Moppin' Sauce), 1 tbsp.	.30
Hawaiian *(Lawry's)*, 1 tbsp.	.20
hickory grill *(Adolph's* Marinade in Minutes), 1 tbsp.	.20
honey Dijon *(World Harbors)*, 2 tbsp.	.35
lemon garlic *(Adolph's* Marinade in Minutes), 1 tbsp.	.30
lemon pepper *(Lawry's)*, 1 tbsp.	.10
mesquite *(Adolph's* Marinade in Minutes), 1 tbsp.	.45
red wine *(Lawry's)*, 1 tbsp.	5
and stir-fry sauce *(Mary Rose* Sari), 1 tbsp.	5
teriyaki *(Adolph's* Marinade in Minutes), 1 tbsp.	.20
mayonnaise, *see "Salad Dressings," page 247*	
mesquite *(S&W)*, 1 tbsp.	.10
mint sauce *(Crosse & Blackwell)*, 1 tsp.	5
miso, soy, 1 tbsp.:	
(Eden Organic Hacho)	.35
with barley *(Eden* Organic Mugi)	.25
with brown rice *(Eden* Organic Genmai)	.25
sweet white *(Eden* Organic Shiro)	.35
mushroom sauce *(House of Tsang)*, 1 tbsp.	.10
mustard, prepared, 1 tsp., except as noted:	
(Boar's Head Deli)	0
(French's Deli)	5
(French's Yellow)	0
(Grey Poupon Classic Deli/Spicy)	5
(Gulden's Spicy)	0
(Kraft Pure)	0
all varieties *(Hebrew National* Deli)	0
all varieties *(Nance's)*	.15
Chinese *(House of Tsang)*, 1 pkt.	.15
Dijon *(Bornier* Genuine)	5
Dijon *(French's)*	5
Dijon *(Grey Poupon)*	5

Condiments & Sauces, mustard, prepared *(cont.)*
Dijon *(Roland* Extra Strong) .10
   with honey, *see "honey mustard," above*
   horseradish *(Kraft)* 0
   horseradish or peppercorn *(Grey Poupon)* 5
   hot *(Eden* Organic) 0
mustard blend *(Best Foods/Hellmann's Dijonnaise),* 1 tsp. 5
olive, *see "Olives," page 123*
orange sauce, mandarin *(Ka-Me),* 2 tbsp. 80
Oriental sauce *(see also specific sauce listings):*
   (House of Tsang Chow Chow), 1 tsp. 5
   (House of Tsang Imperial), 1 tbsp. 25
   (House of Tsang Namasu), 1 tsp. 10
   brown, spicy *(House of Tsang),* 1 tsp. 15
   hot and spicy *(House of Tsang* Hunan), 1 tsp. 5
oyster and shrimp sauce *(Try Me* Caribbean Clipper), 1 tsp. . . .10
peanut sauce, cooking *(Kylin Singapore Satay),* ¼ cup 60
peanut sauce, Oriental *(House of Tsang Bangkok Padang),*
   1 tbsp. 45
pepper, white *(McCormick),* ¼ tsp. 2
pepper, white *(Tone's),* ¼ tsp. 0
pepper sauce, hot:
   (Durkee RedHot), 1 tsp. 0
   (Frank's Original Red Hot), 1 tsp. 0
   (Gebhardt), 1 tsp. 0
   (Goya), 1 tsp. 0
   (Pickapeppa), 1 tbsp. 18
   (Tabasco), 1 tsp. 0
   (Try Me Cajun/Tennessee Sunshine), 1 tsp. 0
   (Try Me Tiger), 1 tsp. 10
   jalapeño or garlic *(Tabasco),* 1 tsp. 0
   hot or original *(Hunt's),* 1 tsp. 0
   in vinegar *(Goya),* 1 tsp. 0
peppers, condiment, *see "Vegetables, Canned or in Jars,"*
   page 103
picante sauce *(see also "Salsa," page 151),* 2 tbsp.:
   (Pace) 10
   all varieties *(Hunt's* Homestyle) 10
   all varieties *(Old El Paso* Thick 'n Chunky) 10
   black bean or black-eyed pea *(Arthur's)* 15
   garlic, with corn and honey *(Arthur's)* 15
   hot *(Chi-Chi's)* 10

hot *(Sun-Vista)* 10
hot or mild *(Arthur's)* 10
jalapeño, zesty, hot, medium, or mild *(Rosarita)* 10
medium *(Chi-Chi's)* 10
medium *(Nalley* Superba) .10
mesquite *(Arthur's)* 10
mild *(Chi-Chi's)* 10
mild *(Gracias* Picante Superba) 5
mild *(Nalley* Superba) 5
mild *(Sun-Vista)* 5
pizza sauce, ¼ cup:
   (Contadina) 25
   (Contadina Chunky) 30
   (Contadina Pizza Squeeze) 35
   (Pastorelli Italian Chef) 40
   (Prince Traditional) 20
   (Progresso) 35
   (Ragu Quick) 40
   with cheese, Italian *(Contadina)* 30
   with cheese, Italian *(Contadina Pizza Squeeze)* 40
   with cheese, three *(Contadina* Chunky) 35
   mushroom *(Contadina* Chunky) 30
   pepperoni *(Contadina)* .30
plum sauce *(Ka-Me)*, 2 tbsp. 80
plum sauce *(La Choy)*, 1 tbsp. 25
raisin sauce *(Reese)*, ¼ cup 150
remoulade sauce *(Zararain's)*, ¼ cup 80
salsa, *see "Salsa," page 150*
sandwich dressing, 2 tbsp.:
   garden onion, bell pepper, or jalapeño salsa *(Vlasic*
     Sandwich Zesters) 15
   Italian tomato or mushroom and onion *(Vlasic Sandwich*
     Zesters) 10
sandwich sauce, ¼ cup, except as noted:
   (Hunt's Manwich Bold) 60
   (Manwich Original) 30
   (Hunt's Manwich Thick & Chunky) 45
   barbecue *(Hunt's Manwich)* 60
   Mexican *(Hunt's Manwich)* 25
   sloppy joe *(Del Monte* Original/Hickory Flavor) 70
   sloppy joe *(Green Giant)* 50
   sloppy joe *(Heinz)*, ½ cup 70

Condiments & Sauces, sandwich sauce *(cont.)*
   sloppy joe *(Hormel Not-So-Sloppy Joe* Sauce) 70
   sloppy joe *(Libby's),* ⅓ cup 45
   sloppy joe, and meat *(Green Giant)* 200
sandwich spread:
   (Blue Plate), 1 tbsp. 75
   (Durkee Famous), 1 tbsp. 60
   (Hellmann's), 1 tbsp. .50
   (Kraft Spread & Burger Sauce), 1 tbsp. 50
   (Loma Linda), ¼ cup .80
seafood marinade, lemon butter dill *(Ken's Steak House),*
   1 tbsp. 50
seafood sauce, cocktail, ¼ cup, except as noted:
   (Bookbinder's Restaurant Style) 70
   (Crosse & Blackwell) 110
   (Del Monte) 100
   (Heinz) 60
   (Heluva Good) 40
   (Maull's), 2 tbsp. 45
   (Nalley) 65
   (S&W), 1 tsp. 20
   (Sauceworks) 60
   hot and spicy *(Bookbinder's)* 70
shrimp sauce *(Crosse & Blackwell),* ¼ cup 110
soup base *(Goya* Recaito), 1 tsp. 3
soup base *(Goya* Sofrito), 1 tsp. 5
soy sauce, 1 tbsp., except as noted:
   (La Choy) 10
   (La Choy Lite) 15
   (House of Tsang), .5-oz. pkt. 5
   (House of Tsang Light/Low Sodium) 5
   (Kikkoman/Kikkoman Light) 10
   dark *(House of Tsang)* .10
   ginger flavor *(House of Tsang)* 20
   ginger or mushroom flavor *(House of Tsang* Low Sodium) . . .10
   hot *(Try Me Dragon Sauce),* 1 tsp. 5
   shoyu *(Eden* Organic/Traditional Imported) 15
   shoyu *(Eden* Reduced Sodium) 10
   tamari *(Eden* Organic Domestic) 15
   tamari *(Eden* Organic Imported) 10
steak sauce, 1 tbsp.:
   (A.1.) 15

(A.1. Bold) 20
(A.1. Thick and Hearty) 25
(Alanna Irish) 15
(Heinz Traditional) 10
(Heinz 57) 15
(HP) 15
(Hunt's) 10
(Maull's) 20
(Texas Best) 15
(Trappey's Great American) 16
and burger *(Try Me Bullfighter)* 15
Caribbean style *(Tabasco)* 15
garlic peppercorn *(Lea & Perrins)* 25
New Orleans style *(Tabasco)* 10
New Orleans style *(Trappey's Chef-Magic)* 10
sweet, mild *(Maull's)* 20
sweet, spicy *(Lea & Perrins)* 25
stir-fry sauce, 1 tbsp., except as noted:
(House of Tsang Classic) .25
(House of Tsang Saigon Sizzle) 40
(House of Tsang Szechuan Spicy) 20
(Ka-Me) 10
(Ken's Steak House) 20
(Kikkoman) 15
(Lawry's) 25
(S&W Oriental) 20
garlic and ginger *(Rice Road)* 25
honey *(Ken's Steak House)* 20
lemon *(Rice Road)* 16
mandarin soy *(La Choy)*, ½ cup 70
and marinade *(Mary Rose* Halu) 25
and rib, garlic *(Mi-Kee)* .30
sesame and ginger *(Rice Road)* 15
spicy *(La Choy* Szechwan), ½ cup 85
sweet and sour *(House of Tsang)* 35
sweet and sour, spicy *(La Choy)*, ½ cup 140
teriyaki *(La Choy)*, ½ cup 95
teriyaki *(Rice Road)* 20
Stroganoff sauce, beef *(Lawry's)*, 1 tbsp. 20
sweet and sour sauce, 2 tbsp., except as noted:
(Contadina) 40
(House of Tsang) 30

Condiments & Sauces, sweet and sour sauce *(cont.)*
   (House of Tsang) .5-oz. pkt. 20
   (Kikkoman) 35
   (Kraft) 80
   (La Choy) 60
   (Sauceworks) 60
   (Woody's) 70
   (World Harbors Maui Mountain) 60
   concentrate *(House of Tsang)*, 1 tsp. 10
   chicken *(Gold's Dip'n Joy)*, 1 tbsp. 30
   duck sauce *(Ka-Me)* 80
   duck sauce *(La Choy)* 60
   duck sauce, all varieties *(Gold's)* 60
Szechwan sauce *(Ka-Me)*, 1 tbsp. 20
Szechwan sauce, cooking *(Kylin Chili & Tomato)*, ¼ cup 50
taco sauce, 1 tbsp., except as noted:
   (Chi-Chi's Thick & Chunky) .10
   (Hunt's Manwich), ¼ cup 30
   (Lawry's Chunky) 10
   (Lawry's Sauce'n Seasoner) .15
   (Pancho Villa), 2 tbsp. 15
   all varieties *(Old El Paso)* 5
   green *(La Victoria)* 0
   red *(La Victoria)* 5
tahini, sesame *(Joyva)*, 2 tbsp. 200
tamari sauce, *see "soy sauce," above*
tamarind pulp *(Frieda's Tamarindo)*, 1 oz. 68
tandoori paste, mild *(Patak's)*, 2 tbsp. 30
tartar sauce, 2 tbsp.:
   (Bookbinder's) 120
   (Heinz) 140
   (Hellmann's/Best Foods) 140
   (Hellmann's/Best Foods Low Fat) 40
   (Nalley) 190
   (Sauceworks) 100
   lemon herb flavor *(Sauceworks)* 150
teriyaki sauce, 1 tbsp., except as noted:
   (House of Tsang Korean Teriyaki) 30
   (La Choy/La Choy Lite) 20
   (Rice Road) 15
   barbecue *(Mary Rose Sumi)* 30
   baste and glaze *(Kikkoman)* 50

baste and glaze, with honey and pineapple *(Kikkoman)* 80
cooking, and marinade *(S&W/S&W Lite)* 25
hot *(La Choy* Chun King) 20
hot *(Mountain Harbors Maui Mountain)*, 2 tbsp. 70
marinade *(Lawry's)* 20
marinade and *(Kikkoman)* 15
marinade and *(Lea & Perrins)* 15
marinade and *(World Harbors Maui Mountain)*, 2 tbsp. 70
light *(Kikkoman)* 15
Thai sauce *(World Harbors* Nong Khai), 2 tbsp. 40
vinegar, 1 tbsp.:
    all varieties *(Progresso)* 0
    all varieties *(Regina)* 0
    all varieties *(S&W)* 0
    balsamic *(Pastorelli Italian Chef)* 5
    red wine *(Pastorelli Italian Chef)* 2
wine, cooking, 2 tbsp.:
    (La Vina Gold) 2
    all varieties except Marsala and sherry *(Holland House)* . . .20
    Marsala *(Holland House)* 35
    red or white *(La Vina)* 2
    sherry *(Holland House)* 45
Worcestershire sauce, 1 tsp.:
    (French's) 0
    (Heinz) 0
    (Lea & Perrins) 5
    white wine *(Lea & Perrins)* 0
    wine and pepper *(Try Me)* 0

BARBECUE SAUCES, two tablespoons, except as noted
See also "Condiments & Sauces" and "Seasonings, Dry & Mixes"

---

                                                calories

(Heinz Buffalo Wing) 15
(Heinz Thick & Rich Old Fashioned) 35
(Hunt's Light) 25
(Hunt's Original) 40
(Hunt's Original Bold) 45
(KC Masterpiece Original) 60
(Kraft Char-Grill) 60
(Kraft Original) 40

Barbecue Sauces *(cont.)*
(Kraft Original Extra Rich) 50
(Kraft Thick'N Spicy Original) 50
(Lea & Perrins Original/Bold & Spicy) 50
(Maull's) 40
(Mississippi) 60
(Open Pit Original) 50
(Woody's Cook-In') 50
all varieties *(Healthy Choice)* 25
all varieties *(Stubb's Legendary)* 25
Buffalo wing *(Heinz)* 15
Cajun *(Luzianne)* 110
Dijon, mild *(Hunt's)* 40
Dijon and honey *(Lawry's)* 60
garlic *(Kraft)* 40
garlic and herb *(Lea & Perrins)* 40
hickory:
   (Hunt's Bold) 45
   (Open Pit/Open Pit Thick and Tangy) 50
   and brown sugar *(Hunt's)* 75
   or honey hickory *(Hunt's)* 40
   hot *(Kraft)* 40
   with onion bits *(Kraft)* 50
hickory smoke:
   (Kraft) 40
   (Kraft Thick'N Spicy) 50
   (Open Pit) 50
honey:
   (Heinz Thick & Rich) .45
   (Kraft) 50
   (Kraft Thick'N Spicy) 60
   Dijon *(KC Masterpiece)* 50
   mustard *(Hunt's)* 45
   and spice *(Open Pit* Thick and Tangy) 45
hot *(Kraft)* 40
hot *(Open Pit)* 50
hot and spicy *(Hunt's)* .45
Italian *(Porino's)* 40
Italian seasonings *(Kraft)* 45
jalapeño *(Maull's)* 60
Kansas City style:
   (Kraft) 45

(Kraft Thick'N Spicy) 60
(Maull's) 60
mesquite *(Hunt's)* 40
mesquite *(Open Pit)* 50
mesquite smoke *(Kraft)* 40
mesquite smoke *(Kraft Thick'N Spicy)* 50
mild *(Hunt's)* 40
onion *(Open Pit/Open Pit* Thick and Tangy) 50
onion bits *(Kraft)* 50
onion bits *(Maull's)* 45
Oriental *(House of Tsang* Hong Kong), 1 tsp. 10
Oriental pork *(House of Tsang)* 90
salsa style *(Kraft)* 40
smokey *(Maull's)* 40
sweet *(Maull's* Sweet-N-Mild/*Maull's* Sweet-N-Smokey) 60
sweet *(Open Pit)* 50
sweet and sour *(Lawry's)* 80
sweet and sour *(Open Pit)* 45
teriyaki *(Hunt's)* 45
teriyaki *(Kraft)* 60
and marinade, tropical *(World Harbors Maui Mountain)* 50

PASTA SAUCES, ½ cup, except as noted
*See also "Tomato Paste, Puree, & Sauce," "Condiments &
Sauces," "Pasta Sauces, Refrigerated," and "Sauces, Mixes"*

calories

(Del Monte) 60
(Eden Organic/Organic No Salt/Pizza) 80
(Healthy Choice) 50
(Heinz Buffalo Wing) 15
(Hunt's Homestyle/Old Country) 55
(Hunt's Original) 65
(Paesana Casalinga) 70
(Patsy's Fileto di Pomodoro) 90
(Pomodoro Fresca Solo) 25
(Porino's) 130
(Prego) 140
(Prego Low Sodium) 110
(Prego Extra Chunky Tomato Supreme) 120
(Pritikin Original) 60
(Progresso) 100

Pasta Sauces *(cont.)*
(Ragú Light No Sugar) 60
(Ragú Old World Traditional) .80
Alfredo:
    (Five Brothers) 120
    (Progresso) 300
    (Ragú), ¼ cup 110
    three cheese *(Lawry's)*, 3 tbsp. 70
all varieties, except vegetable primavera *(Ragú Gardenstyle)* . . . 120
cheese, wine, and herbs *(Porino's)* 150
clam:
    creamy *(Progresso)* 100
    red *(Progresso)* 80
    white *(Bookbinder's)* 300
    white *(Progresso)* 130
    white *(Progresso* Authentic) 90
with basil:
    (Barilla) 70
    (Classico Di Napoli) 50
    (Del Monte) 60
    (Del Monte D'Italia) 50
    (Hunt's Classic) 50
    (Porino's) 100
    (Prego) 110
    summer *(Five Brothers)* 60
    zesty *(Prego Extra Chunky)* 110
beef or beef and pork *(Porino's)* 120
cheese:
    four *(Classico* Di Parma) 70
    four *(Del Monte* D'Italia) 60
    three *(Prego)* 100
cheese and garlic, Italian *(Hunt's)* 65
fra diavolo *(Patsy's)* 120
garden:
    (Porino's Chunky) 150
    (Porino's Gardina Fresca) 110
    (Pritikin Chunky) 50
    combination *(Prego Extra Chunky)* 90
    harvest *(Ragú* Light) 50
    style *(Del Monte)* 60
garlic *(Prego Extra Chunky* Supreme) 130
garlic and cheese *(Prego Extra Chunky)* 120

garlic and herb:
    (Del Monte) 60
    (Healthy Choice) .50
    (Hunt's Old Country) 65
garlic and onion:
    (Del Monte) 60
    (Healthy Choice Extra Chunky) 40
    (Hunt's Chunky/Classic) 60
green pepper and mushroom *(Del Monte)* 60
hot *(Pomodoro Fresca* Cayenne) 40
Italian, herb *(Del Monte)* 60
Italian, spice *(Aunt Millie's* Family Style) 90
lobster, rock *(Progresso)* 100
marinara:
    (Aunt Millie's) 70
    (Barilla) 80
    (Colavita) 65
    (Del Monte D'Italia Classic) 50
    (Hunt's Chunky) .60
    (Paesana) 115
    (Patsy's) 120
    (Prego) 110
    (Prince Chunky) .70
    (Prince Traditional) 50
    (Pritikin) 60
    (Progresso) 80
    (Progresso Authentic) 90
    (Ragú Old World) 90
    (Rao's Homemade) 60
    with Burgundy wine *(Five Brothers)* 80
    with pizza paste *(Aunt Millie's)* 70
meat/meat flavor:
    (Aunt Millie's) 80
    (Aunt Millie's Family Style) 100
    (Del Monte) 70
    (Healthy Choice) .50
    (Hunt's Homestyle/Old Country) 55
    (Hunt's Original) .65
    (Prego) 140
    (Progresso) 100
    (Ragú Old World) 90

Pasta Sauces *(cont.)*

with mushrooms:
(Aunt Millie's)	.70
(Aunt Millie's Family Style)	.80
(Del Monte)	.70
(Healthy Choice)	.50
(Healthy Choice Extra Chunky)	.40
(Hunt's Homestyle/Old Country)	.55
(Hunt's Original)	.65
(Prego)	150
(Prego Extra Chunky Supreme)	130
(Prince Chunky)	.70
(Progresso)	.80
(Ragú Old World)	.90
(Weight Watchers)	.60
chunky *(Ragú* Light)	.50
and garlic *(Barilla)*	.80
and garlic *(Healthy Choice* Super Chunky)	.45
and green pepper *(Prego Extra Chunky)*	120
and onion *(Prego Extra Chunky)*	110
Parmesan *(Prego)*	120
and ripe olive *(Classico* Di Sicilia)	.50
sautéed *(Five Brothers)*	.90
with spice, extra *(Prego Extra Chunky)*	120
and sweet peppers *(Healthy Choice* Super Chunky)	.45
and tomato *(Prego Extra Chunky)*	110
olive, black, and mushrooms *(Porino's)*	100
olive, green and black *(Barilla)*	100
with olives and mushrooms *(Classico Di Sicilia)*	.50

onion and garlic:
(Classico Di Sorrento)	.80
(Porino's)	100
(Prego)	110
(Prego Extra Chunky)	110
oregano, zesty *(Prego Extra Chunky)*	130
with Parmesan *(Hunt's* Classic)	.50
with Parmesan *(Prego)*	120

pepper, sweet or red:
and garlic *(Barilla)*	.70
and onion *(Classico* Di Salerno)	.70
and onion *(Porino's)*	100
red *(Del Monte* D'Italia)	.50

spicy *(Barilla)* 80
spicy *(Classico* Di Roma Arrabbiata) 60
with pesto *(Classico* Di Genoa) 110
pesto *(Sonoma)*, ¼ cup 110
sausage, Italian *(Hunt's)* .75
sausage, Italian, and fennel *(Classico* D'Abruzzi) 90
sausage and pepper *(Prego Extra Chunky)* 180
sausage, pepper, and mushroom *(Porino's)* 150
spinach and cheese *(Classico* Di Firenze) 80
sun-dried tomato *(Classico* Di Capri) 80
tomato and herb *(Ragú Light)* 50
vegetable primavera *(Ragú Gardenstyle* Super) 110
with vegetables:
   (Hunt's Chunky) 65
   (Prego Extra Chunky Supreme) 90
   garden, primavera *(Five Brothers)* 70
   Italian *(Healthy Choice* Extra Chunky) 40
   Italian *(Hunt's* Old Country) 65
   primavera *(Healthy Choice* Super Chunky) 45
zucchini and Parmesan *(Classico* Di Milano) 70

PASTA SAUCES, REFRIGERATED
See also "Pasta Sauces"

                                    calories

Alfredo, ¼ cup:
   (Contadina) 180
   (Contadina Light) .80
   (Di Giorno) 230
   (Di Giorno Reduced Fat) 170
cheese, four *(Di Giorno)*, ¼ cup 200
garden vegetable *(Contadina* Fat Free), ½ cup 40
Gorgonzola *(Monterey Pasta Company)*, 4 oz. 400
marinara *(Contadina)*, ½ cup 80
marinara *(Di Giorno)*, ½ cup 100
meat, traditional *(Di Giorno)*, ½ cup 120
olive oil and garlic, with grated cheese *(Di Giorno)*, ¼ cup 370
pesto:
   (Contadina Reduced Fat), ¼ cup 230
   (Di Giorno), ¼ cup 320
   sun-dried tomato *(Contadina)*, ¼ cup 200
   tomato, creamy *(Contadina)*, ½ cup 140

Pasta Sauces, Refrigerated *(cont.)*

primavera *(Tutta Pasta)*, ½ cup .130
puttanesca *(Tutta Pasta)*, ½ cup 100
red bell pepper *(Contadina)*, ½ cup 180
roasted garlic and artichoke *(Monterey Pasta Company)*,
   ½ cup 70
tomato, ½ cup:
   basil *(Contadina Fat Free)* 45
   chunky, with basil *(Di Giorno Light)* 70
   plum, and basil *(Contadina)* .70
   plum, and mushroom *(Di Giorno)* 70
vodka *(Tutta Pasta)*, ½ cup 300

SAUCES, MIXES
*See also "Soups, Mixes," "Condiments & Sauces," "Pasta
Sauces," "Gravies, Mixes," and "Seasonings, Dry & Mixes"*

---

                                         calories

à la king *(Durkee)*, 1 cup* 60
béarnaise *(Knorr)*, ⅒ pkg. 10
cheese:
   (Durkee), ¼ pkg. 25
   (French's), ¼ pkg. 25
   four *(Knorr)*, ⅓ pkg. 70
   nacho *(Durkee)*, ⅕ pkg. 25
chicken teriyaki *(McCormick)*, ¼ pkg. 40
curry *(Knorr)*, ⅕ pkg. 30
demiglace *(Knorr)*, 1 tbsp. 30
fish, lemon butter *(Weight Watchers)*, ¼ cup* 5
hollandaise:
   (Durkee), ⅒ pkg. 10
   (French's), 2 tbsp. 10
   (Knorr), ⅒ pkg. 10
lemon herb *(Knorr)*, 1 tbsp. 30
mushroom *(Knorr)*, ⅕ pkg. 20
Newburg *(Knorr)*, ⅓ pkg. 30
pasta:
   (Knorr Parma Rosa), 2 tbsp. .60
   (Lawry's), 1 tbsp. 35
   Alfredo *(Knorr)*, ⅓ pkg. 60

* Prepared according to package directions

Alfredo *(Spice Islands)*, ½ pkg.	.45
carbonara *(Knorr)*, 2 tbsp.	.70
garlic and herb *(Knorr)*, ⅓ pkg.	.70
garlic and herb *(Spice Islands)*, ¼ pkg.	.15
primavera *(Spice Islands)*, ⅕ pkg.	.30
salad *(Durkee* Pouch), 2 tsp.	.10
peppercorn *(Knorr)*, 2 tsp.	.25

pesto:

(Knorr), ⅓ pkg.	.15
(Spice Islands), ¼ pkg.	.15
creamy *(Knorr)*, ⅕ pkg.	.30
red bell pepper *(Knorr)*, ⅓ pkg.	.30
tomato *(Spice Islands)*, ¼ pkg.	.15
tomato, sun-dried *(Knorr)*, ⅓ pkg.	.45

spaghetti:

(Durkee), ½ cup*	.15
(Durkee Family), 2 tsp.	.20
American style *(Durkee)*, ½ cup*	.15
with mushrooms *(Durkee)*, ½ cup*	.15
zesty *(Durkee)*, 2 tsp.	.20
white *(Knorr)*, ⅛ pkg.	.25

GRAVIES, CANNED OR IN JARS, ¼ cup
See also "Condiments & Sauces"

	calories
au jus *(Franco-American)*	.10
au jus *(Heinz* Homestyle Bistro)	.15

beef:

(Franco-American)	.30
hearty *(Pepperidge Farm)*	.25
savory *(Heinz)*	.25
brown, with onions *(Franco-American)*	.25

chicken:

(Franco-American)	.45
(Heinz Homestyle)	.25
(Heinz Homestyle Fat Free)	.15
cream of *(Pepperidge Farm)*	.30
giblet *(Franco-American)*	.30
golden, with chicken *(Pepperidge Farm)*	.25

* Prepared according to package directions

Gravies, Canned or in Jars, chicken *(cont.)*
   rotisserie *(Pepperidge Farm* Rotissore) 25
mushroom:
   (Franco-American) 20
   (Heinz Homestyle Fat Free) 10
   country or with wine *(Pepperidge Farm)* 30
   creamy *(Franco-American)* 20
onion, roasted, and garlic *(Pepperidge Farm)* 25
onion, zesty *(Heinz* Homestyle) 25
pork *(Franco-American)* .45
pork *(Heinz* Homestyle) .25
Stroganoff *(Pepperidge Farm)* 30
turkey:
   (Franco-American) 25
   (Heinz Homestyle Fat Free) 15
   roasted *(Heinz* Homestyle) 30
   seasoned, with turkey *(Pepperidge Farm)* 30

GRAVIES, MIXES, ¼ cup*, except as noted
See also "Sauces, Mixes" and "Seasonings, Dry & Mixes"

---

	calories
all varieties *(Pillsbury* with Water)	15
au jus *(Durkee/French's)*	5
au jus *(Knorr)*	15
brown:	
(Durkee/French's)	10
(Knorr Classic)	20
(Loma Linda Gravy Quik)	20
(Tone's Cook Up)	15
(Weight Watchers)	5
herb *(Durkee/French's)*	15
chicken:	
(Durkee)	20
(French's)	25
(Loma Linda Gravy Quik)	20
(McCormick)	20
(Pillsbury with Water/Skim Milk)	20
(Weight Watchers)	10
roasted *(Knorr)*	30

* *Prepared according to package directions*

country:
   (Durkee), 1½ tbsp. mix 35
   (French's) 35
   (Loma Linda Gravy Quik) 25
homestyle *(Durkee)* 15
homestyle *(French's)* 10
mushroom:
   (Durkee) 15
   (French's) 10
   (Loma Linda Gravy Quik) 15
   brown *(Durkee)* 15
   hunter *(Knorr)*, 1 tbsp. mix 25
onion:
   (Durkee) 10
   (French's) 15
   (Loma Linda Gravy Quik) 20
   brown *(Durkee)* 15
   brown, Lyonnaise *(Knorr)* 20
pork *(Durkee)* 10
pork *(French's)* 10
sausage *(Durkee/French's)* 35
Swiss steak *(Durkee)* 15
turkey:
   (Durkee/French's) 20
   (McCormick) 20
   roasted *(Knorr)* 25

SEASONINGS, DRY & MIXES
*See also "Vegetables, Dried," "Soups, Mixes," "Condiments &
Sauces," "Barbecue Sauces," "Sauces, Mixes," "Gravies,
Mixes," and "Pure Herbs & Spices"*

---

                                     calories
adobo *(Durkee)*, ¼ tsp. 0
Alfredo seasoning mix *(Lawry's)*, 1½ tbsp. 35
all-purpose seasoning *(Aromat)*, ¼ tsp. 0
au jus seasoning mix *(Durkee/French's* Roasting Bag), ⅛ pkg. . .10
barbecue seasoning *(Durkee)*, ¼ tsp. 0
beef seasoning mix:
   ground *(Durkee* Pouch), ¼ pkg. 25
   marinade *(Durkee* Pouch), ⅒ pkg. 0
   marinade *(Lawry's)*, ¾ tsp. 0

Seasonings, Dry & Mixes, beef seasoning mix *(cont.)*

pot roast *(McCormick Bag 'n Season)* 1 tbsp.	.10
spare rib *(McCormick Bag 'n Season)* 1 tbsp.	.30
stew *(Adolph's* Meal Makers), approx. 1 tbsp.	.20
stew *(Durkee)*, ¹⁄₉ pkg.	.10
stew *(Durkee* Roasting Bag), ¹⁄₁₀ pkg.	.15
stew *(Lawry's)*, 2 tsp.	.20
Swiss steak *(McCormick Bag 'n Season)*, 1 tsp.	.15
bouillabaisse seasoning mix *(Knorr* Recipe), 1 tbsp.	.20
bourguignonne seasoning mix *(Knorr)*, 1 tbsp.	.35

burrito seasoning mix:

(Durkee Pouch), ¹⁄₁₀ pkg.	.35
(Lawry's), 1 tbsp.	.35
(Old El Paso), 2 tsp.	.15
butter salt *(Durkee)*, ¹⁄₂ tsp.	0
Cajun seasoning *(Tone's)*, ¹⁄₄ tsp.	0
Cajun seasoning, fish, meat, or poultry *(Durkee)*, ¹⁄₄ tsp.	0
Cantonese seasoning mix *(House of Tsang* Cantonese), 4 tbsp.	120
celery salt *(Tone's)*, 1 tsp.	6
charcoal seasoning *(Durkee)*, ¹⁄₄ tsp.	0

chicken seasoning/coating mix:

(Durkee/French's Roasting Bag), ¹⁄₆ pkg.	.20
(McCormick Bag 'n Season), 1 tbsp.	.20
(Shake'n Bake Original Recipe), ¹⁄₈ pkg.	.40
barbecue *(Durkee* Roasting Bag), ¹⁄₆ pkg.	.30
barbecue glaze *(Shake'n Bake)*, ¹⁄₈ pkg.	.45
Buffalo wing, Cajun or garlic and herb *(Durkee)*, ¹⁄₈ pkg.	.15
Buffalo wing, hot, screaming hot, or mild *(Durkee)*, ¹⁄₈ pkg.	.20
cacciatore *(Durkee Easy)*, ¹⁄₁₀ pkg.	.10
coq au vin *(Knorr* Recipe), 1 tbsp.	.30
country *(Durkee* Roasting Bag), ¹⁄₆ pkg.	.35
Dijonne *(Knorr* Recipe), ¹⁄₆ pkg.	.30
extra crispy *(Oven Fry)*, ¹⁄₈ pkg.	.60
homestyle flour *(Oven Fry)*, ¹⁄₈ pkg.	.40
hot, spicy *(McCormick Bag 'n Season)*, 1 tbsp.	.30
hot and spicy *(Shake'n Bake)*, ¹⁄₈ pkg.	.40
Mexican salsa *(Durkee Easy)*, ¹⁄₁₀ pkg.	.10
mushroom *(Durkee Easy)*, ¹⁄₈ pkg.	.15
Southwest, marinade *(Lawry's)*, 1 tsp.	5
stir-fry *(McCormick)*, ¹⁄₆ pkg.	.20
sweet and sour *(Durkee Easy)*, ¹⁄₉ pkg.	.20
chili powder *(Gebhardt)*, ¹⁄₄ tsp.	1

chili powder *(Tone's)*, 1/4 tsp. 0
chili seasoning mix:
    (Adolph's Meal Makers), approx. 1 tbsp. 30
    (Durkee), 1/5 pkg. 30
    (Durkee Pot-O), 1/8 pkg. 30
    (Gebhardt Chili Quik), 2 tbsp. 30
    (Lawry's), 1 tbsp. 25
    (Lawry's Tex-Mex), 2 tbsp. 50
    (McCormick), approx. 4 tsp. 30
    (Mick Fowler's 2-Alarm Family), 2 tbsp. 50
    (Mick Fowler's 2-Alarm Kit), 3 tbsp. 60
    (Old El Paso), 1 tbsp. 25
    mild *(Durkee)*, 1/5 pkg. 30
    Texas red *(Durkee)*, 1/3 pkg. 45
country coating mix *(Shake'n Bake)*, 1/8 pkg. 35
curry powder *(Tone's)*, 1/4 tsp. 0
enchilada seasoning mix:
    (Durkee), 1 1/2 tsp. 10
    (Lawry's), 2 tsp. 20
    (Old El Paso), 2 tsp. 10
fajita seasoning mix:
    (Lawry's), 2 tsp. 15
    (Old El Paso), 1 tbsp. 30
    beef *(Durkee* Easy), 1/6 pkg. 15
fish seasoning/coating mix *(see also "seafood seasoning,"*
    below)
    (Shake'n Bake), 1/4 pkt. 70
    Cajun *(Tone's)*, 1 tsp. 12
    lemon butter *(Durkee/French's* Roasting Bag), 1/4 pkg. 30
    lemon pepper dill *(Durkee Easy)*, 1/6 pkg. 20
    tomato basil *(Durkee Easy)*, 1/7 pkg. 15
garlic seasoning:
    granulated or minced *(Tone's)*, 1/4 tsp. 5
    pepper *(Lawry's)*, 1/4 tsp. 0
    pepper *(Tone's)*, 1/4 tsp. 0
    powder *(McCormick)*, 1/4 tsp. 3
    powder *(Tone's)*, 1/4 tsp. 5
    salt *(Durkee* California), 1/2 tsp. 0
    salt *(Lawry's)*, 1/4 tsp. 0
    salt *(Morton)*, 1/2 tsp. 2
    salt *(Tone's)*, 1/4 tsp. 0
glaze, tangy honey or honey mustard *(Shake'n Bake)*, 1/8 pkg. . .45

Seasonings, Dry & Mixes *(cont.)*

goulash seasoning mix *(Knorr* Recipe), 1⅓ tbsp. 35
guacamole seasoning *(Lawry's),* ½ tsp. 5
gyro seasoning *(Casbah),* ¹⁄₁₀ pkg. 64
herbs, mixed *(Lawry's* Pinch of Herbs), ¼ tsp. 0
hummus mix *(Casbah),* 1 oz. 120
Italian herb coating mix *(Shake'n Bake),* ⅛ pkg. 40
lemon pepper:
  (Lawry's), ¼ tsp. 0
  (Tone's), ¼ tsp. 0
  marinade seasoning *(Adolph's* Marinade in Minutes),
    ½ tsp. 10
marinade, *see specific listings*
meat loaf seasoning mix:
  (Adolph's Meal Makers), approx. 1 tbsp. 30
  (Durkee Pouch), ⅑ pkt. .20
  (Durkee/French's Roasting Bag), ⅛ pkg. 15
  (Lawry's), 1 tbsp. 35
meat marinade seasoning mix *(Lawry's* Carne Asada), 1 tsp. 5
meat seasoning *(Aromat),* ¼ tsp. 0
meat tenderizer, unseasoned *(Tone's),* 1 tsp. 7
meatball seasoning mix, Italian *(Durkee* Pouch), ⅕ pkt. 20
menudo seasoning mix *(Gebhardt),* ¼ tsp. 0
mesquite marinade seasoning *(Adolph's* Marinade in Minutes),
  ¾ tsp. 10
mesquite seasoning *(Tone's),* ¼ tsp. 0
Mexican seasoning:
  (Chi-Chi's Mix), 1 tsp. .10
  (Tone's), 1 tsp. 6
  with coriander or saffron *(Goya),* ¼ tsp. 0
monosodium glutamate *(Tone's),* 1 tsp. 0
mustard herb mix *(Knorr),* 1 tbsp. 4
onion salt *(Durkee* California), ½ tsp. 0
onion salt *(Tone's),* 1 tsp. 1
Oriental 5-spice *(Tone's),* 1 tsp. 9
Parmesan herb marinade seasoning *(Adolph's* Marinade in
  Minutes), ¾ tsp. 10
pepper, flavored, *see specific listings*
pickling spice *(Tone's),* 1 tsp. 10
pizza pepper *(Lawry's),* ¼ tsp. 0
pizza seasoning *(Tone's Presti's),* ¾ tsp. 10
popcorn seasoning *(Tone's),* ¼ tsp. 0

pork seasoning/coating mix:
    (Durkee/French's Roasting Bag), 1/6 pkg. 25
    (Shake'n Bake Original Recipe), 1/8 pkg. 40
    barbecue glaze *(Shake'n Bake),* 1/8 pkg. 35
    batter, frying *(House of Tsang),* 4 tbsp. 140
    chops *(McCormick Bag 'n Season),* 2 tsp. 15
    extra crispy *(Oven Fry),* 1/8 pkg. 60
    hot and spicy *(Shake'n Bake),* 1/8 pkg. 45
    sparerib *(Durkee* Roasting Bag), 1/7 pkg. 25
pot roast seasoning mix, 1/6 pkg., except as noted:
    (Durkee Roasting Bag) .15
    (French's Roasting Bag) 20
    (Lawry's), 1 tsp. 5
    onion *(French's* Roasting Bag) 25
    sauerbraten *(Knorr)* .35
potato salad seasoning *(Tone's),* 1 tsp. 5
potato seasoning *(see also "Vegetable Dishes, Mixes,"*
    page 117):
    cheddar, savory or California onion *(Lipton Recipe*
        Secrets), 1 tbsp. 60
    garlic herb *(Lipton Recipe Secrets),* 1 tbsp. 50
rice seasoning mix, fried *(Durkee),* 1/4 pkg. 15
rice seasoning mix, Mexican *(Lawry's),* 1 1/2 tbsp. 40
salad seasoning *(McCormick),* 1/2 tsp. 0
salad topper *(McCormick Salad Toppins),* 1 1/3 tbsp. 35
salad topper, all varieties *(Pepperidge Farm),* 1 tbsp. 35
salsa seasoning *(Lawry's),* 1/2 tsp. 5
salt, regular, 1/4 tsp.:
    (McCormick Season-All) 0
    (Morton Lite) 0
    iodized/non-iodized *(Morton)* 0
    kosher *(Morton)* 0
salt, flavored, *see specific listings*
salt, seasoned, 1/4 tsp.:
    (House of Tsang Hong King) 0
    (Lawry's) 0
    (Morton) 0
    (Morton Nature's Seasons) . . . . <1
    red pepper *(Lawry's)* 0
salt substitute:
    (Morton), 1/4 tsp. 0
    seasoned *(Lawry's* Salt Free), 1/4 tsp. 0

Seasonings, Dry & Mixes, salt substitute *(cont.)*
seasoned *(Morton),* 1 tsp. 2
seasoned or unseasoned *(Adolph's),* ¼ tsp. 0
sandwich sauce seasoning mix, sloppy joe *(Lawry's),* 1 tsp. . . .15
sausage seasoning, pork *(Tone's),* 1 tsp. 12
seafood seasoning:
   (Old Bay), ½ tsp. 0
   (Tone's), 1 tsp. 10
   marinade, lemon herb or scampi *(Adolph's* Marinade in
      Minutes), ½ tsp. 10
seasoning *(Ac'cent),* ⅛ tsp. 0
seasoning *(Sa-son Ac'cent/Sa-son con Ajo Cebolla/con
   Azafran/con Culantro),*¼ tsp. 0
seaweed, *see "Vegetables, Dried," page 114*
sesame seed seasoning, regular, garlic, or seaweed *(Eden
   Organic Sesame Shake),* ½ tsp. 10
shrimp spice *(Tone's Craboil),* 1 tsp. 10
stew seasoning, *see "beef seasoning mix," above*
Stroganoff mix *(Durkee),* ⅛ pkg. 10
Swiss steak seasoning mix *(Durkee/French's* Roasting Bag),
   ⅑ pkg. 10
taco seasoning *(Tone's),* 2 tsp. .20
taco seasoning mix:
   (Durkee Pouch), ⅛ pkg. 15
   (Durkee Pouch Family), 1/16 pkg. 10
   (Lawry's), 1 tbsp. 25
   (McCormick), 2 tsp. 20
   (Old El Paso), 2 tsp. 20
   (Old El Paso 40% Less Sodium), 2 tsp. 15
   (Pancho Villa), 2 tsp. 20
   chicken *(Lawry's),* 2 tsp. 20
   mild *(Durkee* Pouch), ⅛ pkg. 15
   salad *(Durkee* Pouch), ⅙ pkg. 20
   salad *(Lawry's),* 1 tsp. 15
tahini sauce mix *(Casbah),* 1 oz. 160
tenderizer, all varieties *(Adolph's* 100% Natural), ¼ tsp. 0
teriyaki seasoning mix:
   beef *(Durkee),* 1 tbsp. 30
   marinade seasoning *(Adolph's* Marinade in Minutes),
      1½ tsp. 15
   stir-fry *(Adolph's* Meal Makers), approx. 1 tbsp. 30

tofu seasoning mix:

    all varieties, except Mandarin and Szechwan stir-fry
      (TofuMate), ¼ pkg. 15

    breakfast scramble *(Fantastic* Classics), 2½ tbsp. 60

    Mandarin stir-fry *(TofuMate)*, ¼ pkg. 30

    Szechwan stir-fry *(TofuMate)*, ¼ pkg. 25

turkey seasoning, with gravy *(McCormick Bag 'n Season)*,
    1 tsp. 15

PURE HERBS & SPICES, ¼ teaspoon, except as noted
See also "Seasonings, Dry & Mixes"

	calories
allspice *(McCormick)*	2
basil:	
(McCormick)	<1
dried, leaf *(Tone's)*	0
frozen *(Seabrook)*, 1 tbsp., ¼ oz.	2
bay leaf, dried *(McCormick)*, 1 leaf	<1
bay leaf, dried *(Tone's)*, 2 leaves	0
caraway seed *(McCormick)*	4
cardamom:	
(McCormick)	4
ground *(Tone's)*, 1 tsp.	6
seed *(Spice Islands)*, 1 tsp.	6
celery, flake or seed *(Tone's)*, 1 tsp.	9
chervil *(McCormick)*	<1
chives, freeze-dried *(McCormick)*	<1
chives, freeze-dried *(Tone's)*	0
cilantro, *see "coriander," below*	
cinnamon *(McCormick)*	2
cinnamon *(Tone's)*	5
clover seed, sprouted *(McCormick)*	1
coriander:	
dried *(McCormick)*	<1
ground *(McCormick)*	2
seed *(McCormick)*	3
(Tone's Cilantro)	0
cumin seed, ground *(McCormick)*	3
cumin seed, ground *(Tone's)*	0
dill:	
seed *(McCormick)*	3

Pure Herbs & Spices, dill *(cont.)*

weed, dried *(McCormick)* 1
weed, dried *(Tone's)* 0
ginger, ground *(McCormick)* 2
mace *(McCormick)* 2
marjoram *(McCormick)* 1
mustard seed *(McCormick)* 2
nutmeg, ground *(McCormick)* 3
onion powder *(McCormick)* 3
onion powder *(Tone's)* 5
paprika *(McCormick)* 2
parsley, dried *(McCormick)* . . . . <1
poppy seed *(McCormick)* 4
rosemary, dried *(McCormick)* 2
sage *(McCormick)* 1
savory, ground *(McCormick)* 2
savory, summer *(Tone's)*, 1 tsp. 4
sesame seed, raw *(McCormick)* 2
shallot, freeze-dried *(McCormick)* 3
spearmint, dried *(McCormick)* 1
tarragon, dried *(McCormick)* 1
thyme, dried *(McCormick)* 4
turmeric, dried *(McCormick)* 2

Chapter 16

PUDDINGS, CUSTARDS, AND GELATINS

PUDDING, READY-TO-SERVE, four ounces, except as noted
See also "Custards, Puddings, & Pie Filling, Mixes" and
"Gelatin & Gelatin Desserts"

calories

banana:
    (Del Monte Snack), 3.5-oz. cup 120
    (Hunt's Snack Pack) 160
    (Jell-O Snack) 170
    (Thank You), ½ cup 200
    nondairy *(Imagine)* 150
butterscotch:
    (Del Monte Snack), 3.5-oz. cup 120
    (Hunt's Snack Pack) 150
    (Rich's), 3 oz. 140
    (Swiss Miss) 160
    (Thank You), ½ cup 160
    nondairy *(Imagine)* 150
chocolate:
    (Del Monte Snack), 3.5-oz. cup 130
    (Del Monte Snack Fat Free), 3.5-oz. cup 90
    (Hunt's Snack Pack) 170
    (Hunt's Snack Pack Fat Free) 100
    (Jell-O Snack) 160
    (Jell-O Free Snack) 100
    (Rich's), 3 oz. 140
    (Swiss Miss) 170
    (Thank You), ½ cup 190
    or chocolate fudge *(Swiss Miss* Fat Free) 100
    nondairy *(Imagine)* 170
chocolate fudge:
    (Del Monte Snack), 3.5-oz. cup 130
    (Hunt's Snack Pack) 170
    (Swiss Miss) 175
    (Thank You), ½ cup 180

Pudding, Ready-to-Serve, chocolate fudge *(cont.)*
  parfait *(Swiss Miss)* 160
chocolate marshmallow *(Hunt's Snack Pack)* 155
chocolate swirl:
  caramel *(Hunt's Snack Pack)* 170
  caramel *(Swiss Miss)* 170
  caramel or vanilla *(Jell-O Snack)* 160
  caramel or vanilla *(Jell-O Free Snack)* 100
  milk *(Hunt's Snack Pack)* 160
  vanilla *(Swiss Miss)* 170
chocolate vanilla parfait *(Swiss Miss)* 160
lemon:
  (Hunt's Snack Pack) 160
  (Thank You), ½ cup 170
  nondairy *(Imagine)* 150
rice *(Thank You)*, ½ cup 160
S'mores swirl *(Hunt's Snack Pack)* 150
tapioca:
  (Del Monte Snack), 3.5-oz. cup 120
  (Hunt's Snack Pack) 150
  (Hunt's Snack Pack Fat Free) 95
  (Jell-O Snack) 140
  (Swiss Miss) 140
  (Swiss Miss Fat Free) 100
  (Thank You), ½ cup 160
vanilla:
  (Del Monte Snack), 3.5-oz. cup 120
  (Del Monte Snack Fat Free), 3.5-oz. cup 90
  (Hunt's Snack Pack) 160
  (Hunt's Snack Pack Fat Free) 95
  (Jell-O Snack) 160
  (Jell-O Free Snack) 100
  (Rich's), 3 oz. 140
  (Swiss Miss) 160
  (Swiss Miss Fat Free) 100
  (Thank You), ½ cup 160
vanilla chocolate:
  parfait *(Swiss Miss)* 160
  parfait *(Swiss Miss Fat Free)* 100
  swirl *(Jell-O Snack)* 170
  swirl *(Jell-O Free Snack)* 100

CUSTARDS, PUDDINGS, & PIE FILLINGS, MIXES, ½ cup*,
except as noted
See also "Pudding, Ready-to-Serve," "Gelatin & Gelatin Desserts," and "Pie Fillings, Canned"

	calories
banana *(Jell-O Sugar/Fat Free)*	70
banana cream *(Jell-O)*	140
banana cream *(Jell-O Instant)*	150
butter pecan *(Jell-O Instant)*	160
butterscotch:	
(Jell-O)	160
(Jell-O Instant)	150
(Jell-O Sugar/Fat Free)	70
chocolate:	
(D-Zerta)	60
(Jell-O)	150
(Jell-O Instant)	160
(Jell-O Sugar Free)	80
(Jell-O Sugar/Fat Free)	80
*(My*T*Fine)*	90
milk *(Jell-O)*	150
milk *(Jell-O Instant)*	160
white *(Jell-O Fat Free)*	140
chocolate fudge:	
(JellO)	150
(Jell-O Instant)	160
(Jell-O Sugar/Fat Free)	80
chocolate mousse, dark or milk, dry *(Alsa)*, 2 tbsp.	80
chocolate mousse, white, dry *(Alsa)*, 2 tbsp.	70
coconut cream *(Jell-O)*	150
coconut cream *(Jell-O Instant)*	160
custard *(Jell-O Americana)*	140
custard, tropical *(Goya Tembleque)*	100
flan:	
(Alsa Creme Caramel), 1⅓ tbsp. mix, 1 tbsp. caramel	110
(Goya)	100
(Jell-O)	140
with caramel *(Goya)*	190
lemon *(Jell-O)*	140

* Prepared according to package directions

Custards, Puddings, & Pie Fillings, Mixes *(cont.)*

lemon *(Jell-O* Instant) 150
pistachio *(Jell-O* Instant) 160
pistachio *(Jell-O* Sugar/Fat Free) 70
rennet *(Junket)*, 1 tablet 1
rice:
    (Goya) 90
    (Jell-O Americana) 160
    all varieties *(Lundberg* Elegant), ½ cup mix 70
    cinnamon and raisin *(Uncle Ben's)*, 1.5 oz. 160
tapioca *(Jell-O Americana)* 140
vanilla:
    (Jell-O) 140
    (Jell-O Instant) 160
    (Jell-O Sugar Free) 80
    (Jell-O Sugar/Fat Free) 70
    French *(Jell-O* Instant) 150

GELATIN & GELATIN DESSERTS
See also "Pudding, Ready-to-Serve" and "Custards, Puddings, & Pie Fillings, Mixes"

	calories
gelatin, unflavored *(Knox)*, 1 pkt.	25

gelatin dessert, all flavors, 3½-oz. cup, except as noted:
    (Del Monte Snack) 70
    (Hunt's Snack Pack) 100
    (Jell-O Snacks) .80
    (Jell-O Sugar Free Snacks), 3.2 oz. 10
    (Kraft Handi-Snacks) 80
gelatin dessert mix*, ½ cup, except as noted:
    all flavors *(Jell-O* Sugar Free) 10
    all flavors *(Jell-O)* 80
    strawberry *(D-Zerta)* 10
    strawberry *(Jell-O 1-2-3)*, ⅔ cup 130
gelatin drink mix, orange *(Knox)*, 1 pkt. 40

* *Prepared according to package directions*

Chapter 17

CAKES, COOKIES, PIES, AND PASTRIES

DESSERT CAKES
See also "Dessert Cakes, Frozen," "Dessert Cakes, Mixes," "Dessert Pies, Frozen or Refrigerated," "Dessert Pies, Mixes," "Snack Cakes & Pastries," and "Miscellaneous Desserts"

	calories
apple-spice crumb *(Entenmann's* Fat Free), 1/8 cake	130
banana:	
(Awrey's Sheet), 1/24 cake	350
(Entenmann's Fat Free), 1/8 cake	150
chocolate chip *(Awrey's* Marquise), 1/16 cake	310
crunch *(Entenmann's)*, 1/8 cake	220
crunch *(Entenmann's* Fat Free), 1/8 cake	140
Black Forest torte *(Awrey's)*, 1/12 cake	350
blueberry crunch *(Entenmann's* Fat Free), 1/8 cake	140
Boston creme *(Awrey's)*, 1/16 cake	190
butter *(Entenmann's)*, 1/6 loaf	220
butter, French crumb *(Entenmann's)*, 1/8 cake	210
carrot:	
(Entenmann's), 1/8 cake	290
(Entenmann's Fat Free), 1/8 cake	170
cream cheese iced *(Awrey's)*, 1/16 cake	390
supreme *(Awrey's* Sheet), 1/24 cake	400
cherries cordial *(Awrey's* Marquise), 1/16 cake	240
chocolate:	
crunch *(Entenmann's* Fat Free), 1/8 cake	130
fudge *(Entenmann's)*, 1/6 cake	310
fudge iced *(Entenmann's* Fat Free), 1/6 cake	210
German *(Awrey's* Sheet), 1/24 cake	340
German, layer *(Awrey's)*, 1/16 cake	360
loaf *(Entenmann's* Fat Free), 1/8 cake	130
mocha iced *(Entenmann's* Fat Free), 1/6 cake	200
peanut *(Awrey's* Marquise), 1/16 cake	330
tropical *(Awrey's* Marquise), 1/16 cake	230
white iced, layer *(Awrey's)*, 1/16 cake	270

Dessert Cakes *(cont.)*
chocolate, double:
    (Awrey's Sheet), 1/24 cake 310
    (Awrey's Torte), 1/12 cake 340
    3 layer *(Awrey's)*, 1/16 cake 310
    2 layer *(Awrey's)*, 1/16 cake 250
coconut buttercream *(Awrey's* Sheet), 1/24 cake 380
coconut buttercream layer *(Awrey's)*, 1/16 cake 360
coffee:
    (Awrey's Long John), 1/12 cake 190
    cheese *(Entenmann's)*, 1/9 cake 190
    cheese, crumb *(Entenmann's)*, 1/8 cake 210
    cinnamon apple *(Entenmann's* Fat Free), 1/9 cake 130
    crumb *(Entenmann's)*, 1/10 cake 250
crunch *(Entenmann's* Fat Free), 1/6 cake 220
crunch, Louisiana *(Entenmann's)*, 1/9 cake 310
danish:
    cake, Black Forest *(Entenmann's* Fat Free), 1/9 cake 130
    cake, raspberry cheese *(Entenmann's* Fat Free), 1/9 cake . . . 140
    ring, cinnamon filbert *(Entenmann's)*, 1/6 cake 270
    ring, pecan or walnut *(Entenmann's)*, 1/8 cake 230
    twist, apricot *(Entenmann's* Fat Free), 1/8 cake 150
    twist, cinnamon apple *(Entenmann's* Fat Free), 1/8 cake 140
    twist, lemon *(Entenmann's* Fat Free), 1/8 cake 130
    twist, raspberry *(Entenmann's)*, 1/8 cake 220
    twist, raspberry *(Entenmann's* Fat Free), 1/8 cake 140
devil's food, marshmallow iced *(Entenmann's)*, 1/6 cake 350
espresso, French *(Awrey's* Marquise), 1/16 cake 320
fruit *(Hostess)*, 1/12 cake 510
golden:
    crumb, French *(Entenmann's* Fat Free), 1/8 cake 140
    fudge, thick *(Entenmann's)*, 1/6 cake 330
    fudge iced *(Entenmann's* Fat Free), 1/6 cake 220
    loaf *(Entenmann's* Fat Free), 1/8 cake 120
    loaf, chocolatey chip *(Entenmann's* Fat Free), 1/8 cake 130
lemon layer *(Awrey's)*, 1/16 cake 320
marble loaf *(Entenmann's)*, 1/8 cake 200
marble loaf *(Entenmann's* Fat Free), 1/8 cake 130
Neapolitan *(Awrey's)*, 1/12 cake 360
orange, frosty *(Awrey's* Sheet), 1/24 cake 350
orange layer *(Awrey's)*, 1/16 cake 330
peach, Georgia *(Awrey's* Marquise), 1/16 cake 260

pound, golden *(Awrey's)*, ⅙ cake 250
raisin loaf *(Entenmann's)*, ⅛ cake 220
raisin loaf *(Entenmann's Fat Free)*, ⅛ cake 140
raspberry and cream *(Awrey's* Marquise), ⅟₁₆ cake 260
raspberry nut *(Awrey's* Marquise), ⅟₁₆ cake 310
sour cream chip-nut loaf *(Entenmann's)*, ⅛ cake 240
sponge, uniced *(Awrey's)*, ⅟₂₄ cake 190
strawberry supreme *(Awrey's* Marquise), ⅟₁₆ cake 240
strawberry torte supreme *(Awrey's)*, ⅟₁₂ cake 270
yellow, lemon iced, 2 layer *(Awrey's)*, ⅟₁₆ cake 290
yellow, white iced *(Awrey's* Sheet), ⅟₂₄ cake 360

DESSERT CAKES, FROZEN
*See also "Dessert Cakes" and "Snack Pastries & Pies, Frozen
or Refrigerated"*

                                                              calories

Boston creme *(Mrs. Smith's)*, ⅛ cake 170
Boston creme *(Pepperidge Farm)*, ⅛ cake 260
carrot *(Pepperidge Farm* Deluxe), ⅛ cake 310
cheesecake:
    (Sara Lee Original Cream Cheese), ¼ of 19-oz. cake 330
    French *(Sara Lee)*, ⅕ cake 410
    strawberry *(Amy's)*, 4 oz. 290
    strawberry, French *(Sara Lee)*, ⅙ cake 320
chocolate:
    double, layer *(Sara Lee)*, ⅛ cake 260
    fudge *(Amy's)*, 3.25 oz. 320
    fudge or German, layer *(Pepperidge Farm)*, ⅙ cake 300
    fudge stripe layer *(Pepperidge Farm)*, ⅙ cake 290
    German, layer *(Sara Lee)*, ⅛ cake 280
    mousse *(Pepperidge Farm)*, ⅛ cake 250
    mousse *(Sara Lee)*, ⅕ cake 400
coconut layer *(Pepperidge Farm)*, ⅙ cake 300
coconut layer *(Sara Lee)*, ⅛ cake 280
coffee:
    (Sara Lee Reduced Fat), ⅙ cake 180
    crumb *(Sara Lee)*, ⅛ cake 220
    raspberry *(Sara Lee)*, ⅙ cake 200
devil's food, layer *(Pepperidge Farm)*, ⅙ cake 290
golden layer *(Pepperidge Farm)*, ⅙ cake 290
golden layer *(Sara Lee)*, ⅛ cake 270

Dessert Cakes, Frozen *(cont.)*
lemon mousse *(Pepperidge Farm)*, ⅛ cake 250
pineapple cream *(Pepperidge Farm)*, ⅑ cake 240
pound:
    (Goya), ¼ cake 280
    (Sara Lee Reduced Fat*)*, ¼ cake 280
    butter *(Pepperidge Farm)*, ⅕ cake 290
    butter *(Sara Lee* All Butter*)*, ¼ cake 320
    chocolate swirl *(Sara Lee)*, ¼ cake 330
    strawberry swirl *(Sara Lee)*, ¼ cake 290
strawberry cream *(Pepperidge Farm)*, ⅑ cake 230
strawberry stripe layer *(Pepperidge Farm)*, ⅙ cake 310
vanilla layer *(Pepperidge Farm)*, ⅙ cake 290

DESSERT CAKES, MIXES
See also "Dessert Cakes" and "Snack Cakes, Mixes"

                                                   calories
angel food:
    (Duncan Hines), 1/12 cake* 130
    (Gold Medal), ¼ pkg. mix 170
    (Pillsbury Moist Supreme), 1/12 cake* 140
    (SuperMoist), 1/12 pkg. mix 130
    chocolate swirl or confetti *(SuperMoist)*, 1/12 pkg. mix 150
    lemon custard or white *(SuperMoist)*, 1/12 pkg. mix 140
    strawberry *(Duncan Hines)*, 1/12 cake* 130
banana:
    (Duncan Hines Supreme*)*, 1/12 pkg. mix 180
    (Duncan Hines Supreme*)*, 1/12 cake* 250
    (Pillsbury Moist Supreme), 1/12 pkg. mix 180
    (Pillsbury Moist Supreme), 1/12 cake* 260
    no-cholesterol recipe *(Duncan Hines* Supreme*)*, 1/12 cake* . 240
butter pecan:
    (SuperMoist), 1/12 pkg. mix 180
    (SuperMoist), 1/12 cake* 250
    no-cholesterol recipe *(SuperMoist)*, 1/12 cake* 210
butter recipe:
    (Pillsbury Moist Supreme), 1/12 pkg. mix 170
    (Pillsbury Moist Supreme), 1/12 cake* 260
    chocolate *(Pillsbury Moist Supreme)*, 1/12 pkg. mix 180

---

* Prepared according to package directions

chocolate *(Pillsbury Moist Supreme)*, 1/12 cake* 270
chocolate *(SuperMoist)*, 1/12 pkg. mix 190
chocolate *(SuperMoist)*, 1/12 cake* 270
fudge *(Duncan Hines)*, 1/10 pkg. mix 220
fudge or golden *(Duncan Hines)*, 1/10 cake* 320
golden *(Duncan Hines)*, 1/10 pkg. mix 230
yellow *(SuperMoist)*, 1/12 pkg. mix 170
yellow *(SuperMoist)*, 1/12 cake* 260
butterscotch:
  (Duncan Hines), 1/12 pkg. mix 180
  (Duncan Hines), 1/12 cake* 250
  no-cholesterol recipe *(Duncan Hines)*, 1/12 cake* 240
caramel:
  (Duncan Hines), 1/12 pkg. mix 180
  (Duncan Hines), 1/12 cake* 250
  no-cholesterol recipe *(Duncan Hines)*, 1/12 cake* 240
carrot:
  (Pillsbury Moist Supreme), 1/12 pkg. mix 180
  (Pillsbury Moist Supreme), 1/12 cake* 260
  (SuperMoist), 1/10 pkg. mix 210
  (SuperMoist), 1/10 cake* 300
  no-cholesterol recipe *(SuperMoist)*, 1/10 cake* 250
cheesecake, 1/6 cake*:
  (Jell-O Homestyle) 360
  (Jell-O Real) 350
  blueberry *(Jell-O)* 320
  cherry *(Jell-O)* 330
  strawberry *(Jell-O)* 340
cherry, wild, vanilla:
  (Duncan Hines), 1/12 pkg. mix 180
  (Duncan Hines), 1/12 cake* 250
  no-cholesterol recipe *(Duncan Hines)*, 1/12 cake* 240
chip, cherry:
  (SuperMoist), 1/10 pkg. mix 210
  (SuperMoist), 1/10 cake* 280
  richer recipe *(SuperMoist)*, 1/10 cake* 300
chip, rainbow *(SuperMoist)*, 1/12 pkg. mix 180
chip, rainbow *(SuperMoist)*, 1/12 cake* 250
chocolate *(see also "fudge," below)*:
  (Pillsbury Moist Supreme), 1/12 pkg. mix 180

---

* *Prepared according to package directions*

Dessert Cakes, Mixes, chocolate *(cont.)*
    (Pillsbury Moist Supreme), 1/12 cake* 250
    caramel nut *(Pillsbury Bundt),* 1/16 pkg. mix 180
    caramel nut *(Pillsbury Bundt),* 1/16 cake* 290
    caramel nut *(Pillsbury Streusel Swirl),* 1/16 pkg. mix 200
    caramel nut *(Pillsbury Streusel Swirl),* 1/16 cake* 260
    chip *(SuperMoist),* 1/12 pkg. mix 180
    chip *(SuperMoist),* 1/12 cake* 280
    chip, no-cholesterol recipe *(SuperMoist),* 1/12 cake* 210
    dark *(Pillsbury Moist Supreme),* 1/12 pkg. mix 180
    dark *(Pillsbury Moist Supreme),* 1/12 cake* 250
    fudge or milk *(SuperMoist),* 1/12 pkg. mix 180
    fudge or milk *(SuperMoist),* 1/12 cake* 250
    milk, no-cholesterol recipe *(SuperMoist),* 1/12 cake* 210
    mocha *(Duncan Hines),* 1/12 pkg. mix 180
    mocha *(Duncan Hines),* 1/12 cake* 290
    mocha, no-cholesterol recipe *(Duncan Hines),* 1/12 cake* . . . 280
    swirl, double *(SuperMoist),* 1/12 pkg. mix 180
    swirl, double *(SuperMoist),* 1/12 cake* 250
    swirl, double, no-cholesterol recipe *(SuperMoist),* 1/12 cake* . 230
    Swiss *(Duncan Hines),* 1/12 pkg. mix 180
    Swiss *(Duncan Hines),* 1/12 cake* 290
    Swiss, no-cholesterol recipe *(Duncan Hines),* 1/12 cake* 280
chocolate, German:
    (SuperMoist), 1/12 pkg. mix 180
    (SuperMoist), 1/12 cake* 250
    (Pillsbury Moist Supreme), 1/12 pkg. mix 180
    (Pillsbury Moist Supreme), 1/12 cake* 250
    no-cholesterol recipe *(SuperMoist),* 1/12 cake* 220
coffee *(Aunt Jemima* Easy Mix), 1/3 cup mix 170
date nut roll *(Dromedary),* 1/3 pkg. mix 200
devil's food:
    (Duncan Hines), 1/12 pkg. mix 180
    (Duncan Hines), 1/12 cake* 290
    (Pillsbury Moist Supreme), 1/12 pkg. mix 180
    (Pillsbury Moist Supreme), 1/12 cake* 270
    (Robin Hood Pouch), 1/5 pkg. mix 190
    (Robin Hood Pouch), 1/5 cake* 310
    (SnackWell's), 1/6 pkg. mix 190
    (SnackWell's), 1/6 cake* 200

* *Prepared according to package directions*

(SuperMoist), 1/12 pkg. mix 180
(SuperMoist), 1/12 cake* 240
(SuperMoist Light), 1/10 pkg. mix 210
(SuperMoist Light), 1/10 cake* 230
(Sweet Rewards Reduced Fat), 1/12 pkg. mix 170
(Sweet Rewards Reduced Fat), 1/12 cake* 220
no-cholesterol recipe *(Duncan Hines)*, 1/12 cake* 280
no-cholesterol recipe *(SuperMoist)*, 1/12 cake* 200
no-cholesterol recipe *(SuperMoist* Light), 1/10 cake* 210
no-cholesterol recipe *(Sweet Rewards* Reduced Fat),
   1/12 cake* 210
fudge:
   Dutch dark *(Duncan Hines)*, 1/12 pkg. mix 180
   Dutch dark *(Duncan Hines)*, 1/12 cake* 290
   Dutch dark, no-cholesterol recipe *(Duncan Hines)*,
      1/12 cake* 280
   hot *(Pillsbury Bundt)*, 1/16 pkg. mix 220
   hot *(Pillsbury Bundt)*, 1/16 cake* 350
   swirl *(Pillsbury Moist Supreme)*, 1/12 pkg. mix 200
   swirl *(Pillsbury Moist Supreme)*, 1/12 cake* 250
gingerbread, *see "Sweet Breads, Mix," page 25*
lemon:
   (Duncan Hines Supreme), 1/12 pkg. mix 180
   (Duncan Hines Supreme), 1/12 cake* 250
   (Pillsbury Moist Supreme), 1/10 pkg. mix 210
   (Pillsbury Moist Supreme), 1/10 cake* 300
   (SuperMoist), 1/12 pkg. mix 180
   (SuperMoist), 1/12 cake* 250
   lower-fat recipe *(Duncan Hines* Supreme), 1/12 cake* . . . 200
   no-cholesterol recipe *(Duncan Hines)*, 1/12 cake* 240
   no-cholesterol recipe *(SuperMoist)*, 1/12 cake* 220
lime, key:
   (Duncan Hines), 1/12 pkg. mix 180
   (Duncan Hines), 1/12 cake* 250
   no-cholesterol recipe *(Duncan Hines)*, 1/12 cake* 240
marble, fudge:
   (Duncan Hines), 1/12 pkg. mix 180
   (Duncan Hines), 1/12 cake* 250
   (SuperMoist), 1/12 pkg. mix 180
   (SuperMoist), 1/12 cake* 250

* *Prepared according to package directions*

Dessert Cakes, Mixes, marble fudge *(cont.)*
　　no-cholesterol recipe *(Duncan Hines)*, ¹/₁₂ cake* 240
　　no-cholesterol recipe *(SuperMoist)*, ¹/₁₂ cake* 220
orange:
　　(Duncan Hines Supreme), ¹/₁₂ pkg. mix 180
　　(Duncan Hines Supreme), ¹/₁₂ cake* 250
　　no-cholesterol recipe *(Duncan Hines* Supreme), ¹/₁₂ cake* . 240
(Pillsbury Moist Supreme Funfetti), ¹/₁₂ pkg. mix 190
(Pillsbury Moist Supreme Funfetti), ¹/₁₂ cake* 240
pineapple:
　　(Duncan Hines Supreme), ¹/₁₂ pkg. mix 180
　　(Duncan Hines Supreme), ¹/₁₂ cake* 250
　　no-cholesterol recipe *(Duncan Hines* Supreme), ¹/₁₂ cake* . 240
pound:
　　(Betty Crocker), ¹/₈ pkg. mix 270
　　(Dromedary), ¹/₈ pkg. mix 260
　　(Martha White), ¹/₄ cup mix 270
　　(Martha White), ¹/₄ cake* 300
raspberry:
　　(Duncan Hines), ¹/₁₂ pkg. mix 180
　　(Duncan Hines), ¹/₁₂ cake* 250
　　no-cholesterol recipe *(Duncan Hines)*, ¹/₁₂ cake* 240
spice:
　　(Duncan Hines), ¹/₁₂ pkg. mix 180
　　(Duncan Hines), ¹/₁₂ cake* 250
　　(SuperMoist), ¹/₁₂ pkg. mix 180
　　(SuperMoist), ¹/₁₂ cake* 250
　　no-cholesterol recipe *(Duncan Hines)*, ¹/₁₂ cake* 280
　　no-cholesterol recipe *(SuperMoist)*, ¹/₁₂ cake* 220
strawberry:
　　(Duncan Hines Supreme), ¹/₁₂ pkg. mix 180
　　(Duncan Hines Supreme), ¹/₁₂ cake* 250
　　(Pillsbury Moist Supreme), ¹/₁₂ pkg. mix 180
　　(Pillsbury Moist Supreme), ¹/₁₂ cake* 260
　　no-cholesterol recipe *(Duncan Hines* Supreme), ¹/₁₂ cake* . . 240
　　cream cheese *(Pillsbury Bundt)*, ¹/₁₆ pkg. mix 190
　　cream cheese *(Pillsbury Bundt)*, ¹/₁₆ cake* 300
　　swirl *(SuperMoist)*, ¹/₁₀ pkg. mix 200
　　swirl *(SuperMoist)*, ¹/₁₀ cake* 290
　　swirl, no-cholesterol recipe *(SuperMoist)*, ¹/₁₀ cake* 250

* *Prepared according to package directions*

swirl:
　　party *(SuperMoist)*, ¹/₁₂ pkg. mix 180
　　party *(SuperMoist)*, ¹/₁₂ cake* 250
　　party, no-cholesterol recipe *(SuperMoist)*, ¹/₁₂ cake* 220
　　peanut butter chocolate *(SuperMoist)*, ¹/₁₂ pkg. mix 180
　　peanut butter chocolate *(SuperMoist)*, ¹/₁₂ cake* 240
　　peanut butter chocolate, no-cholesterol recipe
　　　　(SuperMoist), ¹/₁₂ cake* 210
　　white chocolate *(SuperMoist)*, ¹/₁₂ pkg. mix 180
　　white chocolate *(SuperMoist)*, ¹/₁₂ cake* 250
　　white chocolate, no-cholesterol recipe *(SuperMoist)*,
　　　　¹/₁₂ cake* 210
vanilla, French:
　　(Duncan Hines), ¹/₁₂ pkg. mix 180
　　(Duncan Hines), ¹/₁₂ cake* 250
　　(Pillsbury Moist Supreme), ¹/₁₀ pkg. mix 220
　　(Pillsbury Moist Supreme), ¹/₁₀ cake* 300
　　(SuperMoist), ¹/₁₂ pkg. mix 180
　　(SuperMoist), ¹/₁₂ cake* 250
　　no-cholesterol recipe *(Duncan Hines)*, ¹/₁₂ cake* 240
　　no-cholesterol recipe *(SuperMoist)*, ¹/₁₂ cake* 210
vanilla, golden:
　　(SuperMoist), ¹/₁₂ pkg. mix 180
　　(SuperMoist), ¹/₁₂ cake* 280
　　no-cholesterol recipe *(SuperMoist)*, ¹/₁₂ cake* 220
white:
　　(Duncan Hines), ¹/₁₂ pkg. mix 180
　　(Duncan Hines), ¹/₁₂ cake* 240
　　(Pillsbury Moist Supreme/Plus), ¹/₁₀ pkg. mix 220
　　(Pillsbury Moist Supreme/Plus), ¹/₁₀ cake* 280
　　(SnackWell's), ¹/₆ pkg. mix 200
　　(SnackWell's), ¹/₆ cake* 210
　　(SuperMoist), ¹/₁₂ pkg. mix 180
　　(SuperMoist), ¹/₁₂ cake* 230
　　(SuperMoist Light), ¹/₁₀ pkg. mix 210
　　(SuperMoist Light), ¹/₁₀ cake* 210
　　(Sweet Rewards Reduced Fat), ¹/₁₂ pkg. mix 170
　　(Sweet Rewards Reduced Fat), ¹/₁₂ cake* 210
　　Olympic party *(SuperMoist)*, ¹/₁₂ pkg. mix 180
　　Olympic party *(SuperMoist)*, ¹/₁₂ cake* 240

* Prepared according to package directions

Dessert Cakes, Mixes, white *(cont.)*

    Olympic party, richer recipe *(SuperMoist)*, ¹/₁₂ cake* 250
    sour cream *(SuperMoist)*, ¹/₁₀ pkg. mix 210
    sour cream *(SuperMoist)*, ¹/₁₀ cake* 280
    richer recipe *(SuperMoist)*, ¹/₁₂ cake* 250
    whole egg recipe *(Duncan Hines)*, ¹/₁₂ cake* 250
    whole egg recipe *(Sweet Rewards* Reduced Fat)*, ¹/₁₂ cake* . . 210
white 'n fudge swirl *(Pillsbury Moist Supreme)*, ¹/₁₂ pkg. mix . . . 200
white 'n fudge swirl *(Pillsbury Moist Supreme)*, ¹/₁₂ cake* 250
yellow:
    (Duncan Hines), ¹/₁₂ pkg. mix 180
    (Duncan Hines), ¹/₁₂ cake* 250
    (Pillsbury Moist Supreme), ¹/₁₂ pkg. mix 180
    (Pillsbury Moist Supreme), ¹/₁₂ cake* 240
    (Robin Hood Pouch)*, ¹/₅ pkg. mix 190
    (Robin Hood Pouch)*, ¹/₅ cake* 280
    (SnackWell's), ¹/₆ pkg. mix 200
    (SnackWell's), ¹/₆ cake* 210
    (SuperMoist), ¹/₁₂ pkg. mix 170
    (SuperMoist), ¹/₁₂ cake* 240
    (SuperMoist Light)*, ¹/₁₀ pkg. mix 210
    (SuperMoist Light)*, ¹/₁₀ cake* 230
    (Sweet Rewards Reduced Fat)*, ¹/₁₂ pkg. mix 170
    (Sweet Rewards Reduced Fat)*, ¹/₁₂ cake* 220
    no-cholesterol recipe *(Duncan Hines)*, ¹/₁₂ cake* 240
    no-cholesterol recipe *(SuperMoist)*, ¹/₁₂ cake* 210
    no-cholesterol recipe *(SuperMoist* Light)*, ¹/₁₀ cake* 210
    no-cholesterol recipe *(Sweet Rewards* Reduced Fat)*,
        ¹/₁₂ cake* 200

DESSERT PIES, FROZEN OR REFRIGERATED
*See also "Dessert Cakes," "Dessert Pies, Mixes," and "Snack
Pastries & Pies, Frozen or Refrigerated"*

---

                                                        calories

apple:
    (Amy's), 8 oz. 280
    (Banquet), ¹/₅ pie 300
    (Mrs. Smith's 8"), ¹/₆ pie 270
    (Mrs. Smith's 9"), ¹/₈ pie 310

* *Prepared according to package directions*

(Mrs. Smith's 10"*)*, 1/10 pie 280
(Mrs. Smith's Old Fashioned 9"*)*, 1/8 pie 350
(Mrs. Smith's Reduced Fat*)*, 1/6 pie 250
(Mrs. Smith's Reduced Fat No Sugar*)*, 1/6 pie 210
(Sara Lee Homestyle*)*, 1/8 pie 330
(Schwan's), 1/12 pie 270
lattice *(Mrs. Smith's)*, 1/5 pie 310
apple, Dutch:
   (Mrs. Smith's 8"*)*, 1/6 pie 320
   (Mrs. Smith's 9"*)*, 1/8 pie 350
   (Mrs. Smith's 10"*)*, 1/10 pie 320
   (Mrs. Smith's Old Fashioned*)*, 1/8 pie 310
apple-cranberry *(Mrs. Smith's)*, 1/6 pie 280
banana cream:
   (Banquet), 1/3 pie 350
   (Mrs. Smith's), 1/4 pie 280
   (Pet-Ritz), 1/4 pie 270
berry or blackberry *(Mrs. Smith's)*, 1/6 pie 280
blueberry *(Mrs. Smith's)*, 1/6 pie 260
Boston cream, *see "Dessert Cakes, Frozen," page 285*
cherry:
   (Banquet), 1/5 pie 290
   (Mrs. Smith's 8"*)*, 1/6 pie 270
   (Mrs. Smith's 9"*)*, 1/8 pie 310
   (Mrs. Smith's 10"*)*, 1/10 pie 280
   (Mrs. Smith's Old Fashioned 9"*)*, 1/8 pie 320
   (Mrs. Smith's Reduced Fat 8"*)*, 1/6 pie 250
   (Mrs. Smith's Reduced Fat No Sugar 8"*)*, 1/6 pie 220
   lattice *(Mrs. Smith's)*, 1/5 pie 320
   or peach *(Schwan's)*, 1/10 pie 320
chocolate cream:
   (Banquet), 1/3 pie 360
   (Mrs. Smith's), 1/4 pie 330
   (Pet-Ritz), 1/4 pie 290
   (Sara Lee), 1/5 pie 500
   French silk *(Mrs. Smith's)*, 1/5 pie 410
coconut cream:
   (Banquet), 1/3 pie 350
   (Mrs. Smith's), 1/4 pie 340
   (Pet-Ritz), 1/4 pie 270
coconut custard, *(Mrs. Smith's)*, 1/5 pie 280
fudge vanilla cream *(Pet-Ritz)*, 1/4 pie 300

Dessert Pies, Frozen or Refrigerated *(cont.)*
lemon:
    cream *(Banquet)*, ⅓ pie 360
    cream *(Mrs. Smith's)*, ¼ pie 300
    cream *(Pet-Ritz)*, ¼ pie 270
    meringue *(Mrs. Smith's)*, ⅕ pie 302
    meringue *(Sara Lee* Homestyle), ⅙ pie 350
mincemeat *(Banquet)*, ⅕ pie 310
mincemeat *(Mrs. Smith's)*, ⅙ pie 300
peach:
    (Banquet), ⅕ pie 260
    (Mrs. Smith's 8"), ⅙ pie 260
    (Mrs. Smith's 9"), ⅛ pie 310
peanut butter chocolate cream *(Pet-Ritz)*, ¼ pie 300
pecan *(Mrs. Smith's 8")*, ⅙ pie 520
pecan *(Mrs. Smith's 10")*, ⅛ pie 500
pumpkin:
    (Banquet), ⅕ pie 250
    (Mrs. Smith's Hearty 8"), ⅕ pie 250
    (Mrs. Smith's Hearty 9"), ⅛ pie 240
    (Schwan's), ¹/₁₀ pie 250
    cream *(Pet-Ritz)*, ¼ pie 270
    custard *(Mrs. Smith's 8")*, ⅕ pie 270
    custard *(Mrs. Smith's 9")*, ⅛ pie 240
    custard *(Mrs. Smith's 10")*, ¹/₁₀ pie 250
raspberry or strawberry-rhubarb *(Mrs. Smith's)*, ⅙ pie 280
strawberry *(Mrs. Smith's)*, ⅕ pie 280

DESSERT PIES, MIXES
*See also "Dessert Cakes," "Dessert Pies, Frozen or
Refrigerated," and "Pie Fillings, Canned"*

---

                                               calories
banana cream *(Betty Crocker)*, ⅑ pkg. mix 160
banana cream *(Betty Crocker)*, ⅑ pie* 250
chocolate silk:
    (Jell-O), ⅙ pie* 310
    French *(Betty Crocker)*, ⅛ pkg. mix 180
    French *(Betty Crocker)*, ⅛ pie* 270

* Prepared according to package directions

coconut cream:
   (Betty Crocker), ⅑ pkg. mix 200
   (Betty Crocker), ⅑ pie* 290
   (Jell-O), ⅙ pie* 330
cookies 'n creme *(Betty Crocker)*, ⅙ pkg. mix 260
cookies 'n creme *(Betty Crocker)*, ⅙ pie* 360
Sunkist lemon supreme *(Betty Crocker)*, ⅑ pkg. mix 270
Sunkist lemon supreme *(Betty Crocker)*, ⅑ pie* 320

SNACK CAKES & PASTRIES, one piece, except as noted
*See also "Dessert Cakes," "Snack Pies," "Snack Pastries &
Pies, Frozen or Refrigerated," "Snack Cakes, Mixes," and
"Cookies"*

---

                                                         calories
(Tastykake Koffee Kake), 2.5-oz. piece 270
(Tastykake Kreme Krimpies), 2 pieces 230
all varieties *(Health Valley Healthy Tarts)* 150
almond twirl *(Aunt Fanny's)* 110
apple, date, or raisin *(Health Valley Bakes)* 70
apple bar *(Health Valley)* 140
apple filled *(Tastykake Krimpets Low Fat)*, 2 pieces 160
apple raisin bar *(SnackWell's)* 130
apricot bar *(Health Valley)* 140
banana:
   (Little Debbie Twins) 250
   (Tastykake Creamies) 170
   bar *(SnackWell's)* 130
Boston creme *(Drake's)* 170
brownie:
   (Hostess Light), 1.4-oz. piece 140
   bar *(Oreo)* 160
   chocolate *(Awrey's Decadent)* 230
   chocolate *(Little Debbie Low Fat)* 190
   chocolate, Bavarian *(Awrey's)* 250
   chocolate cherry, bar *(SnackWell's)* 130
   chocolate peanut *(Awrey's Sensation)* 230
   fudge *(Entenmann's Fat Free)*, ⅒ strip 110
   fudge *(Little Debbie)* 310
   fudge, bar *(SnackWell's)* 130

---

* *Prepared according to package directions*

Snack Cakes & Pastries, brownie *(cont.)*
    fudge filled *(Health Valley)* 110
    fudge, with nuts *(Awrey's)* 190
    fudge, without nuts *(Awrey's)* 200
    fudge nut *(Drake's* Reduced Fat) 170
    fudge nut, chewy *(Awrey's)* 210
    fudge walnut *(Tastykake)* 370
    mini *(Hostess Bites)*, 5 pieces 290
bun, sweet:
    apple *(Entenmann's* Fat Free) 150
    cheese, blueberry or pineapple *(Entenmann's* Fat Free) 140
    cheese, raspberry *(Entenmann's* Fat Free) 160
    cinnamon *(Entenmann's)* 220
    cinnamon raisin *(Entenmann's* Fat Free) 160
    glazed *(Entenmann's* Donut Dippers) 160
    honey *(Aunt Fanny's)*, 3-oz. piece 360
    honey *(Aunt Fanny's)*, 4-oz. piece 500
    honey *(Grandma's)* 410
    honey *(Little Debbie)*, 3-oz. piece 380
    honey *(Morton)*, 2.3-oz. piece 290
    honey *(Morton* Mini), 1.3-oz. piece 160
    honey, applesauce filled *(Aunt Fanny's)* 330
    honey, banana, chocolate, or vanilla creme filled *(Aunt
       Fanny's)* 350
    honey, glazed *(Hostess)* 320
    honey, glazed or iced *(Tastykake)* 350
    honey, iced *(Aunt Fanny's)* 350
    honey, iced *(Hostess)* 390
    honey, raspberry filled *(Aunt Fanny's)* 350
butterscotch iced *(Tastykake Krimpets)*, 2 pieces 210
cheesecake *(Boar's Head* New York), 4-oz. piece 380
cheesecake bar, all varieties *(Health Valley)* 160
cherry pocket *(Tastykake)* 370
chocolate:
    (Devil Dogs), 1.6-oz. piece 170
    (Ding Dongs), 1.3-oz. piece 160
    (Funny Bones), 2 pieces 300
    (Ho-Hos), 3 pieces 380
    (Hostess Choco-Diles) 240
    (Hostess Choco Licious), 2 pieces 370
    (Ring Dings), 2 pieces 320
    (Suzy Q's), 2 pieces 450

(Tastykake Creamies) 180
(Tastykake Juniors) 360
(Tastykake Kandy Kakes), 3 pieces 270
(Yodels), 2 pieces 280
fingers *(Aunt Fanny's)*, 2 pieces 290
chocolate chip *(Chips Ahoy)* 150
chocolate chip *(Little Debbie)* 280
cinnamon roll *(see also "bun, sweet," above):*
(Awrey's Homestyle) 270
(Hostess) 210
glazed *(Weight Watchers)* 200
cinnamon twirl *(Aunt Fanny's)* 110
coconut covered:
(Sno Balls), 2 pieces 350
(Tastykake Juniors) 320
(Tastykake Kandy Kakes), 3 pieces 260
coconut twirl *(Aunt Fanny's)* 110
coffee cake:
(Drake's) 130
(Drake's Low Fat) 100
(Little Debbie) 230
crumb *(Hostess)*, 2 pieces 360
crumb *(Hostess* Light), 2 pieces 260
cupcake:
(Tastykake Kreme Kup), 2 pieces 190
(Yankee Doodles), 2 pieces 220
apple filled *(Tastykake Koffee Kake* Low Fat), 2 pieces 160
buttercreme, iced *(Tastykake)*, 2 pieces 250
buttercreme, iced, mini *(Tastykake)*, 2 pieces 110
chocolate *(Aunt Fanny's)*, 2 pieces 310
chocolate *(Hostess)*, 2 pieces 360
chocolate *(Hostess* Light), 2 pieces 270
chocolate *(Tastykake)*, 2 pieces 220
chocolate *(Tastykake)*, 3 pieces 330
chocolate, creme *(Tastykake* Low Fat), 2 pieces 200
chocolate, iced, creme *(Tastykake)*, 2 pieces 250
chocolate, iced, creme, mini *(Tastykake)*, 2 pieces 110
chocolate, iced, creme, vanilla, mini *(Tastykake)*, 2 pieces . . . 110
creme *(Tastykake Koffee Kake)*, 2 pieces 80
creme, mini *(Tastykake Koffee Kake)*, 2 pieces 110
lemon filled *(Tastykake Koffee Kake* Low Fat), 2 pieces 160
orange *(Aunt Fanny's)*, 2 pieces 310

Snack Cakes & Pastries, cupcake *(cont.)*

orange *(Hostess)*, 2 pieces 320
raspberry filled *(Tastykake Koffee Kake* Low Fat), 2 pieces . 160
vanilla, creme *(Tastykake* Low Fat), 2 pieces 210
Danish:
all varieties *(Awrey's* Petite) 130
apple *(Awrey's* Grande) 450
apple, cheese, cinnamon swirl, or strawberry *(Awrey's)* 300
cheese *(Awrey's* Grande) 480
cheese *(Tastykake* Pocket) 410
cheese, cherry or lemon *(Awrey's* Marquise) 350
cheese, cinnamon *(Awreys* Marquise) 470
cheese, raspberry swirl *(Awrey's* Grande) 400
cinnamon swirl *(Awrey's* Grande) 420
strawberry *(Awrey's* Grande) 460
date bar *(Health Valley)* 140
date nut pastry *(Awrey's)* 130
devil's food *(Little Debbie Devil Cremes)* 370
donut:
plain *(Awrey's)*, 1.5-oz. piece 170
plain *(Awrey's)*, 2-oz. piece 240
plain *(Hostess* Jumbo), 1.2-oz. piece 140
plain *(Hostess* Old Fashion) 170
plain *(Tastykake* Assorted) 180
assorted *(Hostess)* 200
blueberry *(Hostess)*. 210
cinnamon *(Hostess)* 110
cinnamon *(Tastykake* Assorted) 210
cinnamon and sugar *(Entenmann's* Variety Pack) 310
coconut top *(Awrey's)* 210
crumb *(Entenmann's)* 260
crumb *(Entenmann's* Variety Pack) 420
crumb *(Hostess)* 130
crumb *(Hostess Gems)*, 6 pieces, 3 oz. 320
crunch *(Awrey's)* 280
crunch top *(Awrey's)* 160
devil's food crumb *(Entenmann's)* 250
frosted, chocolate *(Awrey's)*, 1.75-oz. piece 200
frosted, chocolate *(Awrey's)*, 2.5-oz. piece 300
frosted, chocolate *(Hostess)*, 1.4-oz. piece 180
frosted, chocolate *(Hostess* Jumbo), 2-oz. piece 260
frosted, chocolate *(Hostess Gems)*, 6 pieces, 3 oz. 390

frosted, chocolate, chocolate *(Awrey's)*, 1.75-oz. piece 190
frosted, chocolate, chocolate *(Awrey's)*, 2.5-oz. piece 280
frosted, chocolate, custard bismarck *(Awrey's)* 350
frosted, chocolate, mini *(Entenmann's)*, 2 pieces 270
frosted, chocolate, rich *(Entenmann's)* 280
frosted, chocolate, rich *(Entenmann's Variety Pack)* 400
frosted, chocolate, rich *(Tastykake)* 270
frosted, chocolate, rich, mini *(Entenmann's Popettes)*,
    3 pieces 210
frosted, chocolate, rich, mini *(Tastykake)*, 4 pieces 270
frosted, chocolate, rich, with raspberry *(Entenmann's)* 260
frosted, chocolate, ring *(Awrey's)* 350
frosted, chocolate, sour creme *(Awrey's)* 430
glazed *(Entenmann's Popems)*, 6 pieces 240
glazed *(Hostess)* 150
glazed *(Hostess Old Fashion)* 250
glazed *(Hostess Party)* 260
glazed *(Hostess Whirl)* 180
glazed, buttermilk *(Entenmann's)* 270
glazed, chocolate *(Entenmann's Popems)*, 4 pieces 200
glazed, honey, devil's food *(Awrey's)* 310
glazed, honey, ring *(Awrey's)* 310
glazed, honey wheat *(Hostess Old Fashion)* 250
glazed, orange *(Tastykake)* 220
glazed, sour creme *(Awrey's)* 420
honey wheat *(Tastykake)* 230
honey wheat, mini *(Tastykake)*, 6 pieces 280
powdered sugar *(Awrey's)*, 1.5-oz. piece 170
powdered sugar *(Awrey's)*, 2.25-oz. piece 390
powdered sugar *(Entenmann's Softee)* 220
powdered sugar *(Hostess)*, 1-oz. piece 110
powdered sugar *(Hostess Jumbo)*, 1.3-oz. piece 160
powdered sugar *(Hostess Gems)*, 6 pieces, 3 oz. 350
powdered sugar *(Tastykake Assorted)* 210
powdered sugar, jelly bismarck *(Awrey's)* 320
powdered sugar, mini *(Tastykake)*, 6 pieces 290
powdered sugar, raspberry filled *(Hostess O's)* 230
sour creme, plain *(Awrey's)* 370
sprinkle topped *(Awrey's)* 160
vanilla iced *(Awrey's Long John)* 380
vanilla iced, jelly bismarck *(Awrey's)* 320
white, iced *(Awrey's)* 200

Snack Cakes & Pastries *(cont.)*

frosty *(Tastykake Kandy Kakes)*, 3 pieces 260
fudge, frosted *(Little Debbie)* 270
fudge, rounds *(Little Debbie)* 290
golden, bar *(SnackWell's)* 130
golden, creme-filled:
    (Hostess Dessert Cup) 90
    (Little Debbie Golden Cremes) 280
    (Sunny Doodles), 2 pieces 220
    (Sunny Doodles Reduced Fat), 2 pieces 180
    (Twinkies), 2 pieces 300
    (Twinkies Light), 2 pieces 260
jelly filled *(Tastykake Krimpets)*, 2 pieces 190
jelly filled *(Tastykake Krimpets* Low Fat), 2 pieces 180
lemon filled *(Tastykake Krimpets* Low Fat), 2 pieces 180
peanut butter *(Tastykake Kandy Kakes)*, 3 pieces 280
pecan roll *(Little Debbie Spinwheels)* 220
pecan twirl *(Aunt Fanny's)* 100
pound:
    (Aunt Fanny's) 250
    (Awrey's) 210
    (Tastykake) 320
raisin bar *(Health Valley* Fat Free) 140
raspberry fingers *(Aunt Fanny's)*, 2 pieces 280
sprinkled *(Tastykake* Creamies) 150
stick, dunking:
    (Aunt Fanny's), 1.4-oz. piece 190
    (Aunt Fanny's), 1.65-oz. piece 230
    (Little Debbie) 250
    (Tastykake Stix) 190
    cherry or chocolate *(Aunt Fanny's)* 180
    twin sticks *(Awrey's)*, 2.75-oz. piece 330
strawberry, iced *(Tastykake Krimpets)*, 2 pieces 210
strawberry shortcake *(Little Debbie)* 290
strudel, apple *(Entenmann's)*, ¼ piece 310
Swiss roll *(Little Debbie)* 320
vanilla:
    (Little Debbie) 380
    (Tastykake Creamies) 190
    fingers *(Aunt Fanny's)*, 2 pieces 290
zebra *(Little Debbie)* 380

SNACK PIES, one piece, except as noted
*See also "Snack Cakes & Pastries" and "Snack Pastries &
Pies, Frozen or Refrigerated"*

	calories
(Tastykake Tastyklair)	410
all flavors except cherry *(Hostess)*	440
apple:	
(Aunt Fanny's), 3.5-oz. piece	400
(Aunt Fanny's), 4-oz. piece	460
(Drake's), 2 pies, 4-oz. piece	400
(McMillin's), 3.5-oz. piece	390
(McMillin's), 4-oz. piece	460
(Pet-Ritz)	430
(Tastykake)	290
French *(Tastykake)*	360
pocket *(Tastykake)*	380
banana cream *(Aunt Fanny's)*	400
berry:	
(Aunt Fanny's), 3.5-oz. piece	380
(Aunt Fanny's), 4-oz. piece	430
(McMillin's), 3.5-oz. piece	390
(McMillin's), 4-oz. piece	440
blueberry *(Pet-Ritz)*	450
blueberry *(Tastykake)*	320
Boston creme:	
(Aunt Fanny's), 3.5-oz. piece	370
(Aunt Fanny's), 4-oz. piece	440
(McMillin's), 3.5-oz. piece	370
(McMillin's), 4-oz. piece	440
cherry:	
(Aunt Fanny's), 3.5-oz. piece	350
(Aunt Fanny's), 4-oz. piece	400
(Drake's), 2 pies, 4-oz. piece	420
(Hostess)	450
(McMillin's), 3.5-oz. piece	380
(McMillin's), 4-oz. piece	430
(Pet-Ritz)	450
(Tastykake)	320
chocolate creme:	
(Aunt Fanny's), 3.5-oz. piece	390
(Aunt Fanny's), 4-oz. piece	450

Snack Pies, chocolate creme *(cont.)*
   pudding *(McMillin's)*, 3.5-oz. piece 380
   pudding *(McMillin's)*, 4-oz. piece 450
coconut:
   creme *(Aunt Fanny's)*, 3.5-oz. piece 390
   creme *(Aunt Fanny's)*, 4-oz. piece 440
   creme *(Tastykake)* 390
   pudding *(McMillin's)*, 3.5-oz. piece 380
   pudding *(McMillin's)*, 4-oz. piece 440
lemon:
   (McMillin's), 3.5-oz. piece 360
   (McMillin's), 4-oz. piece 410
   (Pet-Ritz) 450
   (Tastykake) 320
   creme *(Aunt Fanny's)*, 3.5-oz. piece 360
   creme *(Aunt Fanny's)*, 4-oz. piece 420
marshmallow, banana *(Little Debbie)* 320
marshmallow, chocolate *(Little Debbie)* 320
oatmeal creme *(Little Debbie)* 300
peach:
   (Aunt Fanny's), 3.5-oz. piece 380
   (Aunt Fanny's), 4-oz. piece 430
   (McMillin's), 3.5-oz. piece 370
   (McMillin's), 4-oz. piece 420
   (Tastykake) 300
peanut butter cream *(McMillin's)* 450
pineapple *(Tastykake)* 290
pineapple cheese *(Tastykake)* 320
pumpkin:
   (Aunt Fanny's) 420
   (McMillin's) 420
   (Tastykake) 330
raisin creme *(Little Debbie)* 270
strawberry:
   (Aunt Fanny's), 3.5-oz. piece 370
   (Aunt Fanny's), 4-oz. piece 420
   (McMillin's), 3.5-oz. piece 370
   (McMillin's), 4-oz. piece 420
   (Tastykake) 310
vanilla:
   creme *(Aunt Fanny's)*, 3.5-oz. piece 350
   creme *(Aunt Fanny's)*, 4-oz. piece 400

pudding *(McMillin's)*, 3.5-oz. piece 360
pudding *(McMillin's)*, 4-oz. piece 400

SNACK PASTRIES & PIES, FROZEN OR REFRIGERATED, one
piece, except as noted
*See also "Dessert Cakes, Frozen," "Dessert Pies, Frozen or
Refrigerated," "Snack Cakes & Pastries," "Snack Pies," and
"Miscellaneous Desserts"*

---

	calories
baklava, wheat *(Cedar's)*	190

baklava, white *(Cedar's)* 210
brownie:
   à la mode *(Weight Watchers)* 190
   chocolate frosted *(Weight Watchers)* 100
   parfait, double fudge *(Weight Watchers)* 190
   peanut butter fudge *(Weight Watchers)* 110
bun, sweet:
   apple cinnamon, iced *(Pillsbury)* 150
   caramel *(Pillsbury)* 170
   cinnamon *(Pepperidge Farm)* 250
   cinnamon *(Sara Lee* Deluxe Roll) 320
   cinnamon, iced *(Pillsbury)* 150
   cinnamon, iced *(Schwan's)* 240
   cinnamon raisin or orange, iced *(Pillsbury)* 170
   honey *(Rich's)* 240
cheesecake:
   French style *(Weight Watchers)* 180
   New York style *(Weight Watchers)* 150
   triple chocolate *(Weight Watchers)* 200
chocolate caramel mousse, triple *(Weight Watchers)* 200
chocolate chip cookie dough sundae *(Weight Watchers)* 180
chocolate mocha pie *(Weight Watchers)* 170
chocolate mousse *(Weight Watchers)* 190
chocolate pastry, dark or milk *(Pepperidge Farm* Clouds),
   2 pieces 580
chocolate raspberry royale *(Weight Watchers)* 190
churro, cinnamon *(Tio Pepe's)*, 1-oz. piece 110
danish, apple or raspberry *(Pepperidge Farm)* 210
danish, cheese *(Pepperidge Farm)* 230
donut, glazed *(Rich's)* 130

Snack Pastries & Pies, Frozen or Refrigerated *(cont.)*
dumpling:
    apple *(Pepperidge Farm)* 290
    cherry *(Pepperidge Farm)* 280
    peach *(Pepperidge Farm)* 300
éclair, chocolate:
    (Rich's) 190
    (Weight Watchers) 150
    triple *(Weight Watchers)* 160
fudge cake, double *(Weight Watchers)* 190
Mississippi mud pie *(Weight Watchers)* 160
praline toffee crunch parfait *(Weight Watchers)* 190
strawberry parfait royale *(Weight Watchers)* 180

SNACK CAKES, MIXES, one piece*, except as noted
*See also "Dessert Cakes, Mixes," "Snack Cakes & Pastries,"
and "Cookies, Refrigerated & Mixes"*

---

                                                       calories
brownie:
    (Arrowhead Mills) 110
    (Arrowhead Mills) Fat Free/Wheat Free 120
    (Betty Crocker), 1/20 pkg. mix 130
    (Betty Crocker) 180
    (Sweet Rewards Reduced Fat), 1/20 pkg. mix 120
    (Sweet Rewards Reduced Fat) 150
    no-cholesterol recipe *(Sweet Rewards* Reduced Fat) 140
    no-cholesterol/reduced-fat recipe *(Betty Crocker)* 160
brownie, blonde, with white chocolate chunks:
    (Duncan Hines), 1/12 pkg. mix 140
    (Duncan Hines) 170
brownie, caramel:
    (Betty Crocker), 1/18 pkg. mix 130
    (Betty Crocker) 190
    no-cholesterol recipe *(Betty Crocker)* 160
brownie, cheesecake swirl *(Pillsbury* Thick 'n Fudgy), 1/16 pkg.
    mix 130
brownie cheesecake swirl *(Pillsbury* Thick 'n Fudgy) 170
brownie, chocolate:
    dark, with *Hershey's* syrup *(Betty Crocker)*, 1/18 pkg. mix . . . 130

---

* *Prepared according to package directions*

dark, with *Hershey's* syrup *(Betty Crocker)* 190
dark, with *Hershey's* syrup, no-cholesterol/reduced-fat
  recipe *(Betty Crocker)* 160
German *(Betty Crocker)*, 1/18 pkg. mix 160
German *(Betty Crocker)* 220
German, no-cholesterol recipe *(Betty Crocker)* 190
chip *(Betty Crocker)*, 1/18 pkg. mix 140
chip *(Betty Crocker)* 220
chip, no-cholesterol recipe *(Betty Crocker)* 180
chunk *(Betty Crocker)*, 1/20 pkg. mix 130
chunk *(Betty Crocker)* 190
chunk, no-cholesterol/reduced-fat recipe *(Betty Crocker)* . . . 160
chunk, milk *(Duncan Hines)*, 1/20 pkg. mix 140
chunk, milk *(Duncan Hines)* 170
chunk, milk, no-cholesterol recipe *(Duncan Hines)* 160
brownie, cookies and cream:
  (Betty Crocker), 1/18 pkg. mix 140
  (Betty Crocker) 200
  no-cholesterol recipe *(Betty Crocker)* 180
brownie, dark 'n chunky *(Duncan Hines)*, 1/20 pkg. mix 140
brownie, dark 'n chunky *(Duncan Hines)* 160
brownie, dark 'n fudgy:
  (Duncan Hines), 1/18 pkg. mix 120
  (Duncan Hines) 170
  no-cholesterol recipe *(Duncan Hines)* 160
brownie, devil's food *(SnackWell's)* 140
brownie, frosted:
  (Betty Crocker), 1/20 pkg. mix 150
  (Betty Crocker) 210
  no-cholesterol/reduced-fat recipe *(Betty Crocker)* 180
brownie, fudge:
  (Betty Crocker), 1/12 pkg. mix 140
  (Betty Crocker) 190
  (Betty Crocker Family Size), 1/18 pkg. mix 140
  (Betty Crocker Family Size) 200
  (Betty Crocker Light) 130
  (Martha White Chewy Family Size), 1/20 pkg. mix 120
  (Martha White Chewy Family Size) 180
  (Martha White Chewy Snack Size), 1/10 pkg. mix 120
  (Martha White Chewy Snack Size) 160
  (Martha White Moist 'n Fudgy), 1/20 pkg. mix 130
  (Martha White Moist 'n Fudgy) 150

Snack Cakes, Mixes, brownie, fudge *(cont.)*

    (Mother's Best Chewy), ¹⁄₁₀ pkg. mix 120
    (Mother's Best Chewy) 160
    (Robin Hood/Gold Medal Pouch), ¹⁄₁₀ pkg. mix 120
    (Robin Hood/Gold Medal Pouch) 170
    (SnackWell's) 150
    (Sweet Rewards Low Fat), ¹⁄₁₈ pkg. mix 130
    chewy *(Duncan Hines* 19.8 oz.), ¹⁄₁₈ pkg. mix 130
    chewy *(Duncan Hines* 19.8/12.9 oz.) 160
    chewy *(Duncan Hines* 12.9 oz.), ¹⁄₁₂ pkg. mix 130
    dark chocolate *(Betty Crocker),* ¹⁄₁₈ pkg. mix 130
    dark chocolate *(Betty Crocker)* 190
    dark chocolate, no-cholesterol recipe *(Betty Crocker)* 160
    double *(Duncan Hines),* ¹⁄₂₀ pkg. mix 140
    double *(Duncan Hines)* 170
    double, no-cholesterol recipe *(Duncan Hines)* 160
    hot *(Betty Crocker),* ¹⁄₁₈ pkg. mix 130
    hot *(Betty Crocker)* 190
    hot, no-cholesterol recipe *(Betty Crocker)* 160
    low-fat *(Betty Crocker),* ¹⁄₁₈ pkg. mix 130
    no-cholesterol/reduced-fat recipe *(Betty Crocker* Family
      Size) 170
brownie, Mississippi mud *(Duncan Hines),* ¹⁄₂₀ pkg. mix 130
brownie, Mississippi mud *(Duncan Hines)* 160
brownie, peanut butter candies, with *Reese's Pieces:*
    (Betty Crocker), ¹⁄₁₈ pkg. mix 140
    (Betty Crocker) 200
    no-cholesterol recipe *(Betty Crocker)* 180
brownie, raspberry dark chocolate *(Duncan Hines),*
    ¹⁄₂₀ pkg. mix 120
brownie, raspberry dark chocolate *(Duncan Hines)* 150
brownie, walnut:
    (Betty Crocker), ¹⁄₁₈ pkg. mix 140
    (Betty Crocker) 200
    (Duncan Hines), ¹⁄₂₀ pkg. mix 140
    (Duncan Hines) 170
    (Martha White Delux), ¹⁄₂₀ pkg. mix 140
    (Martha White Delux) 170
    no-cholesterol/reduced-fat recipe *(Betty Crocker)* 170
brownie, white chocolate swirl:
    (Betty Crocker), ¹⁄₁₈ pkg. mix 150
    (Betty Crocker) 210

no-cholesterol/reduced-fat recipe *(Betty Crocker)* 180
cookie bar:
   chunk, milk chocolate *(Duncan Hines)*, 1/27 pkg. mix 110
   chunk, milk chocolate *(Duncan Hines)* 140
   chunk, milk chocolate, no-cholesterol recipe *(Duncan
     Hines)* 130
   double decker *(Duncan Hines)*, 1/30 pkg. mix 100
   double decker *(Duncan Hines)* 130
cupcake:
   angel food, polka dot *(Duncan Hines)*, 1/8 pkg. mix 160
   angel food, polka dot *(Duncan Hines)*, 3 decorated
     cakes* 160
   dirt *(Duncan Hines)*, 1/6 pkg. mix 180
   dirt *(Duncan Hines)*, 2 decorated cakes 300

MISCELLANEOUS DESSERTS, one piece, except as noted
*See also "Dessert Cakes" and "Snack Pastries & Pies, Frozen
or Refrigerated"*

	calories
apple flauta *(Schwan's)*	160

apple fritters, frozen *(Mrs. Paul's)*, 2 pieces 260
apple puff *(Entenmann's)* 260
cobbler, frozen:
   apple *(Marie Callender's)*, 4 1/4 oz. 350
   apple *(Stilwell)*, 1/8 pkg. 240
   apple *(Stilwell Lite)*, 1/8 pkg. 140
   apricot *(Stilwell)*, 1/8 pkg. 240
   berry *(Stilwell)*, 1/8 pkg. 250
   berry *(Stilwell Lite)*, 1/8 pkg. 140
   berry or cherry *(Marie Callender's)*, 4 1/4 oz. 390
   blackberry *(Stilwell)*, 1/8 pkg. 250
   blackberry *(Stilwell Lite)*, 1/8 pkg. 150
   blueberry *(Marie Callender's)*, 4 oz. 340
   blueberry *(Pet-Ritz)*, 1/6 pkg. 280
   cherry *(Stilwell)*, 1/8 pkg. 250
   cherry *(Stilwell Lite)*, 1/8 pkg. 150
   peach *(Marie Callender's)*, 4 1/4 oz. 370
   peach *(Stilwell)*, 1/8 pkg. 240
   peach *(Stilwell Lite)*, 1/8 pkg. 140

* *Prepared according to package directions*

Miscellaneous Desserts, cobbler, frozen *(cont.)*

strawberry *(Stilwell)*, 1/8 pkg. 260
fruit square, apple, frozen *(Pepperidge Farm)* 210
turnover, frozen or refrigerated:

apple *(Pillsbury)*, 2 pieces 350
apple, cherry, or strawberry, mini *(Pepperidge Farm)* 140
apple or raspberry *(Pepperidge Farm)* 330
apple or raspberry, iced *(Pepperidge Farm)* 360
blueberry or peach *(Pepperidge Farm)* 340
cherry *(Pepperidge Farm)* 320
cherry *(Pillsbury)*, 2 pieces 360
cherry, iced *(Pepperidge Farm)* 340
peach cobbler, mini *(Pepperidge Farm)* 160

COOKIES
*See also "Snack Cakes & Pastries" and "Cookies, Refrigerated
& Mixes"*

---

calories

almond:

(Archway Crescents), 2 pieces, .8 oz. 100
(Stella D'Oro Breakfast Treats), .8-oz. piece 100
(Stella D'Oro Chinese Dessert), 1.2-oz. piece 170
(Sunshine Crescents), 4 pieces, 1.1 oz. 150
horn, with chocolate *(Tekrum)*, 2 pieces, 1.3 oz. 194
toast *(Stella D'Oro* Mandel), 2 pieces, 1 oz. 110
amaretti di Saronno, chocolate dipped *(Lazzaroni)*, 4 pieces,
1.1 oz. 140
animal:

(Barnum's Animals), 12 pieces, 1.1 oz. 140
(Sunshine), 14 pieces, 1.1 oz. 140
vanilla *(Barbara's)*, 8 pieces, 1 oz. 130
anisette:

(Stella D'Oro Sponge), 2 pieces, 1 oz. 90
(Stella D'Oro Toast), 3 pieces, 1.2 oz. 130
(Stella D'Oro Toast Jumbo), 1 piece, 1.1 oz. 100
apple:

(Newtons Fat Free), 2 pieces, 1 oz. 100
(Sunshine Golden Fruit), .7-oz. piece 80
bar *(Archway* Nonfat), .7-oz. piece 60
bran *(Archway)*, 1.2-oz. piece 130
cinnamon bar *(Tastykake)*, 1.5-oz. bar 180

pastry *(Stella D'Oro* Low Sodium), .7-oz. piece 80
and raisin *(Archway)*, 1.1-oz. piece 130
raisin *(Health Valley* Fat Free Jumbo), 1 piece 80
raisin bar *(Smart Snackers)*, .75 oz. 70
spice *(Health Valley* Fat Free), 3 pieces 100
apricot, filled *(Archway)*, 1-oz. piece 110
apricot raspberry *(Pepperidge Farm)*, 3 pieces, 1.1 oz. 140
apricot or date delight *(Health Valley* Nonfat), 3 pieces 100
(Archway Bells and Stars), 3 pieces, 1 oz. 150
(Archway Old Fashion Windmill), .75-oz. piece 100
(Archway Party Treats), 3 pieces, 1.1 oz. 140
(Archway Select Assortment), 4 pieces, 1.1 oz. 160
arrowroot *(National)*, 2-oz. piece 20
banana bran *(Archway* Low Fat), 1.2-oz. piece 120
biscotti:
all varieties *(Health Valley)*, 2 pieces, 1.1 oz. 120
almond *(Pepperidge Farm Caruso)*, .7-oz. piece 90
anise *(Pepperidge Farm La Scala)*, .7-oz. piece 90
chocolate dipped *(Pepperidge Farm Figaro)*, .8-oz. piece . . . 110
cranberry pistachio *(Pepperidge Farm Tosca)*, .7-oz. piece . . .90
blueberry *(Archway)*, 1-oz. piece 110
blueberry *(Fruitastic* Bar), 1 bar 40
brown edge wafer *(Nabisco)*, 5 pieces 140
butter *(see also "shortbread," below)*:
(Master Choice Southern Classics), 10 pieces 150
(Peak Freans Petit Beurre), 4 pieces, 1 oz. 130
(Pepperidge Farm Madaillon au Beurre), 4 pieces, 1.2 oz. . . . 150
(Pepperidge Farm Chessman), 3 pieces, .9 oz. 120
(Sunshine), 5 pieces, 1.1 oz. 140
assorted *(Pepperidge Farm* Toy Chest), 3 pieces, .9 oz. 120
sandwich with fudge *(E. L. Fudge)*, 3 pieces, 1.2 oz. 170
butter pecan bites *(Barbara's Small Indulgences)*, 6 pieces . . . 140
caramel apple *(Barbara's* Fat Free Mini), 6 pieces, 1.1 oz. . . . 110
caramel pecan *(Pepperidge Farm)*, .9-oz. piece 130
carrot cake *(Archway)*, 1-oz. piece 120
cherry:
cobbler *(Pepperidge Farm)*, .6-oz piece 70
filled *(Archway)*, 1-oz. piece 110
nougat *(Archway)*, 3 pieces, 1 oz. 150
chocolate:
(Archway Fat Free), 8-oz. piece 90
(Pepperidge Farm Goldfish), 1.1 oz. 140

Cookies, chocolate *(cont.)*

(Stella D'Oro Castelets), 2 pieces, 1 oz.	130
(Stella D'Oro Margherite), 2 pieces, 1.1 oz.	150
brownie *(Entenmann's* Fat Free), 2 pieces	80
brownie nut *(Pepperidge Farm),* 3 pieces, 1.1 oz.	160
caramel or fudge center *(Health Valley* Fat Free), 2 pieces	70
covered *(Ritz),* 3 pieces, 1.1 oz.	150
dark *(Pepperidge Farm* Espirits Noir), .6-oz. piece	90
double *(Barbara's* Fat Free Mini), 6 pieces, 1.1 oz.	90
fudge *(Dare),* .7-oz. piece	97
fudge *(SnackWell's),* 1 oz.	90
fudge, iced *(Tastykake),* 1.3-oz. piece	170
fudge mint *(Grasshopper),* 4 pieces, 1.1 oz.	150
laced *(Pepperidge Farm Pirouette),* 5 pieces, 1.2 oz.	180
milk, peanut butter *(Pepperidge Farm Chocolate Heaven),* 2 pieces	130
with nuts *(Pepperidge Farm Geneva),* 3 pieces, 1.1 oz.	160
orange *(Pepperidge Farm* Chocolat a l'Orange), 2 pieces, 1.1 oz.	150
snaps *(Nabisco),* 7 pieces, 1.2 oz.	140
wafer *(Nabsico* Famous), 5 pieces, 1.1 oz.	140
wafer, light *(Keebler),* 8 pieces, 1.1 oz.	130

chocolate chip/chunk:

(Archway), 1-oz. piece	130
(Archway Bag), 3 pieces	130
(Archway Ice Box), 1-oz. piece	140
(Barbara's), 2 pieces, 1.3 oz.	170
(Chip-A-Roos), 3 pieces, 1.3 oz.	190
(Chips Ahoy! Chewy), 3 pieces, 1.3 oz.	170
(Chips Ahoy! Chunky), .6-oz. piece	80
(Chips Ahoy! Mini), 14 pieces, 1.1 oz.	150
(Chips Ahoy! Real Chocolate), 3 pieces, 1.1 oz.	160
(Chips Ahoy! Reduced Fat), 3 pieces, 1.1 oz.	150
(Chips Deluxe), .5-oz. piece	80
(Chips Deluxe Chocolate Lovers), .6-oz. piece	90
(Chips Deluxe Light), .6-oz. piece	70
(Chips Deluxe Soft 'n Chewy), .6-oz. piece	80
(Dare), .5-oz. piece	77
(Dare Breaktime), .3-oz. piece	37
(Entenmann's), 3 pieces, 1.1 oz.	140
(Grandma's Big), 1.4-oz. piece	190
(Little Debbie), 2 pieces, 1.3 oz.	180

(Pepperidge Farm Old Fashioned), 3 pieces, 1 oz. 140
(Pepperidge Farm Chesapeake), .9-oz. piece 140
(Pepperidge Farm Goldfish), 1.1 oz. 150
(Pepperidge Farm Nantucket), .9-oz. piece 130
(Smart Snackers), 1.06 oz. 140
(SnackWell's Reduced Fat), 13 pieces, 1 oz. 130
(Tastykake), 1.4-oz. piece 180
all varieties *(Health Valley Healthy Chips* Fat Free), 3 pieces . 100
bar *(Tastykake),* 1.5-oz. bar 200
chocolate *(Barbara's),* 2 pieces, 1.3 oz. 150
chocolate, walnut, soft *(Pepperidge Farm),* .9-oz. piece 130
crisps *(Barbara's Small Indulgences),* 6 pieces, 1 oz. 140
drop *(Archway),* 1-oz. piece 140
fudge *(Grandma's* Big), 1.4-oz piece 170
fudge bar *(Grandma's),* 1.5-oz. bar 190
macadamia *(Pepperidge Farm Sausalito),* .9-oz. piece 140
macadamia, soft *(Pepperidge Farm),* .9-oz. piece 130
macadamia, white chunk *(Pepperidge Farm Tahoe),*
    .9-oz. piece 130
mini *(Sunshine),* 5 pieces, 1.1 oz. 160
peanut butter cup *(Chips Deluxe),* .6-oz. piece 90
rainbow *(Chips Deluxe),* .6-oz. piece 80
snaps *(Nabisco),* 7 pieces, 1.1 oz. 150
soft *(Chips Deluxe),* .5-oz. piece 70
soft *(Pepperidge Farm* Chunk), .9-oz. piece 130
sprinkled *(Chips Ahoy!),* 3 pieces, 1.3 oz. 170
striped *(Chips Ahoy!),* .6-oz. piece 80
and toffee *(Archway),* 1-oz. piece 140
toffee *(Pepperidge Farm Charleston),* .9-oz. piece 130
walnut *(Pepperidge Farm Beacon Hill),* .9-oz. piece 130
chocolate sandwich:
    (Elfin Delights Light), 2 pieces, .9 oz. 110
    (E.L. Fudge), 2 pieces, .9 oz. 120
    (Hydrox), 3 pieces, 1.1 oz. 150
    (Hydrox Fat Free), 3 pieces, 1.1 oz. 130
    (Oreo), 3 pieces, 1.2 oz. 160
    (Oreo Reduced Fat), 3 pieces, 1.1 oz. 140
    (Oreo Double Stuf), 2 pieces, 1 oz. 140
    (Pepperidge Farm Bordeaux), 4 pieces, 1 oz. 130
    (Pepperidge Farm Brussels), 3 pieces, 1.1 oz. 150
    (Pepperidge Farm Lido), .6-oz. piece 90
    (Pepperidge Farm Milano), 3 pieces, 1.2 oz. 180

Cookies, chocolate sandwich *(cont.)*
　　(Smart Snackers), 1.06 oz. 140
　　(SnackWell's Reduced Fat), 2 pieces, .9 oz. 100
　　(Vienna Fingers Reduced Fat), 2 pieces, 1 oz. 120
　　chocolate fudge *(Keebler Classic Collection)*, .6-oz. piece . . .80
　　chocolate fudge, double *(Barbara's Cookies & Creme)*,
　　　　2 pieces, .9 oz. 120
　　double *(Pepperidge Farm Milano)*, 2 pieces, 1 oz. 150
　　fudge coated *(Oreo)*, .75-oz piece 110
　　hazelnut *(Pepperidge Farm Milano)*, 2 pieces, .9 oz. 130
　　milk *(Pepperidge Farm Bordeaux)*, 3 pieces, 1.1 oz. 160
　　milk *(Pepperidge Farm Milano)*, 3 pieces, 1.3 oz. 180
　　mint *(Pepperidge Farm Brussels)*, 3 pieces, 1.3 oz. 190
　　mint *(Pepperidge Farm Milano)*, 2 pieces, .9 oz. 140
　　orange *(Pepperidge Farm Milano)*, 2 pieces, .9 oz. 140
　　raspberry or vanilla *(Barbara's Cookies & Creme)*, 2 pieces,
　　　　.9 oz. 120
　　white fudge coated *(Oreo)*, .75-oz. piece 110
cinnamon:
　　apple *(Archway)*, 1-oz. piece 110
　　honey heart *(Archway* Fat Free), 3 pieces, 1.1 oz. 100
　　snaps *(Archway)*, 5 pieces, 1.1 oz. 150
cocoa, Dutch *(Archway)*, 1-oz. piece 120
cocoa, mocha *(Barbara's* Fat Free Mini), 6 pieces, 1.1 oz. . . . 100
coconut *(Dare Breaktime)*, .3-oz. piece 35
coconut macaroon *(Archway)*, .8-oz. piece 90
coffee cake crunch *(Barbara's Small Indulgences)*, 6 pieces,
　　1 oz. 130
cranberry bar:
　　(Archway Fat Free), .75-oz. bar 70
　　(Newtons Fat Free), 2 pieces, 1 oz. 100
　　(Sunshine Golden Fruit), .7-oz. piece 70
Danish *(Nabisco* Import), 5 pieces, 1.2 oz. 170
devil's food cake *(SnackWell's* Fat Free), .6-oz. piece 50
egg biscuit *(see also "kichel," below)*:
　　(Stella D'Oro Jumbo), 2 pieces, .8 oz. 90
　　(Stella D'Oro Low Sodium), 3 pieces, 1.1 oz. 120
　　Roman *(Stella D'Oro)*, 1.2 oz. 140
fig:
　　(Archway Fat Free), .75-oz. piece 80
　　(Fig Newtons), 2 pieces, 1.1 oz. 110
　　(Fig Newtons Fat Free), 2 pieces, 1 oz. 100

(Smart Snackers), .7 oz. 70
(Sunshine Bar), 2 pieces, 1 oz. 110
(Sunshine Golden Fruit Fat Free), .6-oz. piece 60
fortune *(La Choy)*, 4 pieces, 1.1 oz. 110
fruit:
   bar *(Archway* Fat Free), ½ piece, 1 oz. 90
   cake *(Archway)*, 3 pieces, 1-oz. piece 140
   Hawaiian *(Health Valley* Fat Free), 3 pieces 100
   honey bar *(Archway)*, 1-oz. piece 110
   slices *(Stella D'Oro)*, .6-oz. piece 130
fudge:
   (Stella D'Oro Swiss), 2 pieces, .9 oz. 130
   bar *(Tastykake)*, 1.5-oz. bar 190
   bits *(Grandma's)*, 9 pieces 170
   double, cake *(SnackWell's* Fat Free), .6-oz. piece 50
   fudge filled *(Keebler* Truffles), 3 pieces, 1.2 oz. 180
   mint patties *(Sunshine)*, 2 pieces, .8 oz. 130
   nut bar *(Archway)*, 1-oz. piece 110
   nutty *(Grandma's* Big), 1.4-oz. piece 190
   sandwich *(Grandma's)*, 1 pkg. 240
   sandwich *(Grandma's* Value), 3 cookies 180
ginger:
   (Dare Breaktime), .3-oz. piece 34
   (Pepperidge Farm Gingerman), 4 pieces, 1 oz. 120
   snaps *(Archway)*, 5 pieces, 1.1 oz. 140
   snaps *(Nabisco)*, 4 pieces, 1 oz. 120
   snaps *(Sunshine)*, 7 pieces, 1 oz. 130
gingerbread, iced *(Archway)*, 3 pieces, 1.1 oz. 140
gingerbread, iced *(Sunshine)*, 5 pieces, 1 oz. 130
golden bar *(Stella D'Oro)*, 1-oz. piece 110
graham cracker:
   (Bugs Bunny), 10 pieces, 1.1 oz. 140
   (Keebler), 8 pieces, 1 oz. 130
   (Nabisco), 8 pieces, 1 oz. 120
   (Pepperidge Farm Goldfish), 1.1 oz. 150
   all flavors *(Teddy Grahams* Snacks), 24 pieces, 1.1 oz. 140
   amaranth or oat bran *(Health Valley* Fat Free), 11 pieces,
      1 oz. 100
   chocolate *(Bugs Bunny)*, 13 pieces, 1.1 oz. 140
   chocolate *(Keebler)*, 8 pieces, 1.1 oz. 140
   chocolate *(Nabisco* Pure), 3 pieces, 1.1 oz. 160
   cinnamon *(Bugs Bunny)*, 13 pieces, 1.1 oz. 140

Cookies, graham cracker *(cont.)*
  cinnamon *(Honey Maid)*, 10 pieces, 1.1 oz. 140
  cinnamon *(Keebler* Low Fat), 8 pieces, 1 oz. 110
  cinnamon *(Pepperidge Farm Goldfish)*, 1.1 oz. 150
  cinnamon *(SnackWell's* Fat Free Snacks), 20 pieces, 1.1 oz. . 110
  cinnamon *(Sunshine)*, 2 pieces, 1.1 oz. 140
  French vanilla *(Keebler* Light), 8 pieces 110
  fudge coated *(Keebler* Deluxe), 3 pieces 140
  fudge coated *(Keebler* Deluxe Reduced Fat), 3 pieces,
    .9 oz. 120
  fudge coated *(Nabisco* Family Favorites), 3 pieces, 1 oz. . . . 140
  fudge coated, marshmallow filled *(Keebler* S'mores),
    3 pieces, 1.1 oz. 150
  fudge dipped *(Sunshine)*, 4 pieces, 1.2 oz. 170
  honey *(Honey Maid)*, 8 pieces, 1 oz. 120
  honey *(Keebler* Low Fat), 9 pieces, 1.1 oz. 120
  honey *(Sunshine)*, 2 pieces, 1 oz. 120
granola *(Archway* Fat Free), 2 pieces, 1 oz. 100
granola, soft *(Grandma's* Bar), 1.5-oz. bar 180
hazelnut *(Pepperidge Farm)*, 3 pieces, 1.1 oz. 160
hermit *(Archway* Cookie Jar), 1-oz. piece 110
(Heyday Bar), .75-oz. bar 110
kichel *(Stella D'Oro* Low Sodium), 21 pieces, 1 oz. 150
lemon:
  (Sunshine Coolers), 5 pieces, 1.1 oz. 140
  almond *(Barbara's Small Indulgences)*, 6 pieces, 1 oz. 140
  creme *(Dare)*, .7-oz. piece 95
  drop *(Archway)*, 1-oz. piece 110
  frosty *(Archway)*, 1-oz. piece 120
  nuggets *(Archway* Fat Free), 5 pieces, 1 oz. 100
  nut crunch *(Pepperidge Farm)*, 3 pieces, 1.1 oz. 170
  sandwich *(Barbara's Cookies & Creme)*, 2 pieces, .9 oz. . . . 120
  snaps *(Archway)*, 5 pieces, 1.1 oz. 150
marshmallow:
  chocolate *(Mallomars)*, 2 pieces, .9 oz. 120
  chocolate *(Pinwheels)*, 1.1-oz. piece 130
  fudge puffs *(Nabisco)*, .75-oz. piece 90
  fudge twirls *(Nabisco)*, 1.1-oz. piece 130
mint sandwich *(Mystic Mint)*, .6-oz. piece 90
molasses:
  (Archway), 1-oz. piece 110
  (Archway Low Fat), 1-oz. piece 100

(Archway Old Fashion), 1-oz. piece 120
(Archway Super Pak), 1-oz. piece 110
(Grandma's Old Time Big), 1.4-oz. piece 160
crisps *(Pepperidge Farm),* 5 pieces, 1.1 oz. 150
dark *(Archway),* 1-oz. piece 110
drop, soft *(Archway),* 1-oz. piece 110
iced *(Archway* Iowa), 1-oz. piece 140
iced *(Archway* Ohio), 1-oz. piece 110
iced *(Archway* Super Pak), 1-oz. piece 120
mud pie *(Archway),* 1-oz. piece 110
New Orleans cake *(Archway),* 1-oz. piece 110
nut *(Archway* Nutty Nougat), 3 pieces, 1.1 oz. 160
nut *(Little Debbie Nutty Bars),* 2 pieces, 1.2 oz. 180
oatmeal:
(Archway), 1-oz. piece 110
(Dare Breaktime), .3-oz. piece 35
(Keebler Classic Collection), 2 pieces, 1 oz. 150
(Nabisco Family Favorites), .6-oz. piece 80
(Ruth's), 1-oz. piece 120
(Ruth's Golden), 1-oz. piece 120
(Sunshine Country), 3 pieces, 1.2 oz. 170
apple filled *(Archway),* 1-oz. piece 110
apple spice *(Grandma's* Big), 1.4-oz. piece 170
apple spice bar *(Grandma's),* 1.5-oz. bar 170
butterscotch *(Pepperidge Farm),* 3 pieces, 1.2 oz. 170
chewy *(Master Choice),* .6-oz. piece 80
chocolate chip *(Entenmann's* Fat Free), 2 pieces, .8 oz. 80
chocolate chip *(Sunshine),* 3 pieces, 1.3 oz. 170
date filled *(Archway),* 1-oz. piece 110
iced *(Archway),* 1-oz. piece 120
iced *(Sunshine),* 2 pieces, .9 oz. 120
Irish *(Pepperidge Farm),* 3 pieces, 1 oz. 130
pecan *(Archway),* 1-oz. piece 120
raspberry *(Archway* Fat Free), 1-oz. piece 100
oatmeal raisin:
(Archway), 1-oz. piece 110
(Archway Bag), 3 pieces, 1 oz. 130
(Archway Fat Free), 1-oz. piece 100
(Barbara's), 2 pieces, 1.3 oz. 160
(Barbara's Fat Free Mini), 6 pieces, 1.1 oz. 110
(Entenmann's Fat Free), 2 pieces, .8 oz. 80
(Health Valley Fat Free), 3 pieces 100

Cookies, oatmeal raisin *(cont.)*
    (Little Debbie), 2 pieces, 1.3 oz. 170
    (Pepperidge Farm Old Fashioned), 3 pieces, 1.2 oz. 160
    (Pepperidge Farm Soft), .9-oz. piece 110
    (Pepperidge Farm Santa Fe), .9-oz. piece 120
    (Smart Snackers), 1.06 oz. 120
    (SnackWell's Reduced Fat), 2 pieces, 1 oz. 110
    (Tastykake Bar), 1.5-oz. bar 190
    bran *(Archway)*, 1-oz. piece 110
    iced *(Tastykake)*, 1.4-oz. piece 170
peach tart *(Pepperidge Farm)*, 2 pieces, 1.1 oz. 120
peach-apricot *(Stella D'Oro Sodium Free)*, .7-oz. piece 80
peanut *(Archway Jumble)*, 1-oz. piece 130
peanut butter:
    (Archway), 1-oz. piece 140
    (Archway Ol' Fashion), 1-oz. piece 130
    (Grandma's Big), 1.4-oz. piece 190
    (Little Debbie Bar), 1.8-oz. bar 250
    bits *(Grandma's)*, 9 pieces 150
    chip *(Archway)*, 1-oz. piece 140
    chocolate chip *(Grandma's Bar)*, 1.5-oz. bar 210
    chocolate chip *(Grandma's Big)*, 1¼-oz. piece 190
    chunky *(Tastykake Bar)*, 1 piece 240
    fudge *(P. B. Fudgebutters)*, 2 pieces, .8 oz. 130
    graham *(Mr. Peanut P.B. Crisps)*, 1 oz. 140
    graham *(Mr. Peanut P.B. Crisps)*, 1.5-oz. pkg. 210
    patties *(Nutter Butter)*, 5 pieces, 1.1 oz. 160
    sandwich *(Grandma's)*, 5 pieces 210
    sandwich *(Nutter Butter)*, 2 pieces, 1 oz. 130
    sandwich *(Nutter Butter Bites)*, 10 pieces, 1.1 oz. 150
peanut crunch *(Archway)*, 6 pieces, 1.1 oz. 150
pecan:
    (Archway Ice Box), 1-oz. piece 140
    malted nougat *(Archway)*, 3 pieces, 1.1 oz. 160
    shortbread, *see "shortbread," below*
pound cake *(Aunt Bea's)*, .9-oz. piece 110
prune pastry *(Stella D'Oro Sodium Free)*, .7-oz. piece 90
raisin:
    (Dare Sun Maid), .5-oz. piece 52
    (Health Valley Fat Free Jumbo), 1 piece 80
    oatmeal, *see "oatmeal raisin," above*

raspberry:
   (Fruitastic Bar), 1 bar 40
   (Health Valley Fat Free Jumbo), 1 piece 80
   (Newtons Fat Free), 2 pieces, 1 oz. 100
   (Sunshine Oh! Berry), 3 pieces, 1 oz. 120
   centers *(Health Valley* Fat Free), 1 piece 70
   filled *(Archway),* 1-oz. piece 110
   filled *(Pepperidge Farm* Linzer), .8-oz. piece 100
   filled *(Smart Snackers),* .7 oz. 70
   hazelnut *(Pepperidge Farm Chantilly),* .6-oz. piece 80
rocky road *(Archway* Iowa), 1-oz. piece 120
rocky road *(Archway* Ohio), 1-oz. piece 130
sesame *(Stella D'Oro* Regina), 3 pieces, 1.1 oz. 150
shortbread:
   (Lorna Doone), 4 pieces, 1 oz. 140
   (Pepperidge Farm), 2 pieces, .9 oz. 140
   (Simply Sandies), .5-oz. piece 80
   butter *(Dare),* .5-oz. piece 63
   fudge coated *(Nabisco* Family Favorites), 3 pieces, 1.1 oz. . . 160
   fudge striped *(Keebler),* 3 pieces, 1.1 oz. 160
   fudge striped *(Keebler* Reduced Fat), 3 pieces, 1 oz. 130
   fudge striped *(Sunshine),* 3 pieces, 1.1 oz. 160
   pecan *(Pecan Passion),* .6-oz. piece 90
   pecan *(Pecan Sandies),* .6-oz. piece 80
   pecan *(Pecan Sandies* Reduced Fat), .6-oz. piece 70
   pecan *(Pepperidge Farm),* 2 pieces, .9 oz. 140
(Social Tea), 6 pieces, 1 oz. 120
spice, pfeffernuss *(Archway),* 2 pieces, 1.3 oz. 140
spice, pfeffernuss, drops *(Stella D'Oro),* 3 pieces, 1 oz. 120
sprinkles *(Dare Breaktime),* .3-oz. piece 36
(Stella D'Oro Angelica Goodies), .8-oz piece 100
(Stella D'Oro Angel Wings), 2 pieces, .9 oz. 140
(Stella D'Oro Anginetti), 4 pieces, 1.1 oz. 140
(Stella D'Oro Como Delights), 1.1 oz. 140
(Stella D'Oro Holiday Rings and Stars), 3 pieces, 1.2 oz. 140
(Stella D'Oro Holiday Trinkets), 4 pieces, 1.1 oz. 160
(Stella D'Oro Hostess with the Mostest), 3 pieces, 1 oz. 130
(Stella D'Oro Lady Stella Assortment), 3 pieces, 1 oz. 130
(Stella D'Oro Margherite Combination), 2 pieces, 1.1 oz. 140
(Stella D'Oro Royal Nuggets), 1.1 oz. 140
strawberry:
   (Newtons Fat Free), 2 pieces, 1 oz. 100

Cookies, strawberry *(cont.)*

  (Pepperidge Farm), 3 pieces, 1.1 oz. 140
  (Sunshine Oh! Berry Fat Free), 1 oz. 100
  filled *(Archway)*, .9-oz. piece 100
  filled *(Archway* Ohio), 1-oz. piece 110
sugar:
  (Archway), 1-oz. piece 120
  (Archway Fat Free), .75-oz. piece 70
  (Dare), .3-oz. piece 39
  (Keebler Classic Collection), 2 pieces, 1 oz. 140
  (Pepperidge Farm), 3 pieces, 1.1 oz. 140
  soft *(Archway)*, 1-oz. piece 110
  wafer *(Biscos)*, 8 pieces, 1 oz. 140
  wafer, chocolate *(Sunshine)*, 3 pieces, .9 oz. 130
  wafer, peanut butter *(Sunshine)*, 4 pieces, 1.1 oz. 170
  wafer, vanilla *(Sunshine)*, 3 pieces, .9 oz. 130
  waffle *(Biscos)*, 4 pieces, 1.2 oz. 180
(Sunshine Jingles), 6 pieces, 1.1 oz. 150
vanilla:
  (Pepperidge Farm Goldfish), 1.1 oz. 150
  (Stella D'Oro Margherite), 2 pieces, 1.1 oz. 140
  bits *(Grandma's)*, 9 pieces 150
  raspberry tart *(Pepperidge Farm Wholesome Choice)*,
    2 pieces, 1.1 oz. 120
  wafer *(Archway)*, 5 pieces, 1.1 oz. 130
  wafer *(Keebler)*, 8 pieces, 1.1 oz. 150
  wafer *(Keebler* Light), 8 pieces, 1.1 oz. 130
  wafer *(Nilla)*, 8 pieces, 1.1 oz. 140
  wafer *(Sunshine)*, 7 pieces, 1.1 oz. 150
vanilla sandwich:
  (Cameo), 2 pieces, 1 oz. 130
  (Cookie Break), 3 pieces, 1.1 oz. 160
  (Grandma's), 1 pkg. 240
  (Grandma's Value), 3 pieces 150
  (Nabisco Family Favorites), 3 pieces, 1.2 oz. 170
  (Smart Snackers), 1.1 oz. 140
  (SnackWell's Reduced Fat), 2 pieces, .9 oz. 110
  (Vienna Fingers), 2 pieces, 1 oz. 130
  French *(Keebler Classic Collection)*, .6-oz. piece 80
  raspberry or vanilla *(Barbara's Cookies & Creme)*, 2 pieces,
    .9 oz. 120

wafer:
  all flavors *(Grandma's* Value), 4 pieces 160
  fudge *(Keebler Fudge Sticks),* 3 pieces, 1 oz. 150
walnut, black *(Archway* Ice Box), .8-oz. piece 120
wedding cakes *(Archway),* 3 pieces, 1.1 oz. 160

COOKIES, REFRIGERATED & MIXES
See also "Snack Cakes, Mixes" and "Cookies"

	calories

bunny, flag, Halloween, holiday, snowman, sugar, or valentine
  (Pillsbury), 2 pieces* 130
chocolate chip:
  (Duncan Hines), 2 pieces* 170
  (Nestlé/Nestlé Big Batch), 2 tbsp. 140
  (Nestlé Reduced Fat), 2 tbsp. 130
  (Pillsbury Reduced Fat), 1 oz. 110
  (Robin Hood/Gold Medal Pouch), 2 pieces* 170
  (Schwan's), 1 piece* 120
  (SnackWell's), 1 oz. 110
  or chocolate chunk *(Pillsbury),* 1 oz. 130
  oatmeal *(Pillsbury),* 1 oz. 130
  oatmeal *(Robin Hood/Gold Medal* Pouch), 2 pieces* 160
  peanut butter *(Nestlé),* 2 tbsp. 160
  with walnuts *(Pillsbury),* 1 oz. 140
  mix *(Arrowhead Mills),* 1 piece* 80
  mix *(Arrowhead Mills* Wheat Free), 1 piece* 80
chocolate chunk, double *(Robin Hood/Gold Medal* Pouch),
  2 pieces* 150
chocolate fudge *(SnackWell's),* 1 oz. 90
espresso chip, mix *(Arrowhead Mills),* 1 piece* 80
fudge, candy splash *(Duncan Hines),* 2 pieces* 140
gingerbread, mix *(Betty Crocker* Fun Kit), 2 pieces* 150
Heath *(Pillsbury),* 1 oz. 140
M&M's *(Pillsbury),* 1 oz. 130
oatmeal *(Nestlé Scotchies),* 2 tbsp. 140
oatmeal, mix *(Arrowhead Mills),* 1 piece* 70
oatmeal raisin *(Schwan's),* 1 piece* 110
peanut butter:
  (Duncan Hines), 2 pieces* 140

* Prepared according to package directions

Cookies, Refrigerated & Mixes, peanut butter *(cont.)*
    (Pillsbury), 1 oz. 110
    (Robin Hood/Gold Medal Pouch), 2 pieces* 160
Reese's (Pillsbury), 1 oz. 130
sugar:
    (Nestlé), ½″ slice 120
    golden *(Duncan Hines)*, 2 pieces* 150
    golden, no-cholesterol recipe *(Duncan Hines)*, 2 pieces* . . . 140

CAKE FROSTINGS, two tablespoons, except as noted
*See also "Cake Frostings, Mixes," "Cake Decorations," and
"Miscellaneous Sweet Baking Ingredients"*

---

                                                          calories
banana creme *(Pillsbury Creamy Supreme)* 150
butter pecan *(Betty Crocker Creamy Deluxe)* 150
buttercream:
    (Betty Crocker Creamy Deluxe) 150
    (Duncan Hines) 140
    chocolate *(Duncan Hines)* 130
butterscotch *(Duncan Hines)* 140
caramel *(Duncan Hines)* 140
caramel chocolate chip *(Betty Crocker Creamy Deluxe)* 140
caramel pecan *(Pillsbury Creamy Supreme)* 150
cherry *(Betty Crocker Creamy Deluxe)* 140
cherry, wild, vanilla *(Duncan Hines)* 140
chocolate:
    (Betty Crocker Creamy Deluxe) 150
    (Betty Crocker Creamy Deluxe Low Fat) 120
    (Betty Crocker Sweet Rewards), 1 tbsp. 130
    (Betty Crocker Whipped Deluxe) 100
    (Duncan Hines) 130
    (Pillsbury Creamy Supreme) 140
    (Pillsbury Creamy Supreme Funfetti) 140
    chip *(Betty Crocker Creamy Deluxe)* 160
    chip cookie dough *(Betty Crocker Creamy Deluxe)* 160
    chocolate chip *(Betty Crocker Creamy Deluxe)* 150
    dark *(Betty Crocker Creamy Deluxe)* 150
    dark *(Pillsbury Creamy Supreme)* 130
    dark or milk *(Duncan Hines)* 130

* *Prepared according to package directions*

with dinosaurs *(Betty Crocker Creamy Deluxe* Party) 150
fudge *(Martha White)*. 120
fudge or hot fudge *(Pillsbury Creamy Supreme)* 140
fudge or milk *(SnackWell's)* 120
milk *(Betty Crocker Creamy Deluxe)* 150
milk *(Betty Crocker Whipped Deluxe)* 100
milk *(Martha White)* 120
milk *(Pillsbury Creamy Supreme)* 140
milk, low-fat *(Betty Crocker Creamy Deluxe* Low Fat) 120
milk, low-fat *(Betty Crocker Sweet Rewards)*, 1 tbsp. 130
milk, swirl with fudge glaze *(Pillsbury Creamy Supreme)* . . . 140
mocha *(Duncan Hines)* 130
mocha *(Pillsbury Creamy Supreme)*. 140
sour cream or Swiss almond *(Betty Crocker Creamy
Deluxe)* 150
coconut pecan *(Betty Crocker Creamy Deluxe)* 150
coconut pecan *(Pillsbury Creamy Supreme)* 160
cookie *(Pillsbury Creamy Supreme Oreo)*. 150
cream cheese:
(Betty Crocker Creamy Deluxe) 140
(Betty Crocker Whipped Deluxe) 110
(Duncan Hines) 140
(Pillsbury Creamy Supreme) 150
lemon:
(Betty Crocker Creamy Deluxe) 140
(Betty Crocker Whipped Deluxe). 110
cream *(Duncan Hines)* 140
creme *(Pillsbury Creamy Supreme)* 150
rainbow chip *(Betty Crocker Creamy Deluxe)* 160
raspberries or strawberries 'n cream *(Duncan Hines)* 140
strawberry:
(Betty Crocker Whipped Deluxe) 110
cream cheese *(Betty Crocker Creamy Deluxe)* 150
creme *(Pillsbury Creamy Supreme)* 150
vanilla:
(Betty Crocker Creamy Deluxe) 140
(Betty Crocker Whipped Deluxe). 110
(Duncan Hines) 140
(Martha White) 130
*(Pillsbury Creamy Supreme/Pillsbury Creamy Supreme
Funfetti)* 150
(SnackWell's) 130

Cake Frostings, vanilla *(cont.)*

with bears *(Betty Crocker Creamy Deluxe* Party) 140
French *(Pillsbury Creamy Supreme)* 150
French or with stars *(Betty Crocker Creamy Deluxe)* 140
low-fat *(Betty Crocker Creamy Deluxe* Low Fat) 120
low-fat *(Betty Crocker Sweet Rewards)*, 1 tbsp. 130
pink *(Pillsbury Creamy Supreme Funfetti)* 150
swirl, with fudge glaze *(Pillsbury Creamy Supreme)* 150
white:
  (Betty Crocker Whipped Deluxe) 110
  chocolate *(Betty Crocker Creamy Deluxe)* 140
  sour cream *(Betty Crocker Creamy Deluxe)* 150

CAKE FROSTINGS, MIXES
See also "Cake Frostings, Ready-to-Spread"

---

          calories

chocolate:
  (Robin Hood), 2 tbsp. 110
  (Robin Hood), 2 tbsp.* 140
  fudge *(Betty Crocker)*, 3 tbsp. 110
  fudge *(Betty Crocker)*, 2 tbsp.* 140
coconut pecan *(Betty Crocker)*, 3 tbsp. 120
coconut pecan *(Betty Crocker)*, 2 tbsp.* 160
vanilla *(Betty Crocker)*, 3 tbsp. 110
vanilla *(Betty Crocker)*, 2 tbsp.* 130
white *(Betty Crocker)*, 3 tbsp. 100

CAKE DECORATIONS, one teaspoon, except as noted
*See also "Cake Frostings, Ready-to-Spread" and
"Miscellaneous Sweet Baking Ingredients"*

---

          calories

(Dec-A-Cake Dec-A-Cone) 20
confetti or nonpareils *(Dec-A-Cake)* 15
hearts, bats, or pumpkins *(Dec-A-Cake)* 20
party imperials or fruit cocktail *(Dec-A-Cake)*, 9 pieces 15
rainbow *(Dec-A-Cake)* 15
sprinkles:
  (Hershey's Cookies n' Mint), 2 tbsp. 100

---

* Prepared according to package directions

chocolate, milk *(Hershey's)*, 2 tbsp. 140
fun *(Dec-A-Cake)* 20
holiday *(Dec-A-Cake)* 15
peanut butter *(Reese's)*, 2 tbsp. 160
sugar crystals *(Dec-A-Cake)* 15
trims, chocolate or chocolate mint *(Dec-A-Cake)* 15

PIE FILLINGS, CANNED, ⅓ cup, except as noted
See also "Fruit, Canned or in Jars," "Custards, Puddings, &
Pie Fillings, Mixes," "Dessert Pies, Mixes," "Pastry Fillings,
Canned," and "Dessert Toppings & Syrups"

---

                                                            calories
apple:
(Comstock) 100
(Comstock More Fruit) 80
(Lucky Leaf/Lucky Leaf Premium) 90
(Lucky Leaf Lite) 60
(Musselman's 21 oz.) .90
(Musselman's 24 oz.) 100
cinnamon 'n spice *(Comstock* More Fruit) 110
apple-cranberry *(Comstock)* 90
apricot *(Comstock)* 100
apricot or blackberry *(Lucky Leaf)* 90
banana cream *(Comstock)* 130
blackberry *(Comstock)* 110
blueberry:
(Comstock) 100
(Comstock More Fruit) 80
(Lucky Leaf/Lucky Leaf Premium) 100
(Lucky Leaf Lite) 60
(Musselman's) 100
blueberry-cranberry *(Comstock)* 100
cherry:
(Comstock Regular/More Fruit) 90
(Lucky Leaf/Musselman's) 100
(Lucky Leaf/Musselman's Lite) 60
dark sweet *(Comstock)* 100
dark sweet *(Lucky Leaf/Musselman's)* 110
light *(Comstock* Regular/More Fruit) 60
red ruby *(Comstock/Thank You)* 90
cherry-cranberry *(Comstock)* 90

Pie Fillings, Canned *(cont.)*

chocolate cream *(Comstock)* 130
coconut cream *(Comstock)* 120
coconut creme *(Lucky Leaf)* 110
lemon:
   (Comstock) 130
   (Lucky Leaf/Musselman's) 22 oz./25 oz.) 130
   creme *(Lucky Leaf)* 130
mince/mincemeat:
   (Comstock) 170
   (Lucky Leaf) 140
   (None Such) 190
   (S&W), ¼ cup 180
   with brandy and rum *(None Such)* 200
   condensed *(None Such)*, 4 tsp. 150
peach *(Comstock More Fruit)* 80
peach *(Lucky Leaf)* 80
pineapple *(Comstock)* 110
pineapple *(Lucky Leaf/Musselman's)* 100
pumpkin:
   (Comstock), ½ cup 50
   mix *(Comstock)* 90
   mix *(Libby's)*, ½ cup 100
   mix *(Stokely)* 100
raisin *(Comstock/Thank You)* 120
raisin *(Lucky Leaf)* 100
raspberry *(Comstock)* 100
strawberry *(Comstock)* 100
strawberry *(Lucky Leaf/Musselman's)* 80
strawberry-rhubarb *(Lucky Leaf)* 90

PASTRY FILLINGS, CANNED, two tablespoons
See also "Pie Fillings, Canned"

	calories
almond *(Solo)*	120
almond paste *(Solo)*	180
apple, Dutch *(Solo)*	80
apricot, wild blueberry, cherry, or raspberry *(Solo)*	80
date *(Solo)*	100
nut, fancy *(Solo)*	140
pecan *(Solo)*	130

pineapple *(Solo)* 80
poppy seed *(Solo)* 140
prune, plum, or strawberry *(Solo)* 70

PASTRY & PIE CRUSTS
See also "Shells & Wrappers"

---

	calories
fillo pastry, frozen *(Apollo)*, 1/8 pkg.	180

pastry shell:
  (Stella D'Oro), 1-oz. shell 140
  frozen, dough *(Goya* Discos), 1 piece 120
  frozen, patty *(Pepperidge Farm)*, 1 shell 230
  frozen sheet, puff *(Pepperidge Farm)*, 1/6 sheet 200

pie crust:
  chocolate cookie *(Oreo)*, 1/6 crust 140
  chocolate cookie *(Ready Crust)*, 1/8 crust 110
  cookie crumbs *(Nilla)*, 2 tbsp. 70
  cookie crumbs *(Oreo)*, 2 tbsp. 80
  graham *(Honey Maid)*, 1/6 crust 140
  graham, mini *(Ready Crust)*, .8-oz. crust 120
  graham crumbs *(Honey Maid)*, 2 tbsp. 70
  graham crumbs *(Sunshine)*, 2 tbsp. 80
  shortbread *(Ready Crust 9″)*, 1/8 crust 100
  vanilla cookie *(Nilla)*, 1/6 crust 140

pie crust, frozen or refrigerated, 1/8 crust:
  (Pet-Ritz 9″) 80
  (Pet-Ritz 9⅝″) 110
  (Pillsbury) 120
  deep dish *(Pet-Ritz)* 90
  vegetable shortening *(Pet-Ritz)* 80
  vegetable shortening, deep dish *(Pet-Ritz)* 90

pie crust mix:
  (Betty Crocker), 1/8 of 9″ crust* 110
  (Flako), 1/4 cup mix 130
  (Pillsbury), 1/8 of 9″ crust* 100

tart shell, frozen or refrigerated:
  (Oronoque), 3″ shell 140
  (Pet-Ritz), 3″ shell 140
  (Pet-Ritz), 1/4 of 6″ shell 110

---

* *Prepared according to package directions*

Chapter 18

NUT BUTTERS, JAMS, AND JELLIES

NUT BUTTERS, two tablespoons, except as noted
See also "Nuts & Seeds"

	calories
almond, crunchy or creamy *(Roaster Fresh/Roaster Fresh Unsalted)*, 1 oz.	184
cashew *(Roaster Fresh)*, 1 oz.	165
hazelnut *(Roaster Fresh)*, 1 oz.	188
peanut:	
chunky or crunchy *(Adams No-Stir/Adams Natural/ Unsalted)*	200
chunky or crunchy *(Peter Pan/Peter Pan Real)*	190
chunky or crunchy *(Peter Pan Whipped)*	150
chunky or crunchy *(Roasted Honey Nut Skippy Super Chunk)*	190
chunky or crunchy *(Skippy Super Chunk)*	190
chunky or crunchy *(Skippy Super Chunk Reduced Fat)*	190
chunky or crunchy *(Teddie Super)*	190
chunky or crunchy, spread *(Peter Pan Smart Choice)*	195
chunky or creamy *(Arrowhead Mills)*	190
chunky or creamy *(Jif/Simply Jif/Jif Reduced Fat)*	190
chunky or creamy *(Peter Pan Very Low Sodium)*	195
chunky or creamy *(Roaster Fresh/Roaster Fresh Unsalted)*	166
chunky or creamy *(Smucker's Natural/Natural No Salt)*	200
creamy or smooth *(Adams Natural/Unsalted)*	200
creamy or smooth *(Adams No-Stir)*	210
creamy or smooth *(Peter Pan/Peter Pan Real)*	190
creamy or smooth *(Peter Pan Whipped)*	150
creamy or smooth *(Roasted Honey Nut Skippy)*	190
creamy or smooth *(Skippy/Skippy Reduced Fat)*	190
creamy or smooth *(Teddie)*	190
creamy or smooth, spread *(Peter Pan Smart Choice)*	180
unsalted *(Teddie)*	190
and jelly *(Smucker's Goober)*, 3 tbsp.	230
sesame *(Roaster Fresh)*, 1 oz.	168

soy, mix *(Morningstar Farms/Natural Touch* SoyButter) 170
sunflower seed *(Roaster Fresh)*, 1 oz. 160
tahini:
   (Arrowhead Mills), 1 oz. 170
   (Joyva) 200
   (Krinos) 260

JAMS, JELLIES, & PRESERVES, one tablespoon, except as noted

	calories

butter, apple:
   (Apple Time/Lucky Leaf/Musselman's) 30
   (Dutch Girl/Mary Ellen) 35
   (Eden) 20
   (R.W. Knudsen) 35
   (Smucker's/Simply Fruit) 45
   (White House) 35
   spread *(Apple Time)* .25
   spread *(New Morning)* 25
butter, honey *(Downey's)*, ½ oz. 60
butter, peach *(Smucker's)* 45
fruit spreads, all varieties:
   (Kraft Reduced Calorie) 20
   (Polaner) 40
   (R.W. Knudsen) 50
   (Simply Fruit) 40
   (Slenderella Reduced Calorie) 20
   (Smucker's Homestyle) 45
fruit and peanut spread *(Smucker's* Super Spreaders) 40
jams and preserves:
   all varieties *(Knott's Berry Farm)*, 1 tsp. 18
   all varieties *(Smucker's)* 50
   all varieties *(Smucker's* Reduced Sugar) 25
   all varieties *(Smucker's* Light) 20
   all varieties except mango *(Goya)* 45
   all varieties except grape and red plum *(Kraft)* 50
   grape or red plum *(Kraft)* 60
   mango *(Goya)* 46
   orange marmalade *(Crosse & Blackwell)* 60
jellies:
   all fruit flavors *(Knott's Berry Farm)*, 1 tsp. 18

Jams, Jellies, & Preserves, jellies *(cont.)*
   all fruit flavors *(Smucker's)* 50
   all fruit flavors except apple and strawberry *(Kraft)* 50
   apple or strawberry *(Kraft)* 60
   apple mint *(Crosse & Blackwell)* 50
   currant, red *(Crosse & Blackwell)* 60
   grape *(Goya)* 45
   guava *(Goya)* 50
   pepper, mild *(Tabasco)* .60
   pepper, spicy *(Tabasco)* 50

Chapter 19

SYRUPS, TOPPINGS, AND SWEET BAKING INGREDIENTS

SUGAR
See also "Honey, Molasses, & Syrups"

	calories
brown, light or dark *(Domino)*, 1 tsp.	15
cane *(Domino)*, 1 tsp. or 1 pkt.	15
fructose *(Estee)*, 1 tsp.	16
powdered *(Domino)*, ¼ cup	120
powdered, lemon or strawberry flavored *(Domino)*, ¼ cup	110
substitute:	
(Equal), 1 pkt.	4
(NutraSweet), 1 tsp.	2
(Sweet'n Low), 1 pkt.	4

HONEY, MOLASSES, & SYRUPS
See also "Sugar" and "Dessert Toppings & Syrups"

	calories
barley malt syrup *(Eden)*, 1 tbsp.	60
corn syrup, dark or light *(Karo)*, 2 tbsp.	120
honey *(Aunt Sue's/Grandma's/Sue Bee)*, 1 tbsp.	60
honeycomb, strained *(Frieda's)*, 1 oz.	86
maple syrup *(Cary's/Maple Orchard's/MacDonald's* Pure), ¼ cup	210
molasses, 1 tbsp.:	
(Grandma's 4-Star)	50
bead *(La Choy)*	50
blackstrap *(New Morning)*	60
dark or light *(Brer Rabbit)*	60
gold or green *(Grandma's)*	50
pancake and waffle syrup, ¼ cup:	
(Aunt Jemima)	210
(Aunt Jemima Lite)	100

Honey, Molasses, & Syrups, pancake and waffle syrup *(cont.)*
    (Country Kitchen) 200
    (Country Kitchen Lite) 100
    (Golden Griddle) 220
    (Karo) 240
    (Log Cabin) 200
    (Log Cabin Lite) 100
    (Mrs. Richardson's) 210
    (Mrs. Richardson's Lite) 100
    all flavors *(Hungry Jack)* 210
    all flavors *(Hungry Jack* Lite) 100
    butter flavor *(Aunt Jemima* Butterlite) 100
    butter flavor *(Aunt Jemima* Rich) 210
    butter flavor *(Country Kitchen)* 200
    butter flavor or maple *(S&W* Reduced Calorie) 60
rice syrup *(Lundberg Nutra-Farmed/Lundberg* Organic), ¼ cup . . 170

DESSERT TOPPINGS & SYRUPS, two tablespoons, except as noted
See also "Dips," "Pie Fillings, Canned," and "Honey, Molasses, & Syrups"

---

                                          calories

apple syrup *(R.W. Knudsen)*, ¼ cup 150
blackberry syrup *(Knott's Berry Farm)* 120
blueberry syrup *(Knott's Berry Farm)* 120
blueberry syrup *(R.W. Knudsen)*, ¼ cup 150
blueberry syrup *(S&W* Reduced Cal), ¼ cup 60
boysenberry syrup *(Knott's Berry Farm)* 120
butterscotch topping:
    (Kraft) 130
    (Smucker's Sundae) 110
    caramel *(Smucker's* Nonfat/*(Smucker's* Special Recipe) 130
    or butterscotch caramel fudge *(Mrs. Richardson's)* 130
caramel topping:
    (Kraft) 120
    (Mrs. Richardson's Fat Free) 130
    (Smucker's Sundae) 110
    hot *(Smucker's)* 120
caramel dip *(Marie's)* 150
caramel dip *(Marie's* Low Fat) 140
cherries jubilee *(Lucky Leaf/Musselman's)*, ¼ cup 80

cherry syrup, black *(Fox's)* 80
cherry syrup, black *(Fox's No Cal)* 0
chocolate syrup:
   (Fox's No Cal) 0
   (Fox's U-Bet) 120
   (Hershey's) 100
   (Smucker's Sundae) 110
   (Yoo-Hoo) 110
   dark *(Hershey's Special Dark)* 110
   dark *(Smucker's Dove)* 130
   malt *(Hershey's)* 100
   milk *(Smucker's Dove)* 140
chocolate topping:
   (Kraft) 110
   all varieties *(Smucker's Magic Shell)* 220
   caramel *(Hershey's)* 100
   cherry melba *(Dickinson's Black Forest)* 130
   dark chocolate *(Mrs. Richardson's)* 140
   double *(Hershey's)* 110
   fudge, chocolate *(Smucker's)* 130
   fudge, double *(Hershey's)* 120
   fudge, hot *(Hershey's)* 130
   fudge, hot *(Kraft)* 140
   fudge, hot *(Mrs. Richardson's)* 140
   fudge, hot *(Mrs. Richardson's* Fat Free) 110
   fudge, hot *(Smucker's/Smucker's* Special Recipe) . . . 140
   fudge, hot, fat free *(Hershey's)* 100
   fudge, hot, light *(Smucker's)* 90
   mint *(Hershey's)* 110
fruit dip, caramel or chocolate *(Smucker's Fat Free)* 130
fruit glaze, for banana, creamy *(Marie's)* 60
fruit glaze, for blueberries, peaches, or strawberries *(Marie's)* . . .40
fruit syrup, ¼ cup:
   (Smucker's) 210
   light *(Smucker's)* 130
   and maple *(R.W. Knudsen)* 150
grenadine, *see "Cocktail Mixers, Nonalcoholic," page 389*
marshmallow topping:
   (Smucker's) 120
   all varieties *(Marshmallow Fluff)* 60
   creme *(Kraft)* 40
nut topping *(Planters)* 100

Dessert Toppings & Syrups *(cont.)*

peanut butter caramel topping *(Smucker's)* 150
pecan or walnut topping, with syrup *(Smucker's)* 190
pineapple *(Smucker's)* 110
pineapple topping *(Kraft)* 110
raspberry syrup *(Fox's No Cal)* 0
raspberry syrup *(R.W. Knudsen)*, ¼ cup 150
strawberry pie glaze *(Smucker's)* 80
strawberry syrup:
   (Fox's No Cal) 0
   (Hershey's) 100
   (Knott's Berry Farm) 120
   (R.W. Knudsen), ¼ cup 150
   (S&W Reduced Calorie), ¼ cup 60
strawberry topping:
   (Kraft) 110
   (Mrs. Richardson's Fat Free*)* 70
   (Smucker's) 100
   melba *(Dickinson's)* 90
whipped, frozen *(Kraft* Real*)* .20
whipped, nondairy:
   frozen *(Cool Whip* Extra Creamy*)* 30
   frozen *(Cool Whip* Lite*)* 20
   frozen *(Cool Whip* Non-dairy*)* 25
   frozen *(Kraft* Whipped Topping*)* 20
   frozen *(La Crema* Lite*)* 15
   frozen *(Rich's)* 25
   pressurized can *(Rich's)* 25
   mix* *(D-Zerta)* 10
   mix* *(Dream Whip)* 20

MISCELLANEOUS SWEET BAKING INGREDIENTS
See also "Cake Frostings" and "Cake Decorations"

---

                                                 calories

bits, 1 tbsp.:
   holiday *(Hershey's)* 70
   peanut butter *(Reese's)* 70
   toffee *(Skor)* 70

* Prepared according to package directions

cherry, candied, green or red:
  (Paradise/White Swan), .2-oz. piece 15
  (S&W Glace), 5 pieces 80
  and pineapple mix *(Paradise/White Swan)*, 2 tbsp., 1.3 oz. . . 110
cherry, maraschino, green or red *(Haddon House)*, 1 piece . . .10
cherry, maraschino, green or red *(S&W)*, 1 piece 10
chips, 1 tbsp.:
  all flavors *(Hershey's)* 80
  butterscotch *(Nestlé* Morsels) 80
  rainbow *(Nestlé* Morsels) .70
chocolate, baking, bar:
  (Hershey's), ½ of 1-oz. bar 90
  bittersweet *(Ghirardelli)*, 3 squares, 1.5 oz. 210
  bittersweet or semisweet *(Hershey's)*, ½ oz. 80
  milk *(Ghirardelli)*, 3 squares, 1.5 oz. 220
  milk *(Ghirardelli)*, 1 oz. 140
  semisweet *(Baker's)*, 1 oz. 130
  semisweet *(Ghirardelli)*, 3 squares, 1.5 oz. 210
  semisweet *(Nestlé)*, ½ oz. 70
  sweet *(Baker's German)*, ½ oz. 60
  sweet, dark *(Ghirardelli)*, 3 squares, 1.5 oz. 210
  unsweetened *(Baker's)*, 1 oz. 140
  unsweetened *(Ghirardelli)*, 3 squares, 1.5 oz. 210
  unsweetened *(Nestlé)*, ½ oz. 80
  white *(Baker's)*, 1 oz. 160
  white *(Ghirardelli)*, 3 squares, 1.5 oz. 240
  white *(Nestlé)*, ½ oz. 80
chocolate, pre-melted *(Choco Bake)*, ½ oz. 80
chocolate chips or morsels, ½ oz. or 1 tbsp.:
  (Ghirardelli Flickettes) .70
  milk *(Baker's)* 70
  milk *(Ghirardelli)* 70
  milk *(Hershey's Kisses* Mini), 11 pieces, ½ oz. 80
  milk *(M&M's)* 70
  milk or mint *(Nestlé)* 70
  semisweet *(Ghirardelli)* .70
  semisweet *(Hershey's)* 80
  semisweet *(Hershey's* Reduced Fat) 60
  white *(Ghirardelli)* 80
chocolate chunks *(Hershey's* Semisweet), 6 chunks 80
chocolate, semisweet, ½ oz.:
  (Baker's Real) 60

**Miscellaneous Sweet Baking Ingredients, chocolate, semisweet
(cont.)**
    (M&M's). 70
    flavor (Baker's) 70
    plain or mint (Nestlé) 70
citron, candied (S&W), 39 pieces, 1.1 oz. 90
citron, candied, diced (Paradise/White Swan), 2 tbsp., .9 oz. . . .80
coconut, 2 tbsp:
    flaked (Angel Flake). 70
    flaked (Durkee) 80
    flaked (Mounds) 70
    flaked, and almond bits (Almond Joy) 60
    shredded (Baker's Premium) .60
fruit, mixed, candied:
    (S&W Glace), 2 tbsp. 90
    (White Swan), 1 tbsp., .8 oz. 70
    (White Swan Deluxe), 2 tbsp., 1.2 oz. 100
fruit and peel mix (Paradise Old English), 1 tbsp., .8 oz. . . .70
    cake mix (Queen Anne/Paradise Extra Fancy), 2 tbsp.,
    1.2 oz. 100
ginger, candied or crystallized (Frieda's), 1 oz. 96
ginger, candied or crystallized (Paradise/White Swan),
    3 pieces, 1 oz. 100
lemon peel, candied (S&W), 1.1 oz. 80
lemon peel, candied, diced (Paradise/White Swan), 2 tbsp.,
    1 oz. 80
orange peel, candied (S&W), 58 pieces, 1.1 oz. 80
orange peel, candied, diced (Paradise/White Swan), 2 tbsp.,
    1.1 oz. 90
pineapple, candied:
    (Paradise/White Swan), 6 pieces, 1 oz. 90
    assorted (Paradise/White Swan), 2 tbsp., 1 oz. 90
    green (Paradise/White Swan), 7 pieces, 1 oz. 90
    red (Paradise/White Swan), 8 pieces, 1.1 oz. 100
    slices, natural or color (S&W Glace), 2.2 oz. 180
    wedges, natural or color (S&W Glace), 5 pieces, 1 oz. 80

Chapter 20

CANDY AND CHEWING GUM

CANDY	
	calories
(Baby Ruth), 2.1-oz. bar	280
(Baby Ruth Fun Size), 2 bars	200
(Bar None), 1.65-oz. bar	250
(Buncha Crunch), 1.4 oz.	200
butter crunch/almond (Almond Roca), 4 pieces	280
butter rum (Lifesavers), 2 pieces	20
butter rum (Pearson Nips), 2 pieces	60
(Butterfinger), 2.1-oz. bar	280
(Butterfinger Fun Size), 2 bars	200
(Butterfinger BB's), 1.7-oz. bag	230
butterscotch (Brach's Disks), 3 pieces	70
candy cane (Starburst), 1 piece	70
candy corn (Heide/Heide Indian), 1 oz.	110
caramel:	
(Kraft), 5 pieces	170
(Pearson Nips), 2 pieces	60
chocolate (Milk Duds), 1.85-oz. box	230
chocolate (Pom Poms), 1.58-oz. box	200
chocolate (Rolo), 1.9 oz.	220
caramel, with cookies:	
(Twix), 1-oz. piece	140
(Twix King Size), .8-oz. bar	120
(Twix Miniatures), 3 pieces	150
(Twix Singles), 2 bars, 2 oz.	280
(Twix Fun Size), .6-oz. piece	80
caramel, and peanut butter (Hershey's Sweet Escapes),	
1.4-oz. bar	150
cherry, chocolate (Perugina), 1.21 oz.	160
chocolate:	
(Cella's Dark/Milk), 2 pieces, 1 oz.	110
with hazelnuts (Ferraro Rocher), 3 pieces	220
milk, see "chocolate, milk," below	

Candy, chocolate *(cont.)*
  parfait *(Pearson Nips)*, 2 pieces 60
  toffee crisp *(Hershey's Sweet Escapes)*, 1.4-oz. bar 190
chocolate, candy coated:
  (M&M's), 1.5 oz. 210
  (M&M's King Size), ½ bag, 1.6 oz. 220
  (M&M's Singles), 1.68-oz. bag 240
  (M&M's Fun Size), .75-oz. bag 100
  with almonds *(M&M's)*, 1.5 oz. 230
  with almonds *(M&M's Singles)*, 1.3-oz. bag 200
  mini *(M&M's)*, 3 boxes, 1.5 oz. 210
  mini *(M&M's Tube)*, 1.25-oz. tube 170
  peanut butter *(M&M's)*, 1.5 oz. 220
  peanut butter *(M&M's Singles)*, 1.6-oz. bag 240
  peanut butter *(M&M's Fun Size)*, .75-oz. bag 110
  with peanuts *(M&M's)*, 1.5 oz. 220
  with peanuts *(M&M's King Size)*, ½ bag, 1.6 oz. 240
  with peanuts *(M&M's Singles)*, 1.74-oz. bag 250
  with peanuts *(M&M's Fun Size)*, .75-oz. bag 110
chocolate, dark:
  (Dove), ¼ of 6-oz. bar 230
  (Dove Mini), 7 pieces, 1.5 oz. 220
  (Dove Singles), 1.3-oz. bar 200
  (Ghirardelli), 1.25-oz. bar 180
  (Ghirardelli), 1.5 oz. 210
  (Hershey's Special Dark), 1.45-oz. bar 230
  with almonds *(Ghirardelli)*, 1.5-oz. bar 220
  bittersweet *(Toblerone)*, ⅓ of 3.5-oz. bar 180
  with raspberries *(Ghirardelli)*, 4 pieces 210
chocolate, milk:
  (Dove), ¼ of 6-oz. bar 230
  (Dove Doves), .8-oz. piece 130
  (Dove Mini), 7 pieces, 1.5 oz. 230
  (Dove Single), 1.3-oz. bar 200
  (Ghirardelli), 1.25 oz. 220
  (Ghirardelli), 1.25-oz. bar 190
  (Hershey's), 1.55-oz. bar 230
  (Hershey's Hugs), 8 pieces 200
  (Hershey's Miniatures), 5 pieces 230
  (Nestlé), 1.45-oz. bar 220
  (Symphony), 1.5-oz. bar 230
  plain or with almonds *(Hershey's Nuggets)*, 4 pieces 210

plain or with almonds *(Hershey's Kisses)*, 8 pieces 210
with almonds *(Cadbury)*, 9 blocks 220
with almonds *(Ghirardelli)*, 1.25-oz. bar 170
with almonds *(Ghirardelli)*, 1.5 oz. 230
with almonds *(Ghirardelli)*, 2.1-oz. bar 320
with almonds *(Hershey's)*, 1.45-oz. bar 230
with almonds *(Hershey's* Golden), 2.8-oz. bar 450
with almonds *(Hershey's* Golden Solitaire), 2.8-oz. bag 450
with almonds *(Hershey's Hugs)*, 9 pieces 230
with almonds and toffee *(Symphony)*, 1.5-oz. bar 240
with caramel *(Caramello)*, 1.6-oz. bar 220
cookies and cream *(Ghirardelli)*, 1.3 oz. 190
cookies and cream *(Hershey's* Nuggets), 4 pieces 200
with crisps *(Cadbury* Krisp), 9 blocks 200
with crisps *(Crunch)*, 1.55-oz. bar 230
with crisps *(Crunch* Fun Size), 4 bars 200
with crisps *(Ghirardelli)*, 1.25-oz. bar 180
with crisps *(Ghirardelli)*, 2.1-oz. bar 300
with crisps *(Ghirardelli)*, 2.5-oz. bar 360
with crisps *(Krackel)*, 1.4-oz. bar 220
with fruit and nuts *(Chunky)*, 1.4-oz. bar 200
with hazelnuts *(Mon Cheri)*, 3 pieces 260
with honey and nougat *(Toblerone)*, 1/3 of 3.5-oz. bar 180
with macadamias *(Ghirardelli)*, 1.25-oz. bar 190
with macadamias *(Hershey's* Golden), 2.4-oz. bar 380
with peanuts *(Mr. Goodbar)*, 1.75-oz. bar 270
with pecans *(Ghirardelli)*, 4 pieces, 1.5 oz. 230
thins *(Lindt* Swiss), 15 pieces, 1.5 oz. 230
with toffee *(Ghirardelli)*, 4 pieces, 1.5 oz. 220
wafers *(Ghirardelli)*, 11 pieces, 1.5 oz. 210
chocolate mint:
   (Cadbury Mint), 5 blocks 190
   (Ghirardelli), 1.5 oz. 220
   (Ghirardelli), 2.1-oz. bar 310
   (Pearson Nips), 2 pieces 60
   candy coated *(M&M's)*, 1.5 oz. 200
   cookies and *(Hershey's)*, 1.55-oz. bar 230
   cookies and *(Hershey's* Nuggets), 4 pieces 200
   wafers *(Ghirardelli)*, 11 pieces, 1.5 oz. 210
chocolate, white:
   and cookie *(Hershey's Cookies 'n' Creme)*, 1.5-oz. bar 230
   with crisps *(Nestlé White Crunch* Giant), 1/3 of 4.5-oz. bar . . 230

Candy *(cont.)*

raspberry cream *(Ghirardelli)*, 4 pieces, ⅓ oz.	200
coconut, chocolate coated *(Mounds)*, 1.9-oz. bar	250
coconut, chocolate coated, with almonds *(Almond Joy)*, 1.76-oz. bar	240
coffee *(Pearson Nips)*, 2 pieces	60
coffee beans, espresso, chocolate covered, milk chocolate or hazelnut flavor *(Snap!)*, 1.5-oz. pkg.	200
creme egg *(Milky Way)*, 1.2-oz. piece	190
creme egg *(Snickers)*, 1.2-oz. piece	170

fruit flavored:

(Frooties), 12 pieces, 1.3 oz.	150
(Skittles), 1.5 oz.	170
(Skittles Singles), 2.2-oz. bag	250
(Skittles Fun Size), 3 bags, 1.6 oz.	180
chews *(Starburst)*, 8 pieces, 1.4 oz.	160
chews *(Starburst* Singles), 2.1-oz. pack	240
tropical or wild berry *(Skittles)*, 1.5 oz.	170
tropical or wild berry *(Skittles* Singles), 2.2-oz. bag	250
tropical or wild berry *(Skittles Fun Size)*, 2 bags, 1.4 oz.	160
twists *(Starburst)*, 4 pieces, 1.5 oz.	140
twists *(Starburst* Singles), 2-oz. bag	190

fruit flavored, gummed:

(Amazin' Fruit), 1.9 oz.	180
(Brach's Fruit Bunch), 3 pieces, 1.6 oz.	150
(Dots Mini), .7-oz. box	80
(Gummi Savers), 1.5 oz.	130
original or tropical *(Dots)*, 12 pieces, 1.5 oz.	150
original or tropical *(Dots)*, 2.25-oz. box	220
fudge *(Kraft* Fudgies), 5 pieces, 1.4 oz.	180
halvah, chocolate *(Joyva)*, 1.75 oz.	340

hard, all flavors:

(Brach's Sparklers), 3 pieces, .6 oz.	70
(Charms), 2 pieces, .2 oz.	25
(Hershey's Tastetations), 3 pieces	60
(Lifesavers), 2 pieces	20
(Pez), .3-oz. roll	35
(Pez Sugar Free), .3-oz. roll	30
(Tootsie Pop Drops) 1 piece, .2 oz.	20
chocolate dipped *(Bogdon's* Reception Sticks), 1 piece	16
honey *(Bit-O-Honey)*, 1.7-oz. bar	200

jellied:
 (Heide Jujubes), 58 pieces, 1.4 oz. 160
 (Jujyfruits), 15 pieces, 1.4 oz. 160
 spearmint leaves *(Brach's)*, 5 pieces 130
jelly beans, assorted flavors:
 (Jelly Belly), 1 oz. 100
 (Jelly Belly), 35 pieces, 1.4 oz. 140
 (Starburst), 1.5 oz. 150
 (Starburst Singles), 1.25-oz. bag 130
 egg *(Starburst)*, 2-oz. egg 200
licorice:
 (Crows), 12 pieces, 1.5 oz. 150
 (Pearson Nips), 2 pieces 60
 black or cherry *(Nibs)*, 22 pieces 140
 black or strawberry *(Twizzlers)*, 4 pieces 140
 bridge mix *(Goelitz)*, 2 tbsp., 1.4 oz. 150
 cherry *(Twizzlers)*, 4 pieces 150
 cherry *(Twizzler* Pull-n-Peel), 1.3-oz. piece 110
 chocolate *(Twizzlers)*, 5 pieces 140
licorice, candy coated:
 (Good & Fruity), 1.8-oz. box 150
 (Good & Plenty), 1.4 oz. 130
lollipop, all flavors, 1 pop:
 (Astro Pops), 1 oz. 108
 (Blow Pop), .65 oz. 70
 (Blow Pop), .9 oz. 100
 (Blow Pop), 1.3 oz. 150
 (Blow Pop Junior), .5 oz. .50
 (Caramel Apple), .5 oz. 50
 (Caramel Apple), .6 oz. 70
 (Charms), .5 oz. 60
 (Charms Sweet or Sour), .6 oz. 70
 (Dum-Dums), .6 oz. 71
 (Fiesta), .7 oz. 80
 (Lifesavers), .4 oz. 40
 (Mutant Fruitant), .6 oz. 60
 (Save-A-Sucker/Suck An Egg), 1 oz. 110
 (Save-A-Sucker), 2 oz. 200
 (Sugar Daddy), 1.7 oz. 200
 (Sugar Daddy Junior), 3 pops, 1.3 oz. 160
 (Tootsie Pop), .45 oz. 50
 (Tootsie Pop), .6 oz. 60

Candy, lollipop *(cont.)*
   (Tootsie Roll Candy Cane), .5 oz. 50
   (Tootsie Roll Candy Cane), .7 oz. 80
   (Zip-A-Dee-Doo-Da), 3 pops, .5 oz. 60
malted milk balls *(Whoppers)*, 1.4 oz. 190
(Mars), 1.76-oz. bar 240
(Mars Fun Size), 2 bars 190
marshmallow:
   (Funmallows), 4 pieces 110
   (Kraft Jet-Puffed), 5 pieces, 1.2 oz. 110
   mini *(Funmallows)*, ½ cup 100
   mini *(Kraft)*, ½ cup 100
   peanut *(Spangler)*, 6 pieces 163
(Mexican Midgee), 12 pieces, 1.3 oz. 150
(Milky Way Original Miniatures), 5 pieces, 1.5 oz. 190
(Milky Way Original Singles), 2-oz. bar 270
(Milky Way Original *Fun Size)*, 2 bars, 1.4 oz. 180
(Milky Way Dark Miniatures), 5 pieces, 1.45 oz. 180
(Milky Way Dark Singles), 1.76-oz. bar 220
(Milky Way Dark *Fun Size)*, 2 bars, 1.4 oz. 170
(Milky Way Lite Miniatures), 5 pieces, 1.4 oz. 150
(Milky Way Lite Singles), 1.57-oz. bar 170
mint:
   (Lifesavers Cryst-O-Mint), 2 pieces 20
   (Pez Peppermint), 3 pieces 10
   (Tootsie Roll Candy Cane Ball), 1 piece 45
   all flavors *(Lifesavers)*, 3 pieces 20
   all flavors, except iced and vanilla *(Breath Savers)*, 1 piece . . . 0
   butter *(Kraft)*, 7 pieces .60
   chocolate coated *(After Eight)*, 5 pieces 190
   chocolate coated *(Junior* Mints), 16 pieces 160
   chocolate coated *(Junior* Mints), 1.6 oz.-box 180
   chocolate coated *(Junior* Mints Mini), 3 boxes, 1.5 oz. 170
   chocolate coated *(Pearson)*, 5 pieces 150
   chocolate coated *(York* Peppermint Pattie), 1.5-oz. piece . . 150
   chocolate coated *(York* Peppermint Pattie Mini), 3 pieces,
     1.4 oz. 160
   iced/vanilla *(Breath Savers)*, 1 piece 10
   party *(Kraft)*, 7 pieces .60
(Nestlé Turtles), 2 pieces 160
nonpareils *(Ghirardelli)*, 1.4 oz. 190
nonpareils *(Sno-Caps)*, 2.3 oz. 300

nougat *(Brach's)*, 4 pieces 170
nougat *(Charleston Chew* Vanilla), 5 pieces, 1.2 oz. 150
nougat bar, chocolate covered:
   chocolate *(Charleston Chew)*, .35-oz. bar 35
   chocolate, strawberry, or vanilla *(Charleston Chew)*,
     1.9-oz. bar 230
   chocolate, strawberry, or vanilla *(Charleston Chew)*,
     2.5-oz. bar 300
   vanilla *(Charleston Chew)*, .35-oz. bar 45
(Nutrageous), 1.6-oz. bar 240
(Oh Henry!), 1.8-oz. bar 230
(100 Grand), 1.5-oz. bar 200
(Pay Day), 1.85-oz. bar 250
peanut *(Planters)*, 1.6-oz. bar 230
peanut, chocolate coated *(Goobers)*, 1.38 oz. 210
peanut brittle *(Kraft)*, 1.3 oz. 170
peanut butter, chocolate:
   (5th Avenue), 2-oz. bar 280
   candy coated *(Reese's Pieces)*, 1.6 oz.-bag 230
   with cookie *(Twix)*, .9-oz. bar 130
   with cookie *(Twix* Singles), 2 bars, 1.7 oz. 260
   cup *(Reese's)*, 2 pieces, 1.6-oz. pkg. 240
   cup *(Reese's* Crunchy), 2 pieces, 1.6-oz. pkg. 250
peanut butter parfait *(Pearson Nips)*, 2 pieces 60
popcorn, caramel, *see "Popcorn, Popped," page 373*
raisins, chocolate coated *(Raisinets)*, 1.58 oz. 200
raisins, yogurt coated:
   strawberry or vanilla *(Del Monte)*, .9-oz. bag 110
   vanilla *(Del Monte)*, 1-oz. bag 120
   vanilla *(Del Monte)*, 3 tbsp. 130
rock *(Brach's)*, 1 oz. 110
(Snickers King Size), 1/3 bar 170
(Snickers Miniatures), 4 pieces, 1.26 oz. 170
(Snickers Singles), 2.07-oz. bar 280
(Snickers Fun Size), 2 bars, 1.4 oz. 190
(Snickers Munch), 1.4-oz. bar 230
(Sugar Babies), 30 pieces 180
(Sugar Babies Christmas Pouch), 18 pieces, 9.3 oz. 210
(Sugar Babies Pouch), 1.7-oz. bag 190
(Sugar Daddy Chewz), 5 pieces, 1.5 oz. 160
(Sugar Daddy Nuggets), 5 pieces, 1.5 oz. 170
(3 Musketeers), 2.13-oz. bar 260

Candy *(cont.)*
(3 Musketeers Miniature), 7 bars 170
(3 Musketeers Fun Size), 2 bars 140
toffee *(Brach's* Treasures), 3 pieces 80
toffee bar *(Heath),* 1.4 oz. 210
toffee bar *(Skor),* 1.4 oz. 220
(Tootsie Roll Midges), 6 pieces, 1.4 oz. 160
(Tootsie Roll Snack Bar), 2 pieces, 1 oz. 110
wafer, chocolate coated *(Kit Kat),* 1.5-oz. bar 220
wafer, triple chocolate *(Hershey's Sweet Escapes),* 1.4-oz. bar . . 160
(Whatchamacallit), 1.7-oz. bar 250

CHEWING GUM, one piece

	calories
all flavors:	
(Beech-Nut)	.10
(Big Red)	.10
(Care*Free)	.10
(Doublemint/Winterfresh/Wrigley's Spearmint)	.10
(Extra/Winterfresh Sugarfree)	5
(Freedent)	.10
(Fruit Stripe)	.10
(Juicy Fruit)	.10
bubble:	
(Blow Pop Ball)	.45
(Bubble Yum)	.25
(Bubble Yum Sugarless)	.15
(Care*Free)	.10
stick *(Care*Free)*	5

Chapter 21

ICE CREAM, FROZEN YOGURT, AND RELATED CONFECTIONS

ICE CREAM, ½ cup
See also "Ice Cream Bars & Novelties," "Ice Cream Desserts," " 'Ice Cream,' Nondairy," and "Food Chains and Restaurants"

calories

almond:
  butter *(Breyers All Natural)* 170
  praline *(Edy's/Dreyer's Grand)* 170
  Swiss, fudge twirl *(Breyers Light/Lowfat)* 130
  toasted *(Dreyer's Grand)* 150
Amaretto *(Häagen-Dazs DiSaronno)* 260
banana split *(Edy's Grand)* 160
bananas Foster *(Healthy Choice)* 110
(Ben & Jerry's Chubby Hubby) 350
(Ben & Jerry's Chunky Monkey) 300
(Ben & Jerry's Cool Britannia) 260
(Ben & Jerry's Holy Cannoli) 270
(Ben & Jerry's Phish Food) 310
(Ben & Jerry's Rainforest Crunch) 300
(Ben & Jerry's Wavy Gravy) 330
Black Forest *(Healthy Choice)* 120
brownie, blond, sundae *(Ben & Jerry's Low Fat)* . . 190
brownie, fudge:
  (Breyers Blends Sara Lee) 190
  (Healthy Choice) 120
  à la mode *(Healthy Choice)* 120
  chocolate *(Ben & Jerry's)* 250
  double *(Edy's Grand)* 170
  double chocolate *(Schwan's)* 160
  marble *(Breyers Light/Lowfat)* 120
butter crunch *(Schwan's)* 150
butter crunch *(Schwan's Lowfat)* 120

Ice Cream *(cont.)*
butter pecan:
    (Ben & Jerry's) 310
    (Breyers All Natural) 180
    (Breyers Light/Lowfat) 120
    (Edy's/Dreyer's No Sugar) 110
    (Edy's/Dreyer's Grand) 160
    (Edy's/Dreyer's Grand Light) 120
    (Häagen-Dazs) 320
    (Schwan's) 150
    (Sealtest) 160
    crunch *(Healthy Choice)* 120
butterscotch ripple *(Schwan's)* 140
cappuccino *(Breyers Blends Maxwell House)* 170
cappuccino chocolate chunk or mocha fudge *(Healthy Choice)* . . 120
caramel cream, dreamy *(Edy's Grand* Light) 110
caramel praline:
    almond *(Breyers* All Natural) 170
    crunch *(Breyers* Fat Free) 120
    crunch *(Edy's/Dreyer's* Fat Free) 120
cherry:
    blackjack *(Schwan's)* 160
    chocolate chip *(Ben & Jerry's Cherry Garcia)* 240
    chocolate chip *(Edy's Grand)* 150
    chocolate chunk *(Edy's/Dreyer's Grand)* 150
    chocolate chunk *(Healthy Choice)* 110
cherry nut, cherry vanilla, or dark sweet cherry *(Schwan's)* . . . 140
cherry vanilla:
    (Breyers All Natural) 150
    black, swirl *(Edy's/Dreyer's* No Sugar) 90
    black, swirl *(Edy's* Fat Free) 100
Chiquita 'n chocolate *(Edy's/Dreyer's Grand* Light) 110
chocolate:
    (Breyers All Natural) 160
    (Breyers Fat Free) 90
    (Edy's/Dreyer's Grand) 220
    (Häagen-Dazs) 270
    (Schwan's) 140
    (Sealtest) 140
    chunky *(Schwan's)* 160
    hunk, triple *(Healthy Choice)* 110
    triple *(Edy's/Dreyer's* No Sugar) 100

chocolate almond:
  (Breyers Blends Hershey's Almond) 190
  (Schwan's) 150
  fudge *(Edy's/Dreyer's Grand Light)* 120
chocolate brownie chunk *(Edy's/Dreyer's Fat Free)* 120
chocolate chip:
  (Breyers All Natural) 170
  (Edy's/Dreyer's Grand Chips!) 160
  (Schwan's) 150
  (Sealtest) 150
  chocolate *(Häagen-Dazs)* 300
chocolate chip, mint:
  (Breyers All Natural) 170
  (Breyers Light/Lowfat) 110
  (Breyers No Sugar Added) 100
  (Edy's/Dreyer's Grand Chips!) 170
  (Healthy Choice) 120
  (Schwan's Chip and Mint) 150
  (Sealtest) 150
chocolate chip cookie dough:
  (Ben & Jerry's) 270
  (Breyers All Natural) 170
  (Breyers Light/Lowfat) 110
  (Schwan's) 150
  (Sealtest) 160
chocolate cookie, mint *(Ben & Jerry's)* 260
chocolate fudge:
  (Edy's/Dreyer's Fat Free) 120
  (Edy's/Dreyer's Fat Free/No Sugar) 100
  mousse *(Edy's/Dreyer's Grand Light)* 110
  mousse *(Edy's Grand)* 160
  mousse *(Healthy Choice)* 120
  ripple *(Schwan's)* 140
  sundae *(Edy's Grand)* 170
chocolate marshmallow ripple *(Schwan's)* 140
chocolate mumbo jumbo *(Edy's/Dreyer's Grand)* 170
chocolate peanut butter crunch *(Edy's/Dreyer's Fat Free)* . . . 120
coffee:
  (Ben & Jerry's Coffee Coffee Buzz Buzz Buzz) 290
  (Breyers All Natural) 150
  (Edy's/Dreyer's Grand) 140
  (Häagen-Dazs) 270

Ice Cream *(cont.)*

coffee and biscotti *(Ben & Jerry's* Low Fat) 170
coffee fudge *(Edy's/Dreyer's* Fat Free) 110
coffee fudge *(Edy's/Dreyer's* Fat Free/No Sugar) 100
coffee toffee crunch *(Ben & Jerry's* with *Heath)* 280
cookie chunk *(Edy's/Dreyer's* Fat Free) 120
cookies 'n cream:
   (Breyers) 170
   (Edy's/Dreyer's Grand) 160
   (Edy's/Dreyer's Grand Light) 110
   (Häagen-Dazs) 270
   (Healthy Choice) 120
   (Schwan's) 160
   mint *(Breyers* Fat Free) 100
   mint *(Dreyer's Grand* Light) 110
cookie creme de mint *(Healthy Choice)* 130
cookie chunk *(Edy's/Dreyer's* Fat Free) 120
cookie dough *(Edy's/Dreyer's Grand)* 170
cookie dough *(Edy's/Dreyer's Grand* Light) 130
cream, sweet, and cookies *(Ben & Jerry's* Low Fat) 170
espresso chip *(Edy's Grand)* 150
espresso fudge chip *(Dreyer's Grand* Light) 120
French silk *(Edy's/Dreyer's Grand* Light) 120
fudge:
   chunk *(Ben & Jerry's New York Super Fudge Chunk)* 290
   marble *(Edy's/Dreyer's* Fat Free) 110
   marble *(Edy's/Dreyer's* No Sugar) 90
   mint *(Dreyer's* Fat Free) 110
   royal *(Sealtest)* 150
fudge brownie, double *(Edy's/Dreyer's* No Sugar) 100
fudge toffee parfait *(Breyers* Light/Lowfat) 120
heavenly hash *(Sealtest)* 150
ice cream sandwich *(Edy's Grand)* 140
Irish cream *(Häagen-Dazs Baileys)* 270
macadamia brittle *(Häagen-Dazs)* 300
maple nut *(Schwan's)* 150
(Milky Way) 130
mocha fudge:
   (Edy's/Dreyer's No Sugar) 90
   almond *(Dreyer's Grand)* 170
   almond *(Dreyer's Grand* Light) 120
   almond *(Schwan's)* 170

mud pie *(Dreyer's Grand)* 160
Neapolitan *(Dreyer's Grand)* 140
Neapolitan *(Schwan's)* 140
peach *(Breyers All Natural)* 130
peach *(Schwan's)* 130
peanut butter:
   (Breyers Blends Reese's Pieces) 200
   caramel *(Breyers Blends NutRageous)* 200
   cup *(Ben & Jerry's)* 370
   cup *(Breyers Blends Reese's)* 210
   cup *(Edy's Grand* Light Cups!*)* 130
   fudge ripple *(Schwan's)* 150
pecan praline sundae *(Schwan's)* 150
praline:
   almond crunch *(Breyers Light/Lowfat)* 110
   almondine sundae *(Schwan's Lowfat)* 120
   caramel or praline caramel cluster *(Healthy Choice)* 130
   pecan *(Breyers No Sugar)* 110
raspberry ripple *(Schwan's)* 140
raspberry rumble *(Schwan's)* 160
raspberry vanilla swirl *(Edy's/Dreyer's Fat Free/No Sugar)* 90
rocky road:
   (Breyers Light/Lowfat) 120
   (Edy's/Dreyer's Grand) 170
   (Edy's/Dreyer's Grand Light) 110
   (Healthy Choice) 140
   (Schwan's) 150
   deluxe *(Breyers All Natural)* 190
rum raisin *(Häagen-Dazs)* 270
(Schwan's Summer's Dream) 130
(Snickers) 220
strawberry:
   (Breyers All Natural) 130
   (Breyers Fat Free) 90
   (Edy's/Dreyer's Grand Real) 130
   (Edy's/Dreyer's No Sugar) 80
   (Häagen-Dazs) 250
   (Schwan's) 140
   (Schwan's Fat Free/No Sugar Added) 110
   (Sealtest) 130
strawberry shortcake *(Healthy Choice)* 120
tin roof sundae *(Schwan's)* 150

Ice Cream *(cont.)*

toffee bar crunch *(Breyers* All Natural)	170
turtle fudge cake *(Healthy Choice)*	130

vanilla:

(Ben & Jerry's World's Best)	250
(Breyers All Natural)	150
(Breyers Fat Free)	100
(Breyers Light/Lowfat)	130
(Breyers No Sugar)	80
(Edy's/Dreyer's Fat Free)	100
(Edy's/Dreyer's Fat Free/No Sugar)	90
(Edy's/Dreyer's No Sugar)	80
(Edy's/Dreyer's Grand)	150
(Edy's/Dreyer's Grand Avalanche)	170
(Edy's/Dreyer's Grand Light)	100
(Häagen-Dazs)	270
(Healthy Choice)	100
(Schwan's)	140
(Schwan's Fat Free/No Sugar Added)	110
(Schwan's Lowfat)	100
(Sealtest)	140
bean *(Edy's/Dreyer's* Grand)	130
French *(Breyers* All Natural)	170
French *(Breyers* Light/Lowfat)	90
French *(Edy's/Dreyer's* Grand)	160
French *(Schwan's)*	170
French *(Sealtest)*	140

vanilla and black cherry *(Breyers Take Two* All Natural)	150

vanilla caramel:

(Edy's/Dreyer's Fat Free/No Sugar)	100
(Edy's/Dreyer's No Sugar)	90
fudge swirl *(Ben & Jerry's)*	280
vanilla and chocolate *(Breyers Take Two* All Natural)	160
vanilla and chocolate *(Edy's/Dreyer's* Grand)	150
vanilla and chocolate mint patty *(Ben & Jerry's* Low Fat)	180
vanilla chocolate swirl *(Edy's/Dreyer's* Fat Free/No Sugar)	90

vanilla-chocolate-strawberry combination:

(Breyers All Natural)	150
(Breyers Fat Free/No Sugar Added)	90
(Edy's Grand)	140
(Sealtest)	140
vanilla fudge *(Häagen-Dazs)*	280

vanilla fudge twirl:
    (*Breyers* All Natural) 160
    (*Breyers* Fat Free) 110
    (*Breyers* No Sugar Added) 90
vanilla and orange sherbet (*Breyers Take Two* All Natural) 140
vanilla and strawberry (*Breyers Take Two* Fat Free) 90
vanilla Swiss almond (*Häagen-Dazs*) 310
vanilla toffee crunch (*Ben & Jerry's* with *Heath*) 280

ICE CREAM BARS & NOVELTIES, one piece, except as noted
*See also "Ice Cream," "'Ice Cream,' Nondairy," "Ice Cream
Desserts," and "Ice & Sherbet Bars & Cones"*

---

                                                      calories

ice cream bars:
    all flavors (*Fudgsicle* Pop Variety Pack), 1.75-oz. pop 60
    almond (*Breyers*), 4-oz. bar 300
    almond (*DoveBar*), 2.8-oz. bar 280
    almond (*DoveBar* Singles), 3.5-oz. bar 330
    almond (*Good Humor*), 3-oz. bar 180
    almond (*Good Humor*), 3.75-oz. bar 230
    almond (*Klondike*) 310
    (*Ben & Jerry's Chunky Monkey* Peace Pop) 360
    (*Butterfinger*) 190
    caramel cream swirl with toffee chips (*DoveBar*) 280
    caramel crunch (*Klondike*) 300
    cherry royale (*Dove Bite Size*), 5 bars 340
    chocolate (*Klondike*) 280
    chocolate (*Nestlé Crunch*) 200
    chocolate (*3 Musketeers*), 1.6-oz. bar 150
    chocolate (*3 Musketeers* Singles), 2.2-oz. bar 190
    chocolate, chocolate dipped (*Good Humor* Choco Taco) . . . 320
    chocolate, dark chocolate coated (*DoveBar*), 2.8-oz. bar . . . 260
    chocolate, dark chocolate coated (*DoveBar*), 3.5-oz. bar . . . 330
    chocolate, dark chocolate coated (*Häagen-Dazs*),
        3.2-oz. bar 320
    chocolate, dark chocolate coated (*Häagen-Dazs* Single),
        4-oz. bar 400
    chocolate, double (*Dove Bite Size*), 5 bars 330
    chocolate candy center (*Good Humor* Crunch) 280
    chocolate cookie dough (*Ben & Jerry's* Peace Pop) 420
    chocolate dip (*Weight Watchers*) 100

Ice Cream Bars & Novelties, ice cream bars (cont.)

chocolate éclair (Col. Crunch)	160
chocolate éclair (Good Humor), 3.75-oz. bar	220
chocolate éclair (Good Humor Eclair), 3-oz. bar	170
chocolate malt (Schwan's Push-Ems)	.90
chocolate mousse (Weight Watchers)	.40
chocolate pudding (Schwan's)	160
chocolate sundae crunch (Schwan's)	170
coffee (Klondike)	290
coffee and almond crunch (Häagen-Dazs), 3-oz. bar	290
coffee and almond crunch (Häagen-Dazs Single), 3.7-oz. bar	360
cookies 'n cream (Edy's/Dreyer's)	250
(Cool Creations Mickey Mouse), 2.5-oz. bar	120
(Cool Creations Mickey Mouse), 4-oz. bar	170
fudge, double (Supersicle)	150
fudge stick (Schwan's)	110
fudge stick (Schwan's Trim Creations)	.50
(Good Humor WWF)	200
Irish creme cordial with dark chocolate (Dove Bite Size), 5 bars	340
(Klondike Krispy)	300
(Klondike Krunch), 3-oz. bar	200
(Klondike Krunch), 3.75-oz. bar	250
(Milky Way)	140
mint, green, and chocolate fudge truffle swirl (DoveBar)	290
mocha cashew crunch (DoveBar)	260
(Nestlé Crunch Crunch King)	270
(Nestlé Crunch Reduced Fat)	130
peanut butter (Reese's NutRageous)	240
peanut butter (Schwan's P-Nut Butter Creme)	170
peanut stick (Schwan's)	200
peppermint with dark chocolate (DoveBar)	290
peppermint with dark chocolate (Dove Bite Size Party), 5 bars	360
raspberry cordial (Schwan's)	210
root beer float (Schwan's)	.80
(Schwan's)	200
(Schwan's Healthy Creation Creme Bar)	.70
(Schwan's Rainbow Stick)	.90
(Schwan's Gold 'N' Nugit)	250
(Schwan's Krispie Krunch Bar)	120

(Schwan's Silver Mint) 160
(Snickers Singles) 200
(Snickers Snack Size), 4 bars 390
strawberry shake *(Schwan's Push-Ems)* 90
strawberry shortcake *(Col. Crunch)* 170
strawberry shortcake *(Good Humor)*, 3-oz. bar 160
strawberry shortcake *(Good Humor)*, 3.75-oz. bar 210
toffee, English *(Schwan's)* 200
toffee crunch, English *(Weight Watchers)* 110
toffee crunch, vanilla *(Ben & Jerry's* with *Heath* Peace Pop) . 330
vanilla *(Ben & Jerry's* Peace Pop) 330
vanilla *(Breyers)*, 4-oz. bar 300
vanilla *(Dove Bite Size* Classic), 5 bars 320
vanilla *(Good Humor)*, 2.75-oz. bar 180
vanilla *(Good Humor* Premium), 3-oz. bar 200
vanilla *(Good Humor* Premium), 3.75-oz. bar 220
vanilla *(Klondike* Original) 290
vanilla *(Klondike* Reduced Fat—No Sugar Added) 190
vanilla *(Nestlé Crunch)* 200
vanilla *(Popsicle)* 160
vanilla, French *(Dove Bite Size)*, 5 bars 330
vanilla, brownie *(Ben & Jerry's* Bar) 330
vanilla, white coated *(DoveBar)* 270
vanilla 'n almonds *(Edy's/Dreyer's)* 270
vanilla, with almonds *(Häagen-Dazs)*, 3-oz. bar 300
vanilla, with almonds *(Häagen-Dazs* Single), 3.7-oz. bar . . 370
vanilla, dark chocolate coated *(DoveBar)*, 2.8-oz. bar 260
vanilla, dark chocolate coated *(DoveBar* Single), 3.5-oz. bar . 330
vanilla, dark chocolate coated *(Häagen-Dazs)*, 3.2-oz. bar . . 320
vanilla, dark chocolate coated *(Häagen-Dazs* Single),
  4-oz. bar 390
vanilla, dark chocolate coated *(Klondike)* 290
vanilla, dark or milk chocolate coated *(Milky Way)* 220
vanilla, dark or milk chocolate coated *(Milky Way* Reduced
  Fat) 140
vanilla, ice coated *(Creamsicle* Bar), 2.5-oz. bar 100
vanilla, ice coated *(Creamsicle* Bar), 2.7-oz. bar 110
vanilla, ice coated *(Creamsicle* Pop), 1.75-oz. bar 70
vanilla, ice coated *(Creamsicle* Pop No Sugar Added) 25
vanilla, milk chocolate coated *(DoveBar)*, 2.8-oz. bar 260
vanilla, milk chocolate coated *(DoveBar* Single), 3.5-oz. bar . . 330
vanilla, milk chocolate coated *(Edy's/Dreyer's)* 250

Ice Cream Bars & Novelties, ice cream bars *(cont.)*

vanilla, milk chocolate coated *(Häagen-Dazs)*, 3-oz. bar 280
vanilla, milk chocolate coated *(Häagen-Dazs* Single),
   3.5-oz. bar 330
vanilla and chocolate *(Good Humor* Number 1) 190
vanilla and chocolate *(Snoopy)* 150

ice cream cones:

butter pecan *(Breyers)*, 5-oz. cone 300
chocolate or chocolate dipped *(Drumstick)* 320
chocolate dipped *(Good Humor* Premium Sundae),
   4.6-oz. cone 290
chocolate dipped *(Good Humor* Sundae), 4-oz. cone 230
chocolate dipped, with peanuts *(Good Humor* American
   Glory)* 230
chocolate dipped, with peanuts *(Good Humor* King) 300
chocolate dipped, with peanuts *(Klondike* Sundae) 310
cookies 'n cream *(Edy's/Dreyer's* Sundae) 250
pecan praline *(Schwan's Sundae Cone)* 270
(Schwan's Sundae Cone) 210
(Snickers) 290
vanilla *(Drumstick)* 340
vanilla caramel or vanilla fudge *(Drumstick)* 360
vanilla fudge *(Edy's/Dreyer's* Sundae) 340
vanilla fudge chocolate *(Schwan's Sundae Cone)* 260
vanilla fudge ripple *(Good Humor* Choco Taco) 310

ice cream cups:

chocolate *(Carnation)*, 3 fl. oz. 140
chocolate *(Sealtest)* 140
chocolate malt *(Carnation)*, 12 fl. oz. 270
chocolate malt *(Milky Way)* 220
chocolate shake *(Milky Way* Lowfat) 220
chocolate sundae *(Carnation)*, 5 fl. oz. 210
chocolate sundae or strawberry sundae *(Schwan's)* 120
fudge swirl *(Schwan's* Fat Free) 100
(Good Humor Sundae Twist) 160
peanut butter *(Good Humor* Reese's), 2 oz. 160
peanut butter *(Good Humor* Reese's), 3 oz. 220
strawberry *(Sealtest)* 130
strawberry or vanilla *(Carnation)*, 3 fl. oz. 100
strawberry or vanilla *(Schwan's* Nonfat) 80
strawberry sundae *(Carnation)*, 5 fl. oz. 200
vanilla *(Carnation)*, 5 fl. oz. 170

vanilla *(Schwan's)* 110
vanilla *(Sealtest)* 140
vanilla *(Sealtest* Fat Free) 100
vanilla *(Sealtest* No Sugar Added) 90
vanilla and chocolate *(Breyers)*, 6 oz. 240
vanilla malt *(Carnation)*, 12 fl. oz. 260
ice cream nuggets:
  with chocolate *(Nestlé Crunch)*, 8 pieces 310
  with dark chocolate *(Bon-Bons)*, 5 pieces 190
  with dark chocolate *(Bon-Bons)*, 8 pieces 310
  with milk chocolate *(Bon-Bons)*, 5 pieces 200
  with milk chocolate *(Bon-Bons)*, 8 pieces 330
ice cream sandwiches:
  chocolate chip cookie *(Chipwich* Jr.) 240
  chocolate chip cookie *(Good Humor* Premium), 4-oz. piece . . 280
  chocolate chip cookie *(Good Humor* Premium),
    4.5-oz. piece 290
  cookies and cream *(Cool Creations)* 240
  (Good Humor), 3-oz. piece 160
  (Good Humor American Glory), 3.5-oz. piece 190
  (Good Humor Giant), 5-oz. piece 240
  (Häagen-Dazs) 260
  (Klondike Big Bear), 5-oz. piece 200
  (Klondike Big Bear), 7-oz. piece 300
  (Klondike Big Bear Fat Free) 150
  mini *(Cool Creations)* 110
  Neapolitan *(Good Humor* Giant), 5-oz. piece 260
  (Popsicle) 190
  (Schwan's) 170
  vanilla bars *(Weight Watchers)* 150

ICE CREAM DESSERTS
See also "Ice Cream" and "Ice Cream Bars & Novelties"

calories

ice cream loaf, all varieties *(Viennetta)*, 2.4-oz. slice 190
ice cream pie, grasshopper *(Schwan's)*, ⅛ pie 370
ice cream pie, strawberry cheesecake *(Schwan's)*, ⅛ pie 330

"ICE CREAM," NONDAIRY

calories

"ice cream," 1/2 cup, except as noted:

all flavors (Tofutti Soft Serve)	190
all flavors (Tofutti Soft Serve Lite)	90
all fruit flavors (Tofutti Frutti)	100
better pecan (Tofutti)	220
cappuccino, carob, or cherry vanilla (Rice Dream)	150
carob almond (Rice Dream)	170
chocolate (Rice Dream)	150
chocolate (Tofutti)	180
chocolate cake (Tofutti)	210
chocolate chip or mint chocolate chip (Rice Dream)	170
chocolate fudge (Tofutti Low Fat)	120
cocoa marble fudge (Rice Dream)	150
coffee marshmallow (Tofutti Low Fat)	100
cookies n' dream (Rice Dream)	170
mint carob chip (Rice Dream)	170
Neapolitan (Rice Dream)	150
orange vanilla swirl (Rice Dream)	150
passion island fruit or peach mango (Tofutti Low Fat)	100
strawberry (Rice Dream)	140
strawberry banana (Tofutti Low Fat)	100
vanilla (Rice Dream)	150
vanilla (Tofutti)	190
vanilla (Tofutti Cuties Slice), 1 slice	140
vanilla almond bark (Tofutti)	210
vanilla fudge (Tofutti)	190
vanilla fudge (Tofutti Low Fat)	120
vanilla Swiss almond (Rice Dream)	180
wildberry (Tofutti)	190
wildberry (Tofutti Slice), 1 slice	80
wildberry, chocolate covered (Tofutti Slice), 1 slice	180

"ice cream" bar, 1 piece:

chocolate (Rice Dream)	270
nutty, chocolate or vanilla (Rice Dream)	260
strawberry (Rice Dream)	250
vanilla (Rice Dream)	270

"ice cream" pie, cookie, all flavors (Rice Dream), 1 piece	320
"ice cream" pie, vanilla, chocolate covered (Tofutti Cuties), 1 piece	250

"ice cream" sandwich, chocolate *(Tofutti Cuties)*, 1 piece 130
"ice cream" sandwich, vanilla or wildberry *(Tofutti Cuties)*,
   1 piece 121
"ice cream" stick, 1 piece:
   chocolate *(Tofutti Frutti)* 120
   fudge *(Tofutti* Teddy) 70
   fudge *(Tofutti* Treats) 30

ICES & SHERBET

	calories
ices, Italian, 6 fl. oz.:	
cherry *(Luigi's)*	120
chocolate fudge *(Luigi's)*	150
grape, lemon, or strawberry *(Luigi's)*	110
sherbet, ½ cup, except as noted:	
all flavors *(Breyers)*	120
orange *(Carnation* Cup), 3 fl. oz.	.90
orange *(Carnation* Plastic), 5 fl. oz.	150
orange *(Sealtest)*, 4-oz. cup	130
orange or rainbow *(Schwan's)*	120
pink lemonade, tangerine, or tropical *(Edy's)*	130
strawberry kiwi *(Edy's)*	120
Swiss orange *(Edy's)*	150
sorbet, ½ cup:	
banana strawberry *(Häagen-Dazs)*	140
(Ben & Jerry's Doonesbury)	130
cherry cordial *(Edy's/Dreyer's* Whole Fruit)	160
chocolate *(Häagen-Dazs)*	130
chocolate *(Tofutti)*	.90
coffee *(Tofutti)*	.80
cranberry orange *(Ben & Jerry's)*	130
and cream, orange or raspberry *(Häagen-Dazs)*	190
devil's food *(Ben & Jerry's)*	160
lemon *(Edy's/Dreyer's* Whole Fruit)	140
lemon *(Häagen-Dazs Zesty Lemon)*	120
lemon *(Tofutti)*	.90
mango *(Häagen-Dazs)*	120
mango lime *(Ben & Jerry's)*	130
mango orange *(Edy's/Dreyer's* Whole Fruit)	120
orange-peach-mango *(Tofutti)*	.90
peach *(Edy's/Dreyer's* Whole Fruit)	130

Ices & Sherbet, sorbet *(cont.)*

peach *(Häagen-Dazs Orchard)* 140
piña colada *(Ben & Jerry's)* 140
purple passion fruit *(Ben & Jerry's)* 120
raspberry *(Edy's/Dreyer's Whole Fruit)* 130
raspberry *(Häagen-Dazs)* 120
raspberry *(Tofutti)* 80
strawberry *(Edy's/Dreyer's Whole Fruit)* 120
strawberry *(Häagen-Dazs)* 130
strawberry *(Tofutti)* 80
strawberry kiwi *(Ben & Jerry's)* 130

ICE & SHERBET BARS & CONES, 1 piece
See also "Ice Cream Bars & Novelties"

---

                                                              calories
ice bar:
all flavors *(Popsicle)* 45
all flavors *(Popsicle Sugar Free/Tropical Sugar Free)* . . . 15
all flavors *(Popsicle Super Twin)* 70
bubble gum swirl *(Popsicle)* 55
cappuccino *(Frozfruit)* 140
cherry *(Good Humor Bubble Play)* 110
cherry *(Good Humor Torpedo)* 35
cherry *(Popsicle Bubble Play)* 80
cherry *(Super Mario Bros.)* 120
cherry, lemon, and raspberry *(Good Humor Hyper Stripe)* . . . 80
cherry, lemon, and raspberry *(Popsicle Firecracker)* 40
cherry, lemon, and raspberry *(Supersicle Firecracker)* 80
cherry and pineapple *(Popsicle Big Stick)* 50
(Cool Creations Ice Pop) 50
(Cool Creations Surprise Pop) 60
cotton candy swirl *(Popsicle)* 55
(Ghoulie) 100
(Good Humor Jumbo Jet Star) 80
lemon *(Great White)* 70
lemon and cherry *(Mighty Morphin Power Rangers Zeo)* . . . 100
orange, pineapple, and lemon *(Good Humor Shoot Hoops!)* . . 90
(Popsicle Lick-A-Color), 2-oz. pop 50
(Popsicle Lick-A-Color), 3.5-oz. pop 90
(Popsicle Rainbow), 1.75-oz. pop 45
(Popsicle Rainbow), 3.5-oz. pop 90

(Popsicle Squeeze Ups) 90
(Popsicle Tingle Twister) 45
raspberry (Spider-Man) 100
(Schwan's Pop) 15
(Schwan's Twin Pop) 60
(Supersicle Candy Stripe/Sour Tower) 80
strawberry (Street Sharks) 100
watermelon (Good Humor) .80
ice bar, with fruit or fruit juice:
all flavors (Dole Fruit Juice) 45
all flavors (Dole Fruit Juice No Sugar) 25
all flavors (Dole Fruit 'n Juice), 2.5 oz. 70
all flavors (Minute Maid Fruit Juice), 2.25-oz. bar 60
all flavors (Minute Maid Juice), 1.75-oz. bar 50
all flavors (Popsicle All Natural) 50
all flavors (Popsicle Junior) 120
all flavors (Popsicle Rainbow Jets) 45
all flavors (Popsicle Fantastic Fruity) 60
all flavors (Starburst 12-Pack) 50
all flavors (Starburst Singles) 80
all flavors (Starburst No Sugar Added) 20
banana cream (Frozfruit) 150
cantaloupe (Frozfruit) 60
cherry (Frozfruit) 70
coconut (Dole Fruit 'n Juice), 4 oz. 210
coconut (Edy's/Dreyer's) 160
coconut cream (Frozfruit) 170
cranberry-apple or guava pineapple (Frozfruit) 80
kiwi-strawberry (Frozfruit) 90
lemon (Frozfruit) 90
lemon, iced tea (Frozfruit) 80
lemonade (Dole Fruit 'n Juice), 4-oz. bar 120
lime (Dole Fruit 'n Juice), 4-oz. bar 110
lime (Edy's/Dreyer's) 90
lime (Frozfruit) 90
orange (Frozfruit) 90
orange (Minute Maid), 3.75-oz. bar 90
peach (Edy's/Dreyer's) 140
piña colada, cream (Frozfruit) 170
pineapple (Frozfruit) 80
pine-coconut (Dole Fruit 'n Juice), 4-oz. bar 150
pine-orange-banana (Dole Fruit 'n Juice), 4-oz. bar 110

Ice & Sherbet Bars & Cones, ice bar, with fruit or fruit juice
(cont.)

    raspberry *(Frozfruit)* 80
    raspberry-kiwi *(Edy's/Dreyer's)* 90
    strawberry *(Dole* Fruit 'n Juice), 4-oz. bar 110
    strawberry *(Frozfruit)* .80
    strawberry *(Minute Maid)*, 3.75-oz. bar 120
    strawberry *(Schwan's)* .50
    strawberry cream *(Frozfruit)* 130
    strawberry-banana cream *(Frozfruit)* 140
    tropical *(Frozfruit)* .90
    watermelon *(Frozfruit)* 50
ice cone *(Good Humor* Snow Cone) 60
ice cone, cherry *(Screwball)* 100
sherbet bar/pop:
    chocolate *(Fudgsicle* Bar), 2.5-oz. or 2.7-oz. bar 90
    chocolate *(Fudgsicle* Bar Fat Free), 1.75-oz. bar 60
    chocolate *(Fudgsicle* Bar Sugar Free), 1.75-oz. bar 40
    chocolate *(Weight Watchers Treat)* 100
    orange *(Popsicle Pop Ups)* 80
    orange vanilla *(Weight Watchers Treat)* 40
    (Popsicle Big Stick) 110
    (Popsicle Cyclone) 50
    rainbow *(Popsicle Pop Ups)* 90
    (Schwan's Push-Ems) .90
smoothie bar, strawberry fields *(Dreyer's)* 100
smoothie bar, tropical oasis *(Dreyer's)* 90
sorbet bar, berry, wild *(Häagen-Dazs)* 90
sorbet bar, chocolate *(Häagen-Dazs)* 80
sorbet and yogurt bar:
    banana and strawberry *(Häagen-Dazs)* 90
    chocolate and cherry *(Häagen-Dazs)* 100
    raspberry and vanilla *(Häagen-Dazs)* 90

FROZEN YOGURT, ½ cup
See also "Frozen Yogurt Bars & Cup" and "Yogurt"

                                                 calories
all flavors:
    (Colombo Cooler) 60
    (Dannon Fat Free Soft) 100
    (Dannon Light 'n Crunchy) 110

except black cherry, chocolate, and lemon *(Schwan's)* 110
except caramel praline crunch, cookies in cream,
and vanilla fudge twirl *(Breyers* Fat Free) 100
except chocolate *(Colombo* Slender Sensations) 60
except German chocolate fudge *(Colombo* Nonfat) 100
except peanut butter *(Colombo* Lowfat) 110
banana pudding, homestyle *(TCBY)* 120
butter pecan *(Breyers)* 170
cappuccino *(Ben & Jerry's* No Fat) 140
caramel praline crunch *(Breyers* Fat Free) 120
caramel praline crunch *(Edy's/Dreyer's* Fat Free) 100
cherry:
    black *(Schwan's)* 120
    black, vanilla swirl *(Edy's/Dreyer's* Fat Free) 80
    vanilla *(Häagen-Dazs)* 140
    vanilla, chocolate chip *(Ben & Jerry's* Cherry Garcia) 170
cherry chocolate chunk *(Edy's/Dreyer's)* 110
chocolate:
    (Breyers) 130
    (Colombo Slender Sensations) 70
    (Dannon Fat Free Light) 70
    (Dannon Lowfat Soft) 120
    (Häagen-Dazs) 140
    (Schwan's) 120
    Dutch *(TCBY)* 100
    German chocolate fudge *(Colombo* Nonfat) 110
chocolate brownie chunk *(Edy's/Dreyer's)* 120
chocolate chip:
    cookie dough *(Ben & Jerry's)* 210
    cookie dough *(Breyers)* 150
    mint *(Breyers)* 140
chocolate fudge *(Edy's/Dreyer's* Fat Free) 100
chocolate fudge brownie *(Ben & Jerry's)* 190
chocolate silk mousse *(Edy's/Dreyer's* Fat Free) 90
coffee:
    (Häagen-Dazs) 140
    fudge *(Ben & Jerry's* No Fat) 140
    fudge sundae *(Edy's/Dreyer's* Fat Free) 100
cookies and cream:
    (Breyers Fat Free) 110
    (Edy's/Dreyer's) 120
    (TCBY) 120

Frozen Yogurt *(cont.)*

cookie dough *(Edy's/Dreyer's)* 130
cone crunch, crispy *(TCBY)* 130
lemon *(Schwan's)* 130
marble fudge *(Edy's/Dreyer's Fat Free)* 100
peach *(Breyers)* 120
peach *(TCBY)* 110
peach raspberry trifle *(Ben & Jerry's)* 180
peanut butter:
   (Colombo Lowfat) 120
   (Dannon Lowfat Soft) 120
   fudge sundae *(TCBY)* 110
pecan praline crisp *(TCBY)* 110
raspberry, black, swirl *(Ben & Jerry's No Fat)* 150
raspberry sorbet 'n cream *(Edy's/Dreyer's Fat Free)* 90
strawberry:
   (Breyers) 120
   cheesecake *(Breyers)* 130
   summertime *(TCBY)* 100
toffee crunch:
   (Ben & Jerry's English) 190
   (Edy's/Dreyer's Heath) 120
   bar *(Breyers)* 140
vanilla:
   (Breyers) 130
   (Dannon Fat Free Light) 70
   (Dannon Lowfat Soft) 110
   (Edy's/Dreyer's) 100
   (Edy's/Dreyer's Fat Free) 80
   (Häagen-Dazs) 140
   classic *(TCBY)* 110
   French *(Breyers)* 110
vanilla chocolate swirl *(Edy's/Dreyer's Fat Free)* 80
vanilla, chocolate, and strawberry combination *(Breyers)* 120
vanilla fudge:
   (Häagen-Dazs) 160
   swirl *(Ben & Jerry's No Fat)* 140
   twirl *(Breyers)* 130
   twirl *(Breyers Fat Free)* 110
vanilla raspberry swirl *(Häagen-Dazs)* 130
vanilla raspberry truffle *(Dannon Pure Indulgence)* 150

FROZEN YOGURT BARS & CUP
See also "Yogurt" and "Frozen Yogurt"

calories

bars, 1 piece:
    (Creamsicle) 60
    (Schwan's Push-Ems) 100
    all flavors *(Starburst)* 70
    cherry chocolate chip *(Ben & Jerry's Cherry Garcia)* 260
    chocolate almond *(Frozfruit)* 130
    peach *(Frozfruit)* 100
    and sorbet, see "Ice & Sherbet Bars & Cones," page 356
    strawberry or strawberry-banana *(Frozfruit)* 100
cup, chocolate chip *(Breyers)*, 6 oz. 230

ICE CREAM CONES & CUPS, UNFILLED, one piece

calories

cone:
    (Oreo) 50
    cinnamon *(Teddy Grahams)* .60
    sugar *(Comet)* 50
    waffle *(Comet)* 70
cup *(Comet)* 20

Chapter 22

NUTS, CHIPS, PRETZELS, AND RELATED SNACKS

NUTS & SEEDS,* one ounce, except as noted
See also "Nut Butters" and "Chips, Puffs, & Similar Snacks"

	calories
almonds:	
(Dole)	170
(Planters)	170
honey-roasted *(Planters)*	160
slivered *(Paradise/White Swan)*, ¼ cup, 1.1 oz.	200
slivered *(Planters Gold Measure)*, 2-oz. pkg.	340
tamari-roasted *(Eden)*	170
cashews:	
(Frito-Lay's), 1.5 oz.	270
whole *(Paradise/White Swan)*, ¼ cup, 1.2 oz.	210
honey-roasted *(Planters)*	150
honey-roasted *(Planters)*, 2-oz. pkg.	310
honey-roasted and peanuts *(Planters)*	150
oil-roasted *(Master Choice)*	170
oil-roasted *(Planters)*, 1-oz. pkg.	160
oil-roasted *(Planters)*, 1.5-oz. pkg.	250
oil-roasted *(Planters Fancy)*	170
oil-roasted *(Planters Fancy)*, 2-oz. pkg.	340
oil-roasted *(Planters Halves)*	170
oil-roasted *(Planters Halves Lightly Salted)*	160
oil-roasted *(Planters Munch 'N Go Singles)*, 2-oz. pkg.	330
coquito nuts *(Frieda's)*, 1 oz.	180
macadamia nuts, raw *(Frieda's)*, 1 oz.	196
mixed nuts:	
cashews, with almonds and macadamias *(Planters Select)*	170
cashews, with almonds and pecans *(Planters Select)*	170
dry-roasted *(Planters)*	170

* Shelled, except as noted

honey-roasted *(Planters)* 140
oil-roasted *(Paradise/White Swan)*, ¼ cup, 1.2 oz. 210
oil-roasted *(Planters)* 170
oil-roasted *(Planters* Deluxe/Lightly Salted/Unsalted) 170
oil-roasted, no Brazils *(Planters)*, 3.5-oz. pkg. 170
oil-roasted, no Brazils *(Planters* Lightly Salted) 170
oil-roasted, no peanuts *(Paradise/White Swan* Deluxe),
   ¼ cup, 1.2 oz. 220
sesame, oil-roasted *(Planters)* 150
tamari-roasted *(Eden)* 170
peanuts:
   dry-roasted *(Little Debbie)* 160
   dry-roasted *(Planters)* 160
   dry-roasted *(Planters* Lightly Salted) 170
   dry-roasted *(Planters* Lightly Salted), 1-oz. pkg. 160
   dry-roasted *(Planters* Lightly Salted), 1¾-oz. pkg. 290
   dry-roasted *(Planters* Unsalted) 160
   honey-roasted *(Frito-Lay's)*, ¼ cup 270
   honey-roasted *(Planters)* 160
   honey-roasted *(Smart Snackers)*, .7 oz. 100
   honey-roasted, dry-roasted *(Planters)*, 1.7-oz. pkg. 260
   honey-roasted, oil-roasted *(Planters* Reduced Fat) 130
   hot *(Frito-Lay's)*, ¼ cup 280
   hot and spicy *(Planters Heat)* 160
   hot and spicy *(Planters Heat)*, 1.7-oz. pkg. 290
   hot and spicy *(Planters Heat)*, 2-oz. pkg. 330
   hot and spicy *(Planters Heat Munch 'N Go Singles)*,
      2.5-oz. pkg. 410
   oil-roasted *(Pennant)* 170
   oil-roasted *(Planters)*, 2-oz. bag 340
   oil-roasted *(Planters* Fun Size), 2 bags, 1 oz. 170
   oil-roasted *(Planters* Lightly Salted), 1¾-oz. pkg. 300
   oil-roasted *(Planters* Munch 'N Go) 170
   oil-roasted, cocktail *(Planters/Planters* Lightly Salted/
      Unsalted) 170
   oil-roasted, fancy *(Paradise/White Swan)*, ¼ cup, 1½ oz. . . . 270
   oil-roasted, salted *(Planters)* 170
   oil-roasted, salted *(Planters)*, 1-oz. pkg. 170
   oil-roasted, salted *(Planters)*, 1.7-oz. pkg. 290
   salted *(Frito-Lay's)* 180
   Spanish *(Planters)* 170
   Spanish, raw *(Planters)* 150

Nuts & Seeds, peanuts *(cont.)*
 sweet *(Planters Sweet N Crunchy)* 140
pecans:
 chips *(Planters)*, 2-oz. pkg. 390
 halves *(Planters Gold Measure)*, 2-oz. pkg. 390
 halves or pieces *(Paradise/White Swan)*, ¼ cup, 1 oz. 200
 halves or pieces *(Planters)*, 1 oz. 190
 pieces *(Planters)*, 2-oz. pkg. 390
 honey-roasted *(Planters)*, 1 oz. 180
pine nuts, dried, pignolia *(Krinos)*, .5 oz. 90
pine nuts, dried, pignolia *(Progresso)*, 1 oz. 170
pistachios:
 dried *(Dole)*, 1 oz. 163
 dried *(Sonoma)*, ¼ cup 190
 dried, in shell *(Dole)*, 1 oz. 90
 dry-roasted *(Planters)*, 1 oz. 160
 dry-roasted *(Planters Munch 'N Go Singles)*, 2-oz. pkg. . . . 330
 dry-roasted, in shell *(Planters)*, ½ cup, 1 oz. edible 160
pumpkin seeds, tamari-roasted, spicy *(Eden)* 170
sesame seeds, whole, brown *(Arrowhead Mills)*, ¼ cup 200
sesame seeds, kernels, decorticated *(Arrowhead Mills)*, ¼ cup . . 210
sunflower seeds:
 (Frito-Lay's), ⅓ cup 140
 dried, in shell *(Arrowhead Mills)*, 1 cup, 1.3 oz. edible 180
 dry-roasted, in shell *(Planters)*, ¾ cup, 1 oz. edible 160
 dry-roasted, in shell *(Planters)*, 3-oz. bag, 1.5 oz. edible . . . 240
 dry-roasted, in shell *(Planters Original)*, ¾ cup, 1 oz. edible . 160
 dry-roasted, in shell *(Planters Munch 'N Go)*, .75 oz. edible . 120
 dry-roasted, kernels *(Planters)*, ¼ cup 190
 honey-roasted, kernels *(Planters)*, 1.7 oz. 280
 oil-roasted, kernels *(Planters)*, 1.7 oz. 290
 oil-roasted, kernels *(Planters)*, 2 oz. 340
 oil-roasted, kernels *(Planters Munch 'N Go)*, ¼ cup 200
 barbecued kernels *(Planters)*, 1.7 oz. 290
 barbecued kernels *(Planters Munch 'N Go)*, 3 tbsp. 150
 salted kernels *(Planters)* 170
 tamari-roasted *(Eden)* 170
walnuts, dried:
 (Paradise/Wild Swan), ¼ cup, 1 oz. 190
 black *(Planters)*, 2-oz. pkg. 340
 halves *(Planters)*, ⅓ cup 220

halves *(Planters Gold Measure)*, 2-oz. pkg. 380
pieces *(Planters)*, ¼ cup 190

TRAIL MIX
See also "Fruit Snacks"

	calories
(Eden Fruit & Nuts), 1 oz.	160
(Sonoma), ¼ cup	160
California:	
(Dole), 1.2 oz.	130
(Dole), 2 oz.	220
(Eden Harvest), 1 oz.	130
Hawaiian style *(Dole)*, 1.2 oz.	150
Hawaiian style *(Dole)*, 2 oz.	250
Sierra:	
(Del Monte), .9 oz.	110
(Del Monte), 1 oz.	120
(Del Monte), ¼ cup	150

CHIPS, CRISPS, & SIMILAR SNACKS, one ounce, except as noted
See also, "Crackers," "Nuts & Seeds," "Corn Chips, Puffs, & Similar Snacks," "Popcorn, Popped" and "Pretzels"

	calories
(Zings Chips), 1.8-oz. bag	240
apple cinnamon *(Crunchwells Crumpet Chips)*	110
cheddar *(Old Dutch Multicrisps)*	130
hot and spicy *(Eden* Wasabi), 50 chips, 1.1 oz.	130
mixed *(Terra* Chips)	140
onion:	
(Funyuns)	140
French *(Old Dutch Multicrisps)*	128
french fried *(French's)*, 2 tbsp.	45
pappadum, *see "Crackers," page 44*	
pappadum snack crisps *(Tamarind Tree)*, 30 pieces	140
Parmesan garlic *(Crunchwells Crumpet Chips)*	100
pork rind, ½ oz.:	
(Baken • ets)	80
(Baken • ets Cracklins)	80
(Old Dutch Bac'n Puffs)	80

Chips, Crisps, & Similar Snacks, pork rind *(cont.)*
 hot and spicy *(Baken • ets)* 70
 hot and spicy *(Baken • ets Cracklins)* 80
potato chips and crisps:
 (Barbara's Regular/Ripple/No Salt) 150
 (Barrel O'Fun/Barrel O'Fun Ripple) 150
 (Kettle Chips) 150
 (Kettle Crisps) 110
 (Lay's/Lay's Unsalted) 150
 (Mr. Phipps Crisps) 120
 (Munchos) 150
 (No Fries Original) 110
 (Old Dutch/Old Dutch Ripl) 150
 (Pringles Original) 160
 (Pringles Original Ridges) 150
 (Ridgies Flat/Curlie/Super Crispy) 150
 (Ruffles Reduced Fat) 140
 (Wise Ripple) 150
 all varieties *(Lay's Baked)* 110
 all varieties *(Lay's Wavy)* 160
 all varieties *(Pringles Right)* 140
 all varieties, except cheddar and sour cream *(Ruffles)* 150
 barbecue *(Barbara's)* 160
 barbecue *(Barrel O'Fun)* 145
 barbecue *(Lay's Hickory/Lay's KC Masterpiece)* 150
 barbecue *(Mr. Phipps Crisps)* 130
 barbecue *(Munchos)* 160
 barbecue *(No Fries)* 110
 barbecue *(Old Dutch/Old Dutch Ripl)* 150
 barbecue, honey *(Kettle Crisps)* 110
 barbecue, mesquite *(Krunchers!)* 140
 barbecue, mesquite *(Old Dutch Kettle)* 130
 barbecue, mesquite *(Pringles)* 150
 Caribbean flavor *(Borden Calypso)* 160
 cheddar *(Health Valley Puffs)* 110
 cheddar, New York, with herbs *(Kettle Chips)* 150
 cheddar and sour cream *(Barrel O'Fun Ripple)* 150
 cheddar and sour cream *(Old Dutch)* 160
 cheddar and sour cream *(Old Dutch Ripl)* 150
 cheddar and sour cream *(Pringles)* 150
 cheddar and sour cream *(Ruffles)* 160
 cheddar and sour cream *(Wise)* 150

cheddar and sour cream *(Wise* Super Crispy) 160
cheese *(Pringles Cheez Ums)* 150
dill pickle *(Old Dutch)* 140
honey Dijon *(Kettle* Chips) 150
hot *(Barrel O'Fun)* 150
hot *(Lay's* Flamin') 150
jalapeño *(Krunchers!)* 140
jalapeño, jack *(Kettle* Chips) 140
jalapeño, and cheddar *(Old Dutch)* 130
onion, French *(Old Dutch Ripl)* 150
onion and garlic *(Barrel O'Fun)* 140
onion and garlic *(Borden)* 150
onion and garlic *(Lay's)* 150
onion and garlic *(Old Dutch)* 140
pesto *(Kettle* Crisps) 110
ranch *(Pringles)* 150
ranch, puffs *(Health Valley)* 110
salsa, and cheese *(Lay's)* 160
salsa, with mesquite *(Kettle* Chips) 140
salt and sour *(Barrel O'Fun)* 150
salt and vinegar *(Borden)* 150
salt and vinegar *(Kettle* Chips) 150
salt and vinegar *(Lay's)* 160
salt and vinegar *(Old Dutch)* 130
sour cream and onion *(Barrel O'Fun)* 150
sour cream and onion *(Borden)* 150
sour cream and onion *(Golden Ridges)* 150
sour cream and onion *(Lay's)* 160
sour cream and onion *(Mr. Phipps* Crisps) 130
sour cream and onion *(Old Dutch)* 150
sour cream and onion *(Pringles)* 160
sour cream and onion *(Ruffles* Reduced Fat) 130
yogurt and green onion *(Barbara's/Barbara's* No Salt) 150
yogurt and green onion *(Kettle* Chips) 150
potato sticks:
   (Butterfield), ⅔ cup 150
   (Butterfield), 1.7 oz. 250
   (French's), ¾ cup 180
   (French's), 1 cup 250
   (Pik-Nik Fabulous Fries) 150
   hot *(Chester's* Fries Flamin') 140
   ketchup *(Pik-Nik* Ket-'n Fries), ⅔ cup 160

Chips, Crisps, & Similar Snacks, potato sticks *(cont.)*

shoestring *(Pik-Nik)*, ⅔ cup 160
shoestring *(Pik-Nik)*, 1.75-oz. can 280
shoestring *(Pik-Nik Less Salt)*, ¾ cup, 1.1 oz. 165
shoestring, BBQ or sour cream and cheddar *(Pik-Nik)*,
    ⅔ cup 180
raspberry *(Crunchwells Crumpet Chips)* 110
rice, brown, chips *(Eden)*, 50 chips, 1.1 oz. 150
rice puffs, five flavors *(Eden Arare)*, 30 puffs, 1.1 oz. 110
sea vegetable chips *(Eden)*, 50 chips, 1.1 oz. 140
snack mix:
    (Cheez-It), ½ cup 140
    (Chex Mix), ⅔ cup 130
    (Chex Mix Bold n' Zesty), ½ cup 150
    (Old Dutch Party Mix), ⅔ cup 150
    (Pepperidge Farm Light Season), ½ cup 170
    (Pepperidge Farm Goldfish), ½ cup 170
    cheddar *(Chex Mix)*, ⅔ cup 140
    cheddar, zesty *(Pepperidge Farm Goldfish)*, ½ cup 180
    honey mustard and onion *(Pepperidge Farm)*, ½ cup 180
    nutty, extra *(Pepperidge Farm)*, ½ cup 180
spicy barbecue *(Crunchwells Crumpet Chips)* 100
sweet potato chips, plain or cinnamon *(Terra Chips)*, 1 oz. . . 140
taro chips, spiced *(Terra)*, 1 oz. 130
vegetable chips *(Eden)*, 50 chips, 1.1 oz. 130

CORN CHIPS, PUFFS, & SIMILAR SNACKS, one ounce, except
as noted
*See also "Crackers," "Chips, Crisps, & Similar Snacks,"
"Popcorn, Popped," and "Pretzels"*

---

                                                    calories
(Baked Bugles), 1½ cups 130
(Baked Bugles Single), 1 bag 170
(Barbara's Pinta Chips) 130
(Barrel O'Fun Chip), 1.1 oz. 160
(Bugles), 1⅓ cups 160
(Bugles Single), 1½-oz. bag 230
(Dipsy Doodles) 160
(Fritos King Size/Original/Wild N' Mild) 160
(Fritos Scoops) 150
(Old Dutch Chips), 1.1 oz. 170

(Old Dutch Chips), 1¼-oz. bag 200
(Old Dutch Puffcorn Curls), 1.1 oz. 180
(Planters Chips) 160
all varieties *(Sunchips)* 140
barbecue:
   (Fritos) 150
   (Old Dutch), 1.1 oz. 165
   (Old Dutch), 1¼-oz. bag 190
   (Smart Snackers Curls), ½ oz. 60
blue corn:
   (Barbara's), 1.1 oz. 140
   (Barbara's Pinta Blues) 130
   light salt *(Barbara's* Amazing Bakes) 100
   picante *(Barbara's* Pinta) 130
   salsa *(Barbara's* Pinta) 130
caramel coated *(Old Dutch* Puffcorn) 120
cheese:
   (Cheese Doodles) 150
   (Chee•tos Cheesy Checkers/Crunchy) 150
   cheddar *(Baked Bugles),* 1½ cups 130
   chili, with corn shell *(Combos)* 140
   fried *(Cheese Doodles)* 150
   hot *(Chee•tos* Flamin' Hot) 160
   nacho *(Barbara's* Pinta) 130
   nacho *(Bugles),* 1⅓ cups 160
   nacho *(Combos)* 130
   nacho *(Combos),* 1.7-oz. bag 230
   nacho *(Doodle Twisters)* 160
cheese balls:
   (Barrel O'Fun), 1.1 oz. 160
   (Planters Cheez) 150
   (Planters Cheez), 1-oz. bag 150
   puffed *(Chee•tos)* 160
cheese curls:
   (Barrel O'Fun Baked), 1.1 oz. 160
   (Barrel O'Fun Crunchy), 1.1 oz. 160
   (Chee•tos) 150
   (Old Dutch Crunchy) 130
   (Planters Cheez) 150
   (Planters Cheez), 1¼-oz. pkg. 190
   (Smart Snackers), ½ oz. 70

Corn Chips, Puffs, & Similar Snacks *(cont.)*
cheese puffs:
   (Barbara's Bakes) 160
   (Barbara's Original) 150
   (Barrel O'Fun Light), 1.1 oz. 125
   (Chee•tos) 160
   cheddar *(No Fries)* 110
   cheddar, New York *(Barbara's* Less Fat) 140
   jalapeño *(Barbara's)* 150
   Monterey Jack and green chili *(Barbara's* Less Fat) 140
cheese twists, cheddar *(Jax),* 25 pieces, 1.1 oz. 150
chili cheese *(Fritos)* 160
onion flavor rings *(Borden),* 1-oz. bag 140
pepperoni pizza *(Combos)* 140
pepperoni pizza *(Combos),* 1.7-oz. bag 240
pizza curls *(Smart Snackers),* ½ oz. 60
ranch:
   (Bugles), 1⅓ cups 160
   (Smart Snackers), ½ oz. 60
   puffs *(No Fries)* 110
sour cream and onion *(Bugles),* 1⅓ cups 160
taco *(Taco Bell* Supreme) 140
Texas grill *(Fritos* Honey BBQ/Sizzlin' Fajita) 150
tortilla:
   (Bachman Original), 1.1 oz. 150
   (Mesa) 150
   (Nachips) 150
   (No Fries Natural) 100
   (Old Dutch Restaurant) 140
   (Santitas Chips/Strips) 140
   (Tostitos Baked/Baked Unsalted) 110
   (Tostitos Bite Size) 140
   (Tostitos Crispy Round) 150
   (Tostitos Restaurant) 130
   (Tostitos Restaurant Unsalted/Santa Fe Gold) 140
   (Tyson), 1.2 oz. 170
   (Tyson Yellow Corn), 1.1 oz. 150
   all varieties *(Doritos)* 140
   all varieties *(Doritos* Reduced Fat) 130
   black bean salsa *(Chipitos),* 1.1 oz. 150
   blue corn *(Barbara's* Less Fat) 120
   blue corn *(Kettle* Tias) 140

blue corn, hot salsa *(Barbara's* Less Fat) 120
crisps *(Mr. Phipps)* 130
crisps *(Pepperidge Farm)*, 1.1 oz. 130
5 grain *(Kettle* Tias) 140
lime and chili *(Kettle* Tias) 140
lime and chili *(Tostitos)* 150
ranch *(No Fries)*, 1.1 oz. 110
ranch *(Tostitos* Baked) 120
salsa crisps *(Pepperidge Farm)*, 1.1 oz. 130
salsa and sour cream *(No Fries)*, 1.1 oz. 110
tomato basil *(Kettle* Tias) 140
tostados *(Old Dutch)*, 1.1 oz. 150
white corn *(Barbara's* Less Fat) 120
white corn *(Chipitos* Restaurant Style) 130
white corn *(Durangos)*, 1.1 oz. 150
white corn *(Kettle* Tias) 140
white corn *(Old Dutch)*, 1.1 oz. 150
white corn *(Old El Paso)* 140
white corn *(Santitas* 100%) 140
white corn, ranch *(Barbara's* Less Fat) 120
tortilla, cheese:
cheddar, white *(Barbara's* Less Fat) 120
cheddar jalapeño *(No Fries* Blue Corn), 1.1 oz. 110
chili crisps *(Pepperidge Farm)*, 1.1 oz. 130
nacho *(Barrel O'Fun)* 130
nacho *(Borden)* 150
nacho *(Old Dutch)*, 1-oz. bag 140
nacho *(Old Dutch)*, 1.1 oz. 155
nacho *(Old Dutch)*, 2¼-oz. bag 320
nacho *(Tyson)* 140
nacho, crisps *(Mr. Phipps)* 130
tortilla, flour:
cheese and salsa *(Barrel O'Fun)* 140
nacho *(Barrel O'Fun)* 140
white *(Barrel O'Fun)* 140
white, mini rounds *(Barrel O'Fun)* 150
yellow *(Barrel O'Fun* Tostada) 130
yellow, mini *(Barrel O'Fun* Tostada) 140

POPCORN, UNPOPPED, 2 tablespoons, except as noted
See also "Popcorn, Popped"

---

	calories
(Arrowhead Mills), ¼ cup, 1¾ oz.	180
(Orville Redenbacher Original/White)	90
hot air *(Orville Redenbacher)*	90
microwave:	
(Orville Redenbacher)	120
(Rudenbudders Movie Theater)	180
(Rudenbudders Movie Theater Light)	115
(Smart Pop)	100
(Smart Snackers), 1 oz.	100
butter *(Orville Redenbacher)*	170
butter *(Orville Redenbacher* Light)	120
butter *(Pop•Secret)*, 3 tbsp.	180
butter *(Pop•Secret* Jumbo Pop), 3 tbsp.	170
butter *(Pop•Secret Movie Theater)*, 3 tbsp.	170
butter *(Pop•Secret Movie Theater* Jumbo Pop), 3 tbsp.	170
butter *(Pop•Secret* Single Serving), ¼ cup	230
butter *(Schwan's)*, 3 tbsp.	180
butter, light *(Pop•Secret)*, 3 tbsp.	140
butter, light *(Pop•Secret Movie Theater)*, ¼ cup	160
butter, light *(Pop•Secret* Single Serving), ¼ cup	230
butter, 94% fat free *(Pop•Secret)*, 3 tbsp.	120
butter, real *(Pop•Secret)*, 3 tbsp.	180
caramel *(Orville Redenbacher)*	180
cheddar *(Orville Redenbacher)*	140
cheese, cheddar or nacho *(Pop•Secret)*, 3 tbsp.	180
herb and garlic *(Rudenbudders)*	180
light *(Schwan's* Light), 3 tbsp.	130
natural *(Orville Redenbacher)*	160
natural *(Pop•Secret)*, 3 tbsp.	170
natural, light *(Pop•Secret)*, 3 tbsp.	140
natural, 94% fat free *(Pop•Secret)*, 3 tbsp.	120
zesty *(Rudenbudders)*	180

POPCORN, POPPED
See also "Chips, Crisps, & Similar Snacks," "Corn Chips,
Puffs, & Similar Snacks," and "Popcorn, Unpopped"

	calories
(Barrel O'Fun Canola), 3 cups	145
(Barrel O'Fun Light), 3 cups	110
(Chester's Triple Mix), 1½ cups	140
(Wise Choice), 2½ cups	140
air-popped:	
(Bachman), 2¾ cups	170
(Bachman Lite), 5 cups	120
white or yellow *(Jolly Time)*, 5 cups	100
butter/butter flavor:	
(Borden), 1-oz. bag	150
(Chester's), 3 cups	160
(Smart Snackers), .66 oz.	90
(Smartfood), 3 cups	150
(Smartfood Reduced Fat), 3⅓ cups	130
(Wise Reduced Fat), 3 cups	130
caramel:	
(Barrel O'Fun Fat Free), ¾ cup	120
(Chester's), ¾ cup	130
(Cracker Jack Fat Free), 1 cup, 1 oz.	110
(Smart Snackers), .9 oz.	100
(Wise Fat Free), 1 cup	110
caramel, with peanuts:	
(Barrel O'Fun), ⅔ cup	130
(Cracker Jack), ⅔ cup	120
(Cracker Jack), 1.25-oz. box	150
(Old Dutch), 1 oz.	128
cheddar, white:	
(Barrel O'Fun), 3 cups	185
(Chester's), 3 cups	190
(Smart Snackers), .66 oz.	90
(Smartfood), 2 cups	190
(Smartfood Reduced Fat), 3 cups	140
cheese *(Barrel O'Fun)*, 2½ cups	135
cheese *(Barrel O'Fun* Low Fat), 2½ cups	140
microwave:	
(Jolly Time), 4 cups	160
(Jolly Time Light), 4 cups	100

Popcorn, Popped, microwave *(cont.)*

   butter *(Schwan's)*, 1 cup 35
   cheese, cheddar or nacho *(Pop•Secret)*, 1 cup 30
   cheese, cheddar or nacho *(Pop•Secret)*, 5 cups 150
   light *(Schwan's Light)*, 1 cup 20
   natural *(Pop•Secret)*, 1 cup 35
   natural *(Pop•Secret)*, 4 cups 150
   natural, light *(Pop•Secret)*, 1 cup 25
   natural, light *(Pop•Secret)*, 6 cups 130
   natural, 94% fat free *(Pop•Secret)*, 1 cup 20
   natural, 94% fat free *(Pop•Secret)*, 6 cups 110
microwave, butter flavor:
   (Chester's), 5 cups 200
   (Jolly Time), 4 cups 140
   (Jolly Time Light), 4 cups 80
   (Pop•Secret), 1 cup 35
   (Pop•Secret), 4 cups 150
   (Pop•Secret Jumbo Pop), 1 cup 40
   (Pop•Secret Single Serving), 1 cup 30
   (Pop•Secret Movie Theater), 1 cup 40
   (Pop•Secret Movie Theater Jumbo Pop), 1 cup 40
   light *(Pop•Secret)*, 1 cup 25
   light *(Pop•Secret)*, 6 cups 130
   light *(Pop•Secret Single Serving)*, 1 cup 25
   light *(Pop•Secret Movie Theater)*, 1 cup 25
   light *(Pop•Secret Movie Theater)*, 6 cups 130
   94% fat free *(Pop•Secret)*, 1 cup 20
   94% fat free *(Pop•Secret)*, 6 cups 110
   real *(Pop•Secret)*, 1 cup 35
toffee, butter:
   (Cracker Jack Fat Free), 1 cup, 1 oz. 110
   (Smart Snackers), .9 oz. 110
   (Wise Fat Free), 1 cup 110
   with peanuts *(Cracker Jack)*, 1.25-oz. box 160
   with pecans and almonds *(Cracker Jack)*, 1 oz. 130
toffee crunch *(Smartfood)*, ¾ cup 130
toffee, with nuts *(Franklin)*, ⅔ cup 140

PRETZELS
See also "Chips, Crisps, & Similar Snacks" and "Corn Chips, Puffs, & Similar Snacks"

	calories
(Bachman Thin 'n Right), 12 pieces	120
(Barbara's Honeysweet), 1 oz.	100
(Barrel O'Fun Minis), 1 oz.	105
(Borden Thins/Tiny Thins/Mini/Ultra Thins), 1 oz.	100
(Little Debbie), 1.2 oz.	140
(Mister Salty Mini), 1 oz.	110
(Old Dutch), 1⅛-oz. bag	125
(Pepperidge Farm Goldfish), 45 pieces, 1.1 oz.	120
(Quinlan Beer), 2 pieces, 1 oz.	110
(Quinlan Nuggets), 1.1-oz. bag	130
(Quinlan Party Thins/Sticks), 1 oz.	110
(Quinlan Thin), 1.5-oz. bag	160
(Quinlan Tiny Thins/Mini), 1-oz. bag	110
(Quinlan Ultra Thin), 8 pieces, 1 oz.	110
bagel shaped *(Manischewitz),* 4 pieces, 1 oz.	110
Bavarian *(Barbara's/Barbara's No Salt),* 1 oz.	100
Bavarian *(Rold Gold),* 1 oz.	110
cheese:	
(Handi-Snacks), 1.1-oz. piece	110
cheddar *(Combos),* 1.8-oz. bag	240
cheddar or nacho *(Combos),* 1 oz.	130
nacho *(Combos),* 1.8-oz. bag	230
chips, 1 oz.:	
(Mr. Phipps/Mr. Phipps Lower Sodium), 1 oz.	120
(Mr. Phipps Fat Free), 1 oz.	100
(Mister Salty), 1 oz.	110
(Mister Salty Fat Free), 1 oz.	100
Dutch *(Mister Salty),* 2 pieces, 1.1 oz.	120
honey mustard–onion *(Old Dutch),* 1.1 oz.	140
honey mustard–onion *(Old Dutch),* 2-oz. bag	260
mini *(Barbara's/Barbara's No Salt),* 1 oz.	100
9-grain *(Barbara's),* 1 oz.	100
nuggets *(Bachman Nutzels),* ½ cup, 1 oz.	110
oat bran nuggets *(Smart Snackers),* 1.5 oz.	170
pizza *(Combos Pizzeria),* 1 oz.	130
pizza *(Combos Pizzeria),* 1.8-oz. bag	230

Pretzels *(cont.)*
rods:
   (Bachman), 2 pieces 110
   (Old Dutch), 3 pieces, 1.2 oz. 130
   (Rold Gold), 3 pieces 110
soft:
   (Superpretzel/Superpretzel Added Salt), 2.3-oz. piece 170
   bites *(Superpretzel/Superpretzel* Added Salt), 4 pieces,
      1½ oz. 110
   cheese-filled, cheddar, nacho or pizza
      (Superpretzel Softstix), 2 pieces, 1.8 oz. 140
   cheese-filled, frozen *(Schwan's),* 3 pieces 210
   cinnamon raisin *(Superpretzel),* 2 pieces, 2 oz. 190
   peanut butter and jelly–filled, frozen *(Schwan's),* 3 pieces . . 240
sourdough:
   (Quinlan/Quinlan No Salt), 1 piece 80
   Bavarian or twists *(Barbara's),* 1.1 oz. 110
   hard *(Bachman),* 1 piece 90
   hard *(Rold Gold),* 1 oz. 110
sticks, 1 oz.:
   (Bachman Stix) 100
   (Mister Salty Fat Free) 110
   (Old Dutch) 110
   (Quinlan) 100
   (Rold Gold Fat Free) 110
sticks, sesame *(Barbara's),* 1.1 oz. 110
thins:
   (Bachman Fat Free), 11 pieces 110
   (Old Dutch Fat Free), 1.1 oz. 110
   (Quinlan), 1 oz. 120
   (Rold Gold/Rold Gold Fat Free), 1 oz. 110
twists:
   (Bachman/Bachman Butter), 5 pieces 110
   (Old Dutch), 1 oz. 110
   (Mister Salty), 1 oz. 110
   (Planters), 1 oz. 100
   (Planters), 1½-oz. bag 160
   tiny *(Rold Gold* Fat Free), 1 oz. 100

GRANOLA & SNACK BARS, one bar, except as noted
*See also "Toaster Muffins & Pastries" and "Rice & Grain
Cakes"*

                                                              calories

cereal/granola bars:
  (Health Valley Scones) 180
  (Kudos M&M's) 90
  (Kudos Snickers) 100
  (Rice Krispies Treats) 90
  all varieties *(Grandma's)* 160
  all varieties *(Health Valley Fat Free Granola)* 140
  all varieties *(Health Valley Healthy Breakfast Bakes* Fat
    Free*)* 110
  all varieties *(Health Valley Healthy Cereal Bars No Fat)* 100
  all varieties *(Health Valley Healthy Energy Bars)* 180
  all varieties *(Kellogg's Low Fat)* 80
  all varieties *(Nature Valley)*, 2 bars 200
  all varieties *(Nature Valley Low Fat)* 110
  all varieties *(Nature's Choice Fat Free Granola)* 90
  all varieties *(Nature's Choice Real Fruit)*, 2 bars 100
  all varieties *(Nutri•Grain)* 140
  all varieties *(Quaker Chewy Lowfat)* 110
  with almonds, chewy *(Little Debbie)* 200
  apple, blueberry, or peach filled *(Nature's Choice Fat Free
    Cereal)* 110
  carob chip *(Nature's Choice Granola)* 80
  chocolate chip *(Carnation Chewy)* 150
  chocolate chip *(Little Debbie)* 220
  chocolate chip *(Nature's Choice Grrr-Nola Treats)* 80
  chocolate chip *(Quaker Chewy)* 120
  chocolate chip *(Rice Krispies)* 120
  chocolate chip or fudge *(Kudos Enrobed)* 120
  chocolate chunk *(Carnation Granola)* 140
  cinnamon and oats *(Barbara's Granola)* 260
  cinnamon raisin *(Nature's Choice Granola)* 80
  coconut almond *(Barbara's Granola)* 290
  cranberry, raspberry, or strawberry filled *(Nature's Choice
    Fat Free Cereal)* 110
  fudge dipped, macaroon *(Little Debbie)* 280
  fudge dipped, with peanuts *(Little Debbie)* 270
  oats and honey *(Carnation Granola)* 130

Granola & Snack Bars, cereal/granola bars *(cont.)*
   oats and honey *(Little Debbie)* 210
   oats and honey *(Nature's Choice Granola)* 80
   oatmeal raisin *(Little Debbie)* 160
   oatmeal raisin *(Sweet Success)* 120
   peanut butter *(Barbara's* Granola) 260
   peanut butter *(Kudos* Enrobed) 130
   peanut butter *(Nature's Choice* Granola) 80
   peanut butter chocolate chip *(Carnation* Chewy) 150
   peanut butter chocolate chip *(Quaker Chewy)* 120
   peanut butter and jelly *(Nature's Choice Grrr-Nola)* 80
   popcorn bar, caramel or chocolate *(Pop•Secret)* 70
snack bars:
   (Little Debbie Star Crunch) 280
   all flavors *(Figurines* Diet Bars), 2 bars 220
   blueberry *(Little Debbie Fruit Boosters)* 190
   blueberry *(Sweet Rewards)* 120
   brownie *(Sweet Rewards)* 100
   brownie or chocolate chip *(Sweet Success* Chewy) 120
   chocolate raspberry or peanut butter *(Sweet Success
     Chewy)* 120
   fig *(Little Debbie Figaroos)* 180
   fudge, double *(Sweet Rewards)* 100
   raspberry *(Sweet Rewards)* 120
   strawberry *(Little Debbie Fruit Boosters)* 190
   strawberry *(Sweet Rewards)* 120

Chapter 23

COCOA, COFFEE, SOFT DRINKS, COOLERS, AND MIXERS

COCOA & FLAVORED MIXES, one packet, except as noted
See also "Flavored Milk Beverages"

	calories
all flavors *(Pillsbury* Instant Breakfast)	140
all flavors *(Pillsbury* Instant Breakfast), 1 cup*	220
banana flavor *(Nestlé Quik),* 2 tbsp.	90
chocolate flavor:	
(Nestlé Quik), 2 tbsp.	90
(Nestlé Quik No Sugar), 2 tbsp.	40
all flavors *(Sweet Success)*	90
creamy milk or classic malt *(Carnation Instant Breakfast)*	130
creamy milk or malt *(Carnation Instant Breakfast* No Sugar)	70
fudge shake *(Weight Watchers)*	80
cocoa, powder, 1 tbsp., except as noted:	
sweetened *(Ghirardelli),* 2½ tbsp.	80
unsweetened *(Ghirardelli)*	35
unsweetened *(Hershey's)*	20
unsweetened *(Nestlé* Baking)	15
cocoa mix:	
(Carnation Fat Free)	25
(Carnation No Sugar)	50
(Carnation 70)	70
(Swiss Miss)	140
(Swiss Miss Diet)	20
(Swiss Miss Fat Free)	50
(Swiss Miss Lite)	70
(Swiss Miss Sugar Free), ¼ cup	70
(Weight Watchers)	70
almond mocha *(Swiss Miss* Premiere)	140
chocolate *(Swiss Miss* Sensations)	150

* Prepared with skim milk

Cocoa & Flavored Mixes, cocoa mix *(cont.)*

chocolate, all varieties *(Land O' Lakes)* 160
chocolate, double *(Ghirardelli)* 90
chocolate, hazelnut or mocha *(Ghirardelli)* 90
chocolate, Irish creme or Swiss truffle *(Nestlé)*, 3 tbsp.   . . .90
chocolate, milk *(Carnation)*, 3 tbsp. 110
chocolate, milk *(Swiss Miss)* 110
chocolate, milk *(Swiss Miss* Sugar Free) 50
chocolate raspberry truffle *(Swiss Miss* Premiere) 140
chocolate, rich *(Carnation)*, 3 tbsp. 110
chocolate, rich *(Swiss Miss)* 110
chocolate, rich, with marshmallow *(Carnation)*, 3 tbsp. . . . 110
chocolate, rich, with or without marshmallow *(Nestlé)* 110
chocolate, Suisse truffle or English toffee *(Swiss Miss*
  Premiere) 140
chocolate, white *(Ghirardelli)*, 2 tbsp. 90
chocolate, white *(Swiss Miss)* 110
and cream *(Swiss Miss)* 150
Irish cream *(Land O' Lakes)* 150
mini-marshmallow *(Swiss Miss)* 110
mini-marshmallow *(Swiss Miss* No Sugar) 50
malted milk powder, 3 tbsp.:
  natural *(Kraft)* 80
  natural *(Nestlé* Original) .90
  chocolate *(Kraft)* 90
  chocolate *(Nestlé)* 90
strawberry flavor, powder:
  (Nestlé Quik), 2 tbsp. 90
  creme *(Carnation Instant Breakfast)* 130
  creme *(Carnation Instant Breakfast* No Sugar) 70
vanilla flavor, mix:
  creamy *(Sweet Success)* .90
  French *(Carnation Instant Breakfast)* 130
  French *(Carnation Instant Breakfast* No Sugar) 70

COFFEE, DRY & MIXES, eight fluid ounces*, except as noted
See also "Coffee, Canned or Bottled"

---

                                                                  calories

flavored:
   café Amaretto *(General Foods International)* 60
   café Français *(General Foods International)* 60
   café Vienna *(General Foods International)* 70
   cappuccino *(Nestlé* Instant), 1 pkt. 80
   cappuccino, cinnamon or coffee *(Maxwell House)* 90
   cappuccino, Italian *(General Foods International)* 50
   cappuccino, mocha *(Maxwell House)* 100
   cappuccino, mocha *(Nestlé)*, 1 pkt. 110
   cappuccino, orange *(General Foods International)* 70
   cappuccino, vanilla *(Maxwell House)* 90
   chocolate, Viennese *(General Foods International)* 60
   hazelnut, Belgian *(General Foods International)* 70
   Kahlua Cafe (General Foods International) 60
   mocha, café *(Carnation Instant Breakfast)* 130
   mocha, Suisse *(General Foods International)* 60
   vanilla, French *(General Foods International)* 60
coffee substitute (cereal grain beverage):
   (Natural Touch Kaffree Roma) 10
   (Natural Touch Roma Cappuccino), 3 tbsp. 50
   regular or coffee flavor *(Postum* Instant), 1 tsp. 10

COFFEE, CANNED OR BOTTLED
See also "Coffee, Dry & Mixes"

---

                                                                  calories

(Jamaican Gold), 11 oz. 140
cappuccino, iced:
   (Jamaican Gold), 11 oz. 145
   coffee *(Maxwell House Cappio)*, 8 fl. oz. 130
   mocha or vanilla *(Maxwell House Cappio)*, 8 fl. oz. 140
latte *(Jamaican Gold)*, 11 oz. 140

---

* *Prepared according to package directions*

TEA, BOTTLED & MIXES

---

calories

flavored, lemon, instant *(Lipton)*, 1 tsp. 0
iced, 8 fl. oz., except as noted:
   (Schweppes) 90
   (Snapple) 70
   (Veryfine Chillers) 80
   all fruit flavors *(Apple & Eve)* 100
   all fruit flavors *(Lipton* Chilled) 80
   all fruit flavors, herbal *(R.W. Knudsen* Coolers) 90
   lemon *(Tropicana)* 100
   lemon *(Veryfine* Chillers) 90
   lemon, peach, raspberry, or strawberry *(Snapple)* 100
   mango or passion fruit *(Snapple)* 110
   mint *(Snapple)* 120
   peach or raspberry *(Snapple)*, 11.5 fl. oz. 150
   peach or raspberry *(Tropicana)*, 11.5 fl. oz. 160
   peach-kiwi *(Veryfine* Chillers) 80
   raspberry *(Veryfine* Chillers) 100
iced, mix, lemon flavor *(Lipton)*, 1²/₃ tbsp. 90
iced, mix, without lemon *(Lipton)*, 1²/₃ tbsp. 80

SOFT DRINKS, 12 fl. oz., except as noted
*See also "Fruit & Fruit-Flavored Drinks," "Sports Drinks," and
"Cocktail Mixers, Nonalcoholic"*

---

calories

all varieties *(R.W. Knudsen Fruit TeaZer)* 110
all varieties, sparkling *(Santa Cruz)* 150
apple:
   (R.W. Knudsen Spritzer) 160
   (Welch's Sparkling) 200
   spiced *(Natural Brew)* 170
Amaretto almond *(After the Fall* Spritzer) 150
berry *(After the Fall* Berrymeister Spritzer) 160
birch beer *(Canada Dry)*, 8 fl. oz. 110
boysenberry *(R.W. Knudsen* Spritzer) 160
café mocha *(Natural Brew)* 150
(Canada Dry Hi-Spot/Canada Dry Cactus Cooler)*, 8 fl. oz. 110
cappuccino, iced, *see "Coffee, Canned & Bottled," page 381*

cherry:
    (After the Fall American Pie Spritzer) 150
    (Crush) 200
    (Sundrop) 180
    (Sunkist), 8 fl. oz. 140
    Amaretto *(Natural Brew)* 160
    black *(After the Fall* Spritzer) 170
    black *(Canada Dry)*, 8 fl. oz. 130
    black *(R.W. Knudsen* Spritzer) 170
    black *(Shasta)* 170
    French *(Snapple)*, 8 fl. oz. 120
    spice *(Slice)* 150
    wild *(Canada Dry)*, 8 fl. oz. 110
cherry-lime:
    (Slice) 160
    (Spree) 170
    rickey *(Snapple)*, 8 fl. oz. 110
chocolate drink, *see "Flavored Milk Beverages," page 50*
citrus *(Canada Dry* Half & Half), 8 fl. oz. 110
citrus *(Sunkist)*, 8 fl. oz. 100
club soda:
    (Canada Dry) 0
    (Schweppes) 0
    (Shasta) 0
cola:
    (Canada Dry Jamaica), 8 fl. oz. 110
    (Coca-Cola Classic), 8 fl. oz. 100
    (Juice Fizz Cooler), 8 fl. oz. 110
    (Pepsi/Pepsi Caffeine Free) 150
    (Shasta) 170
    (Shasta), 8 fl. oz. 110
    (Slice) 160
    (Spree) 170
cola, cherry:
    (R.W. Knudsen Spritzer) 170
    (Shasta) 160
    wild *(Pepsi)* 160
cola, ginseng *(Natural Brew)* 170
collins mixer *(Canada Dry)*, 8 fl. oz. 100
collins mixer *(Schweppes)*, 8 fl. oz. 100
cranberry:
    (After the Fall Tart 'n Sweet Spritzer) 170

Soft Drinks, cranberry *(cont.)*
   (R.W. Knudsen Spritzer) 190
   (Shasta) 180
cran-orange *(After the Fall* Tart 'n Sweet Spritzer) 170
cran-raspberry *(After the Fall* Tart 'n Sweet Spritzer) 160
cream/creme:
   (A&W), 8 fl. oz. 110
   (Hires) 180
   (IBC) 180
   (Mug) 170
   (Shasta) 190
   vanilla *(Canada Dry)*, 8 fl. oz. 120
   vanilla *(Crush)* 180
   vanilla *(Natural Brew)* 170
   vanilla *(R.W. Knudsen* Spritzer) 160
   vanilla *(Snapple)*, 8 fl. oz. 130
(Doc Shasta) 160
(Dr Pepper) 160
(Dr. Slice) 140
fruit punch/blend:
   (Canada Dry Tahitian), 8 fl. oz. 150
   (Juice Fizz), 8 fl. oz. 130
   (Juice Fizz Tropical/Wild Red), 8 fl. oz. 120
   (Shasta) 200
   (Slice) 190
   (Sunkist), 8 fl. oz. 130
   (Welch's Sparkling) 210
   tropical *(Spree)* 170
ginger ale:
   (After the Fall Nantucket) 140
   (Canada Dry), 8 fl. oz. 90
   (Canada Dry Golden), 8 fl. oz. 100
   (Natural Brew Outrageous) 170
   (R.W. Knudsen Spritzer) 160
   (Schweppes), 8 fl. oz. 90
   (Shasta) 130
   (Shasta), 8 fl. oz. 90
   cherry *(Canada Dry)*, 8 fl. oz. 100
   cranberry *(After the Fall)* 140
   cranberry or lemon *(Canada Dry)*, 8 fl. oz. 90
   grape, dry *(Schweppes)*, 8 fl. oz. 100
   raspberry *(After the Fall)* 150

raspberry *(Schweppes)*, 8 fl. oz. 100
ginger beer *(Goya)* 190
ginger beer *(Schweppes)*, 8 fl. oz. 100
grape:
    (After the Fall Concord Spritzer) 180
    (Canada Dry Concord), 8 fl. oz. 120
    (Crush) 200
    (Juice Fizz Purple Thunder), 8 fl. oz. 130
    (R.W. Knudsen Spritzer) 170
    (Schweppes), 8 fl. oz. 130
    (Shasta) 190
    (Slice) 190
    (Welch's Sparkling) 200
grapefruit:
    (Schweppes), 8 fl. oz. 110
    (Shasta Ruby Red) 190
    (Spree) 170
    (Wink), 8 fl. oz. 130
    (Wink Diet), 8 fl. oz. 5
guava passion fruit *(Shasta)* 180
kiwi-lime *(R.W. Knudsen* Spritzer) 160
kiwi-strawberry:
    (After the Fall Spritzer) 170
    (Shasta) 170
    (Snapple), 8 fl. oz. 130
lemon:
    bitter or sour *(Schweppes)*, 8 fl. oz. 110
    sour *(Canada Dry)*, 8 fl. oz. 100
    spicy *(After the Fall* Spritzer) 150
lemonade:
    (Country Time), 8 fl. oz. 120
    (Sunkist), 8 fl. oz. 120
    Jamaican *(R.W. Knudsen* Spritzer) 170
    tangerine, kiwi berry, or raspberry *(Country Time)*, 8 fl. oz. . 110
lemon-lime:
    (Schweppes), 8 fl. oz. 100
    (Slice) 150
    (Spree) 170
    or mandarin-lime *(R.W. Knudsen* Spritzer) 170
lime *(After the Fall* Caribbean Spritzer) 170
lime *(Canada Dry* Island), 8 fl. oz. 140
lime-lemon *(Shasta Twist)* 150

Soft Drinks *(cont.)*

lime-lemon *(Shasta Twist)*, 8 fl. oz. 100
mandarin-lime *(Spree)* 170
mandarin-pineapple *(After the Fall* Spritzer) 150
mango *(After the Fall* Hawaiian Spritzer) 180
mango *(R.W. Knudsen* Fandango Spritzer) 190
mango ginger *(After the Fall* Spritzer) 150
(Mountain Dew/Mountain Dew Caffeine Free) 170
orange:
   (After the Fall Icicle Spritzer) 170
   (After the Fall Zudachi Spritzer) 160
   (Canada Dry Sunripe), 8 fl. oz. 140
   (Crush) 200
   (Orangina), 10 fl. oz. 120
   (Shasta) 200
   (Sunkist), 8 fl. oz. 140
   (Welch's Sparkling) 200
   creme *(Natural Brews)* 160
   mandarin *(Slice)* 190
orange passion fruit *(R.W. Knudsen* Spritzer) 160
passion fruit *(Snapple)*, 8 fl. oz. 120
peach:
   (Canada Dry), 8 fl. oz. 120
   (R.W. Knudsen Spritzer) 160
   (Shasta) 170
   (Snapple Melba), 8 fl. oz. 120
   (Sunkist), 8 fl. oz. 120
   (Welch's Sparkling) 220
peach vanilla *(After the Fall* Spritzer) 170
pear *(Kristian Regale* Swedish Sparkler), 8 fl. oz. 100
pineapple:
   (Canada Dry), 8 fl. oz. 110
   (Crush) 200
   (Shasta) 200
   (Slice) 190
   (Sunkist), 8 fl. oz. 140
   (Welch's Sparkling) 210
pineapple-orange *(Shasta)* 180
raspberry:
   (After the Fall Spritzer) 170
   (Snapple Royal), 8 fl. oz. 120
   cream *(Shasta)* 170

red *(R.W. Knudsen* Spritzer) 170
red *(Shasta)* 170
red *(Slice)* 190
root beer:
   (A&W), 8 fl. oz. 110
   (Hires) 180
   (IBC) 168
   (Mug) 160
   (Natural Brews Draft) 180
   (Shasta) 170
   (Snapple Tru), 8 fl. oz. 110
   (Spree) 170
seltzer, all flavors *(Canada Dry)* 0
seltzer, all flavors *(Schweppes)* 0
(7Up) 160
(7Up Cherry) 160
sour mixer *(Canada Dry),* 8 fl. oz. 90
spritzer, *see specific soda listings*
strawberry:
   (After the Fall Twist O' Spritzer) 150
   (Canada Dry California), 8 fl. oz. 110
   (Crush) 180
   (R.W. Knudsen Spritzer) 170
   (Shasta) 190
   (Slice) 170
   (Sunkist), 8 fl. oz. 140
   (Welch's Sparkling) 200
   strawberry peach *(Shasta)* 170
strawberry vanilla *(After the Fall* Spritzer) 160
(Sundrop) 200
(Surge) 170
tangerine spritzer *(After the Fall)* 170
tangerine spritzer *(R.W. Knudsen)* 170
tea, flavored, *see "Tea, Bottled & Mixes," page 382*
tonic:
   (Canada Dry), 8 fl. oz. 100
   (Schweppes), 8 fl. oz. 90
   (Shasta) 170
   with fruit flavors *(Schweppes),* 8 fl. oz. 90
   with lime *(Canada Dry),* 8 fl. oz. 100
vanilla, *see "cream/creme," above*

Soft Drinks *(cont.)*
vanilla bean *(After the Fall* Spritzer) 170
vichy water *(Canada Dry),* 8 fl. oz. 0

SPORTS DRINKS, all flavors
See also "Fruit & Fruit-Flavored Drinks" and "Soft Drinks"

---

calories

(All Sport), 8 fl. oz. 70
(Body Works), 12 fl. oz. 90
(Recharge), 8 fl. oz. 70

MALT & WINE COOLERS

---

calories

malt coolers, 12 fl. oz.:
    berry *(Bartles & Jaymes)* 210
    black cherry *(Bartles & Jaymes)* 200
    Fuzzy Navel *(Bartles & Jaymes)* 230
    iced tea, Long Island *(Bartles & Jaymes)* 250
    mai tai *(Bartles & Jaymes)* 240
    margarita *(Bartles & Jaymes)* 260
    original *(Bartles & Jaymes)* 190
    piña colada *(Bartles & Jaymes)* 270
    peach *(Bartles & Jaymes)* 210
    sangria, red *(Bartles & Jaymes)* 200
    strawberry *(Bartles & Jaymes)* 210
    strawberry daiquiri *(Bartles & Jaymes)* 220
    tropical *(Bartles & Jaymes)* 230
wine coolers, 12 fl. oz.:
    (Bartles & Jaymes Original) 200
    berry, peach, or strawberry *(Bartles & Jaymes)* 220
    black cherry *(Bartles & Jaymes)* 210
    Fuzzy Navel or Long Island iced tea *(Bartles & Jaymes)* . . . 250
    mai tai *(Bartles & Jaymes)* 250
    margarita *(Bartles & Jaymes)* 270
    piña colada *(Bartles & Jaymes)* 280
    strawberry daiquiri *(Bartles & Jaymes)* 230
    tropical *(Bartles & Jaymes)* 240

COCKTAIL MIXERS, NONALCOHOLIC
See also "Soft Drinks"

calories

Bloody Mary:
- bottled *(Mr & Mrs T)*, 8 fl. oz. 40
- canned *(V-8)*, 11.5 fl. oz. 70
- rich and spicy, bottled *(Mr & Mrs T)*, 8 fl. oz. 50

daiquiri:
- bottled *(Holland House/Mr & Mrs T)*, 4 fl. oz. 150
- instant *(Bar-Tenders)*, 2 pkts., 1.2 oz. 30
- banana, frozen, diluted *(Bacardi)*, 8 fl. oz. 140
- strawberry, bottled *(Holland House)*, 3.5 fl. oz. 150
- strawberry or peach, frozen, diluted *(Bacardi)*, 8 fl. oz. . . . 120

grenadine *(Mr & Mrs T)* 80
grenadine *(Rose's)* 90
mai tai, bottled *(Mr & Mrs T)*, 4.5 fl. oz. 140
Manhattan, bottled *(Holland House/Mr & Mrs T)*, 2 fl. oz.   . . .60

margarita:
- bottled *(Holland House/Mr & Mrs T)*, 4 fl. oz. 130
- frozen, diluted *(Bacardi)*, 8 fl. oz. 90
- instant *(Bar-Tenders)*, 2 pkts., .9 oz. 90
- strawberry, bottled *(Holland House/Mr & Mrs T)*, 3.5 fl. oz. . 150

old-fashioned, bottled *(Holland House)*, 2 fl. oz. 80

piña colada:
- bottled *(Holland House/Mr & Mrs T)*, 4.5 fl. oz. 180
- canned *(Goya)*, 1/3 cup 120
- frozen, diluted *(Bacardi)*, 8 fl. oz. 170
- instant *(Bar-Tenders)*, 1.2-oz. pkt. 140

rum runner, raspberry, frozen, diluted *(Bacardi)*, 8 fl. oz. . . . 120
sweet and sour *(Holland House/Mr & Mrs T)*, 4 fl. oz. 100
Tom Collins, bottled *(Holland House)*, 3 fl. oz. 160
vodka sour, instant *(Bar-Tenders)*, 2 pouches, 1.1 oz. 110

whiskey sour:
- bottled *(Holland House)*, 4 fl. oz. 150
- bottled *(Mr & Mrs T)*, 4 fl. oz. 100
- instant *(Bar-Tenders)*, 2 pkts. 130
- instant *(Bar-Tenders Lite)*, 3 pkts. 20
- instant *(Bar-Tenders Slightly Sour)*, 2 pkts. 120

Chapter 24

FOOD CHAINS AND RESTAURANTS

The listings in this section—which are broken down by restaurant rather than by food category—are generally based on one "average" or "standard" serving. The caloric content of a serving may vary slightly according to restaurant location. And, of course, individual orders that result in a change of ingredients or quantity of ingredients will alter the caloric value.

ARBY'S

	calories
breakfast items:	
bacon, 2 strips	90
biscuit, plain	280
blueberry muffin	230
cinnamon-nut Danish	360
croissant, plain	220
egg portion	95
French-Toastix, 6 pieces	430
ham	45
sausage	163
Swiss cheese, ½ oz.	45
table syrup	100
chicken fingers, 2 pieces	290
sandwiches:	
chicken, breaded fillet	536
chicken, Cordon Bleu	623
chicken, grilled, BBQ	388
chicken, grilled, deluxe	430
chicken, roast, club	546
chicken, roast, deluxe, light	276
chicken, roast, deluxe, sesame seed bun	433
chicken, roast, Santa Fe	436
Ham 'n Cheese	359

Ham 'n Cheese melt 329
fish fillet 529
roast beef, *Arby's* Melt with cheddar 368
roast beef, *Arby-Q* 431
roast beef, Bac'n Cheddar deluxe 539
roast beef, Beef 'n Cheddar 487
roast beef, deluxe, light 296
roast beef, giant 555
roast beef, junior 324
roast beef, regular 388
roast beef, super 523
turkey, roast, deluxe, light 260
sandwiches, sub roll:
French dip 475
hot Ham'n Swiss 500
Italian sub 675
Philly Beef 'n Swiss 755
roast beef sub 700
triple cheese melt 720
turkey sub 550
salads:
garden 61
roast chicken 149
side 23
soups:
Boston clam chowder 190
broccoli, cream of 160
cheese, Wisconsin 280
chicken noodle, old fashion 80
chili, *Timberline* 220
potato with bacon 170
vegetable, mixed, lumberjack 90
potatoes:
baked, plain, 11.5 oz. 355
baked, with margarine and sour cream 578
baked, Broccoli 'n Cheddar 447
baked, deluxe 736
cakes, 2 pieces 204
fries, curly 300
fries, curly, cheddar 333
fries, french 246

Arby's (cont.)

sauces and dressings:

Arby's Sauce	.15
barbecue sauce	.30
beef stock au jus	.10
blue cheese dressing	290
buttermilk ranch dressing, reduced calorie	.50
catsup	.16
cheddar sauce	.35
honey French dressing	280
honey mayonnaise, reduced calorie	.70
Horsey Sauce	.60
Italian dressing, reduced calorie	.20
Italian sub sauce	.70
mayonnaise	110
mayonnaise, light	.12
Parmesan cheese sauce	.70
ranch dressing, red	.75
tartar sauce	140
Thousand Island dressing	260

desserts:

apple turnover	330
cheesecake, plain	320
cherry turnover	320
chocolate chip cookie	125
Polar Swirl, Butterfinger	457
Polar Swirl, Heath	543
Polar Swirl, Oreo	482
Polar Swirl, Snickers	511
Polar Swirl, peanut butter cup	517
shake, chocolate	451
shake, jamocha	384
shake, vanilla	360

BASKIN-ROBBINS

	calories
ice cream, deluxe:	
Baby Ruth, ½ cup	170
Baby Ruth, regular scoop	300
banana nut, ½ cup	150
banana nut, regular scoop	260

banana strawberry, ½ cup 130
banana strawberry, regular scoop 240
Baseball nut or black walnut, ½ cup 160
Baseball nut or black walnut, regular scoop 260
blackberry, Oregon, ½ cup 140
butter pecan, ½ cup 160
butter pecan, regular scoop 290
Butterfinger, ½ cup 160
Butterfinger, regular scoop 300
caramel chocolate crunch, ½ cup 160
caramel chocolate crunch, regular scoop 290
cheesecake, blueberry, cherry, New York, or strawberry,
 ½ cup 150
cheesecake, strawberry, regular scoop 270
cherries jubilee, ½ cup 140
cherries jubilee, regular scoop 240
chocolate, ½ cup 150
chocolate, regular scoop 270
chocolate, triple passion, ½ cup 180
chocolate, triple passion, regular scoop 290
chocolate, white, winter, ½ cup 150
chocolate, white, winter, regular scoop 270
chocolate, world class, ½ cup 160
chocolate, world class, regular scoop 280
chocolate almond, ½ cup 180
chocolate almond, regular scoop 310
chocolate cake, German, ½ cup 180
chocolate chip, ½ cup 150
chocolate chip, regular scoop 270
chocolate chip cookie dough, ½ cup 170
chocolate chip cookie dough, regular scoop 300
chocolate fudge, ½ cup 160
chocolate fudge, regular scoop 290
chocolate mousse royale, ½ cup 170
chocolate mousse royale, regular scoop 310
chocolate raspberry truffle, ½ cup 160
chocolate raspberry truffle, regular scoop 280
chocolate ribbon, ½ cup 140
chocolate ribbon, regular scoop 250
Chocoholic's Resolution, ½ cup 170
Chocoholic's Resolution, regular scoop 150
Choc O The Irish, ½ cup 160

Baskin-Robbins, ice cream, deluxe *(cont.)*

Choc O The Irish, regular scoop 280
Chunk A Cherry Burnin' Love, ½ cup 140
Chunk A Cherry Burnin' Love, regular scoop 250
coconut, ½ cup 160
coconut, regular scoop 280
coconut, nutty, ½ cup 170
coconut, nutty, regular scoop 310
cookies 'n cream, ½ cup 170
cookies 'n cream, regular scoop 300
Everyone's Favorite Candy Bar, ½ cup 170
fudge brownie, ½ cup 170
fudge brownie, regular scoop 310
gold medal ribbon, ½ cup 150
gold medal ribbon, regular scoop 270
Heath Bar, ½ cup 170
Heath Bar, regular scoop 300
Here Comes the Fudge, ½ cup 150
jamoca, ½ cup 140
jamoca, regular scoop 250
jamoca, almond fudge, ½ cup 160
jamoca, almond fudge, regular scoop 280
Kahlua and chocolate cream or pecan caramel fudge,
   ½ cup 150
lemon custard, ½ cup 150
lemon custard, regular scoop 260
mint, chocolate chip, ½ cup 150
mint, chocolate chip, regular scoop 270
mint, Martian, ½ cup 160
mint, Martian, regular scoop 260
Mississippi mud, ½ cup 160
Naughty New Year's Resolution, ½ cup 170
Nutty or Nice, ½ cup 160
Nutty or Nice, regular scoop 290
peach, ½ cup 130
peach, regular scoop 240
peanut butter 'n chocolate, ½ cup 180
peanut butter 'n chocolate, regular scoop 330
peanut butter, Reese's, ½ cup 180
peanut butter, Reese's, regular scoop 310
peppermint, ½ cup 150
peppermint, regular scoop 270

peppermint, winter wondermint, ½ cup 150
peppermint, winter wondermint, regular scoop 270
pink bubble gum, ½ cup 150
pink bubble gum, regular scoop 270
pistachio-almond, ½ cup 170
pistachio-almond, regular scoop 300
pralines 'n cream, ½ cup 160
pralines 'n cream, regular scoop 290
pumpkin pie, ½ cup 130
Quarterback Crunch, ½ cup 160
Quarterback Crunch, regular scoop 290
rocky road, ½ cup 170
rocky road, regular scoop 300
rum raisin, ½ cup 140
rum raisin, regular scoop 250
S'mores, ½ cup 170
S'mores, regular scoop 300
strawberry shortcake, ½ cup 160
strawberry shortcake, regular scoop 280
strawberry, very berry, ½ cup 130
toffee, English, ½ cup 160
toffee, English, regular scoop 290
vanilla, ½ cup 140
vanilla, regular scoop 240
vanilla, decorating, ½ cup 140
vanilla, decorating, regular scoop 250
vanilla, French, ½ cup 160
vanilla, French, regular scoop 280
ice cream, light, ½ cup:
  cherry cheesecake or praline dream 110
  chocolate caramel nut 120
  espresso 'n cream 100
ice cream, fat free, ½ cup:
  caramel banana, berry innocent cheesecake, or jamoca
    swirl 110
  chocolate marshmallow 120
  chocolate vanilla twist 100
  soft-serve, caramel praline or vanilla 120
ice cream, no sugar added, ½ cup:
  all flavors except berries 'n banana 100
  berries 'n banana 80

Baskin-Robbins (cont.)
ices, sherbets, and sorbets:
daiquiri ice, ½ cup 110
daiquiri ice, regular scoop 130
grape ice, ½ cup 100
mandarin mimosa sorbet, ½ cup 120
margarita ice, ½ cup 110
The Mask Twist ice, ½ cup 120
orange sherbet, ½ cup 120
orange sherbet, regular scoop 160
peachy keen sorbet, ½ cup 100
rainbow sherbet, ½ cup 120
rainbow sherbet, regular scoop 160
raspberry sherbet, blue, ½ cup 120
raspberry sorbet, red, ½ cup 120
raspberry sorbet, red, regular scoop 140
raspberry-cranberry sorbet, *Rudolph's* red, ½ cup 110
raspberry-cranberry sorbet, *Rudolph's* red, regular scoop . . . 140
raspberry-lemonade sorbet, pink, ½ cup 120
strawberry island delight ice, ½ cup 100
novelties, 1 piece:
Cappy Blast bar, cappuccino 100
Cappy Blast bar, mocha cappuccino 120
chillyburger, regular or mint chocolate chip 220
sundae bar, jamoca almond fudge or pralines 'n cream 280
sundae bar, peanut butter chocolate 340
Tiny Toon bar, vanilla 210
yogurt, frozen, ½ cup:
low-fat, blueberry, cheesecake, chocolate, or vanilla 120
nonfat, all flavors except black cherry, coconut, piña
colada, and vanilla 100
nonfat, black cherry, coconut, or piña colada 110
nonfat, vanilla 80
nonfat, reduced sugar, all flavors except chocolate and
whata banana 90
yogurt, frozen, hard-packed, ½ cup:
brownie madness, Maui, low-fat 140
Caramelcopia 130
Have Your Cake, low-fat 110
Jumpin' Java Bean, nonfat 120
Last Mango In Paradise, nonfat 120
Perils of Praline, low-fat 130

raspberry cheese Louise, low-fat 130
fountain drinks, 1 serving, except as noted:
blueberry strawberry smoothie 150
Cappy Blast 150
Cappy Blast, with whipped cream 170
Capply Blast, nonfat 90
chocolate, *Cappy Blast* 240
chocolate, *Cappy Blast,* with whipped cream 250
chocolate, *Cappy Blast,* lowfat 390
chocolate shake, vanilla ice cream 660
malt powder, 1 oz. 110
orange banana smoothie 120
piña colada, *Paradise Blast* 190
piña colada, *Paradise Blast,* with whipped cream 200
piña colada, *Paradise Blast,* nonfat 140
strawberry banana smoothie 170
strawberry luau, *Paradise Blast* 170
strawberry luau, *Paradise Blast,* with whipped cream 190
strawberry luau, *Paradise Blast,* low-fat 140
cones, 1 piece:
cake cone 25
sugar cone 60
waffle cone, fresh baked 146
waffle cone, large 120
toppings:
butterscotch, 2 oz. 200
chocolate syrup, 2 tbsp. 90
gummy bears, baby, 75 pieces 130
hot fudge, 1 oz. 100
hot fudge, no sugar added, 1 oz. 90
praline caramel, 1 oz. 90
sprinkles, 1/6 oz. 90
strawberry, 1 oz. 60
whipped cream, Rod's, 2 tsp. 30

BOSTON MARKET

calories

entrees:
chicken, half, with skin 630
chicken, quarter, dark meat, no skin 210
chicken, quarter, dark meat, with skin 330

Boston Market, entrees (cont.)

chicken, quarter, white meat, no skin or wing	160
chicken, quarter, white meat, with skin	330
chicken potpie	750
ham, with cinnamon apples	350
meat loaf, and tomato sauce	370
meat loaf, and gravy	390
turkey breast, skinless	170

sandwiches:

chicken	430
chicken, with cheese and sauce	760
chicken salad	680
ham	450
ham, with cheese and sauce	760
ham and turkey club	430
ham and turkey club, with cheese and sauce	890
meat loaf	690
meat loaf, with cheese	860
turkey	400
turkey, with cheese and sauce	710

salads:

Caesar, 10 oz.	520
Caesar, without dressing, 8 oz.	240
Caesar, 4 oz.	210
Caesar, chicken	670
chicken, chunky	390
coleslaw	280
fruit*	70
pasta, Mediterranean	170
tortellini	380

side dishes, soup, and bread:

apples, cinnamon	250
baked beans, BBQ	330
corn, buttered	190
corn bread	200
cranberry relish	370
gravy, chicken, 1 oz.	15
macaroni and cheese	280
potatoes, mashed	180
potatoes, mashed, with gravy	200

* Recipes vary from restaurant to restaurant

potatoes, new 140
rice pilaf 180
soup, chicken 80
soup, chicken tortilla 220
spinach, creamed 300
squash, butternut 160
stuffing 310
vegetables, steamed .35
zucchini 80
desserts:
brownie 450
chocolate chip cookie 340
oatmeal raisin cookie 320

BURGER KING

calories

breakfast items:
A.M. Express jam, grape or strawberry 30
biscuit with bacon, egg, cheese 510
biscuit with sausage 590
Croissan'wich, sausage, egg, cheese 600
French toast sticks 500
hash browns 220
sandwiches:
BK Big Fish 700
BK Broiler chicken 550
cheeseburger 380
cheeseburger, double 600
cheeseburger, double, with bacon 640
chicken sandwich 710
Double Whopper 870
Double Whopper with cheese 960
hamburger 330
Whopper 640
Whopper with cheese 730
Whopper Jr. 420
Whopper Jr. with cheese 460
Chicken Tenders, 8 pieces 310
dipping sauces, 1 oz., except as noted:
A.M. Express 80
barbecue 35

Burger King, dipping sauces *(cont.)*
   Bull's Eye, ½ oz. 20
   honey 90
   ranch 170
   sweet and sour 45
side dishes:
   fries, medium 370
   fries, coated, medium 340
   onion rings 310
salad, without dressing:
   chicken, broiled 200
   garden 100
   side 60
salad dressings, ½ oz.:
   bleu cheese 160
   French 140
   Italian, light 15
   ranch 180
   Thousand Island 140
desserts and shakes:
   Dutch apple pie 300
   shake, chocolate, medium 320
   shake, chocolate, with syrup, medium 440
   shake, strawberry, with syrup, medium 420
   shake, vanilla, medium 300

CAPTAIN D'S

                                             calories

lunches* and platters**:
   chicken, broiled, lunch 503
   chicken, broiled, platter 802
   chicken sandwich 451
   crab, stuffed 91
   fish, broiled, lunch 435
   fish, broiled, platter 734
   fish and chicken, broiled, lunch 478
   fish and chicken, broiled, platter 777

All lunches include rice, vegetable medley, and breadstick
**All platters include rice, vegetable medley, baked potato, salad, and breadstick*

CARL'S JR.

calories

Carl's Jr., breakfast (cont.)

French toast dips, without syrup	410
quesadilla, breakfast	300
sausage, 1 patty	200
scrambled eggs	160
Sunrise Sandwich	370
table syrup, 1 oz.	90
chicken stars, 6 pieces	230

sauces:

barbecue sauce	50
honey sauce	90
mustard sauce	45
salsa	10
sweet n' sour sauce	50

sandwiches:

Big Burger	470
Carl's Catch Fish Sandwich	560
chicken bacon Swiss	670
chicken, barbequed	310
chicken, ranch	580
chicken, Santa Fe	530
chicken club	550
double cheeseburger, 1/3 lb.	660
Double Western Bacon Cheeseburger	970
Famous Big Star hamburger	610
hamburger	200
Hot & Crispy sandwich	400
Super Star hamburger	820
Western Bacon Cheeseburger	870

"Great Stuff" potato:

bacon and cheese	630
broccoli and cheese	530
potato, plain	290
sour cream and chive	430

Entree Salads-To-Go:

chicken	260
garden	50

salad dressing, 2 oz.:

blue cheese	310
French, fat free	70
house	220
Italian, fat free	15

Thousand Island 250
side dishes:
   CrissCut Fries, large 550
   fries, regular 370
   hash brown nuggets 270
   onion rings 520
   zucchini 380
bakery products:
   blueberry muffin 340
   bran muffin 370
   cheese Danish 400
   cheesecake, strawberry swirl 300
   chocolate cake 300
   chocolate chip cookie 370
   cinnamon roll 420
shake, small:
   chocolate 390
   strawberry 400
   vanilla 330

CARVEL

calories

ice cream, soft serve, ½ cup:
   chocolate 180
   chocolate, no fat 90
   vanilla 190
   vanilla, no fat 120
sherbet, all flavors, ½ cup 150
yogurt, soft serve, vanilla, no sugar, ½ cup 100
novelties, 1 piece:
   Brown Bonnet cone 380
   Chipsters 380
   Flying Saucer 240
   ice cream cupcake 210

CHICK-FIL-A

calories

chicken dishes:
   chargrilled, 2.8 oz. 130
   Chick-Fil-A Nuggets, 8-pack 290

Chick-Fil-A, chicken dishes *(cont.)*

Chick-n-Strips, 4 pieces 230
Chick-n-Strips salad 290
salad, chargrilled garden 170
salad plate 290

chicken sandwiches:
regular 290
chargrilled 280
chargrilled, deluxe 290
chargrilled club, without dressing 390
Chick-n-Q 370
deluxe 300
salad, whole wheat 320

side dishes, small:
carrot raisin salad 150
chicken soup, 1 cup 110
coleslaw 130
tossed salad 70
Waffle fries, salted or unsalted 290

desserts:
brownie, fudge nut 350
cheesecake 270
cheesecake, with blueberry or strawberry 290
Icedream, small cone 140
Icedream, small cup 350
lemon pie 280

CHURCH'S CHICKEN

calories

chicken, edible portion:
breast, 2.8 oz. 200
leg, 2 oz. 140
Tender Strip, 1.1 oz. 80
thigh, 2.8 oz. 230
wing, 3.1 oz. 250

sides:
biscuit 250
Cajun rice 130
coleslaw 92
corn on cob 139
fries 210

okra	210
potatoes and gravy	.90
apple pie	280

DAIRY QUEEN/BRAZIER

	calories
DQ Homestyle burgers:	
cheeseburger	340
cheeseburger with bacon, double	610
double cheeseburger, regular or deluxe	540
hamburger	290
hamburger, deluxe double	440
ultimate burger	670
sandwiches:	
chicken fillet, breaded	430
chicken fillet, breaded with cheese	480
chicken fillet, grilled	310
fish fillet	370
fish fillet with cheese	420
hot dog, plain	240
hot dog, with cheese	290
hot dog, with chili	280
hot dog, with chili and cheese	330
chicken strip basket:	
with BBQ sauce	810
with gravy	860
side dishes:	
fries, large	390
fries, regular	300
fries, small	210
onion rings, regular	240
desserts and shakes:	
banana split	510
Blizzard:	
Butterfinger, regular	750
Butterfinger, small	520
chocolate chip cookie dough, regular	950
chocolate chip cookie dough, small	660
chocolate sandwich cookie, regular	640
chocolate sandwich cookie, small	520
Heath, regular	820

Dairy Queen/Brazier, **desserts and shakes**, *Blizzard (cont.)*

    Heath, small 560
    Reese's peanut butter cup, regular 790
    Reese's peanut butter cup, small 590
    strawberry, regular 570
    strawberry, small 400
Buster Bar 450
cone, chocolate, regular 360
cone, chocolate, small 240
cone, chocolate-dipped, regular 510
cone, chocolate-dipped, small 340
cone, vanilla, large 410
cone, vanilla, regular 350
cone, vanilla, small 230
DQ cake, undecorated:
    heart, 1/10 cake 270
    log, 1/8 cake 280
    round, 8", 1/8 cake 340
    round, 10", 1/12 cake 360
    sheet, 1/20 cake 350
DQ caramel and nut bar 260
DQ fudge bar 50
DQ Lemon Freez'r, 1/2 cup 80
DQ sandwich 150
DQ Treatzza Pizza, 1/8 pie:
    Heath or strawberry-banana 180
    M&M 190
    peanut butter fudge 220
DQ vanilla orange bar 60
Dilly bar, chocolate or toffee with *Heath* pieces 210
Dilly bar, chocolate mint 190
Fudge Nut Bar 410
malt, chocolate, regular 880
malt, chocolate, small 650
Misty cooler, strawberry 190
Misty slush, regular 290
Misty slush, small 220
Peanut Buster parfait 730
Queen's Choice Big Scoop, chocolate or vanilla 250
shake, chocolate, regular 770
shake, chocolate, small 560
soft-serve, *DQ*, chocolate, 1/2 cup 150

soft-serve, *DQ,* vanilla, ½ cup 140
Starkiss 80
strawberry shortcake 430
sundae, chocolate, regular 410
sundae, chocolate, small 290
yogurt, *Breeze:*
   Heath, regular 710
   Heath, small 470
   strawberry, regular 460
   strawberry, small 320
yogurt, frozen:
   cone 280
   DQ Nonfat, ½ cup 100
   regular cup 230
   strawberry sundae 300

DENNY'S

calories

breakfast, without bread:
  All American Slam 1,028
  Belgian waffle, plain 304
  Belgian waffle supreme, without bacon or sausage 433
  chicken fried steak and eggs 723
  French Slam 1,029
  French toast, plain, 2 pieces 510
  fresh fruit mix 36
  ham 'n' cheddar omelet 743
  Moons Over My Hammy, without potato 807
  Original *Grand Slam,* without syrup, margarine 795
  pancakes, plain, 3 pieces 491
  pork chop and eggs 555
  porterhouse steak and eggs 1,223
  Scram Slam 974
  Senior Belgian Waffle Slam, without syrup, margarine 399
  Senior Omelette 623
  Senior Starter, without bacon or sausage 336
  Senior Triple Play, without bacon or sausage 537
  sirloin steak and eggs 808
  Slim Slam, with syrup, without topping 638
  Southern Slam 1,065
  Super/Play It Again Slam 1,192

Denny's, breakfast *(cont.)*

tomato juice, 10 oz. 56
topping, blueberry, 3 oz. 106
topping, strawberry, 3 oz. 115
salad, without dressing, except as noted:
   fried chicken 506
   garden chicken delite 119
   grilled chicken Caesar, with dressing 655
   Oriental chicken, with dressing 568
   side Caesar, with dressing 338
   side garden 113
dressings, 1 oz.:
   bleu cheese 124
   Caesar 142
   French 106
   French, reduced calorie 76
   honey mustard, fat free 38
   Italian, creamy 106
   Italian, reduced calorie 23
   Oriental 106
   ranch 101
   Thousand Island 104
condiments, 1.5 oz.:
   BBQ sauce 47
   horseradish sauce 170
   sour cream 91
soup, 8 oz.:
   cheese 293
   chicken noodle 60
   clam chowder 214
   cream of broccoli 193
   cream of potato 222
   split pea 146
   vegetable beef 79
sandwiches, without fries or substitutes:
   bacon Swiss burger 710
   bacon, lettuce, and tomato 634
   Charleston Chicken 566
   chicken melt 520
   club 718
   Delidinger 852
   deluxe grilled cheese 482
   Denny Burger 513

Denny's, sandwiches (cont.)

French dip, without horseradish sauce 531
fried fish 905
grilled chicken 436
Humdinger Hamburger 748
patty melt 694
Super Bird 620

sandwiches, lunch combinations:
turkey breast on multigrain, without soup, salad 476
ham and Swiss on rye, without soup, salad 533

sandwiches, senior, sandwich only:
half grilled cheese 246
ham and Swiss, without fries or substitutes 497
turkey, without fries or substitutes 476

appetizers, without condiments, except as noted:
Buffalo chicken strips 734
Buffalo wings, 12 pieces 856
chicken quesadilla 827
chicken strips, 5 pieces 720
mozzarella sticks, 8 pieces, with sauce 756
onion rings, 7 pieces 439
Sampler 1,120

entrees*:
battered cod, with tartar sauce 732
Charleston Chicken 327
chicken fried steak 265
chicken strip, with honey-mustard dressing 635
Denny Cut Prime Rib, 8 oz., au jus, with horseradish . . . 760
grilled Alaskan salmon 296
grilled breast of chicken 130
liver with bacon and onions 497
pork chop dinner 386
porterhouse steak 708
roast turkey and stuffing 701
shrimp 558
steak and shrimp 645
T-bone steak dinner 530

junior meals, without fries or substitutes:
burger 261

---

* Add bread; choice of salad, soup, or fruit; choice of potato or rice pilaf; and
choice of vegetable

fried fish 465
grilled cheese 375
shrimp basket 291
senior meals*:
   battered cod, without potato or pilaf 465
   chicken fried steak 341
   grilled chicken breast 219
   liver with bacon and onions 322
   pork chop 193
   pot roast 149
   turkey and stuffing 596
sides:
   broccoli in butter sauce, 4 oz. 50
   carrots in honey glaze, 4 oz. 80
   corn in butter sauce, 4 oz. 120
   cornbread stuffing, 2 oz. 182
   french fries, unsalted, 4 oz. 323
   fries, seasoned, 4 oz. 261
   gravy, brown, 1 oz. 13
   gravy, chicken, 1 oz. .14
   gravy, country, 1 oz. .17
   green beans with bacon, 4 oz. 60
   green peas in butter sauce, 4 oz. 100
   potato, baked, plain, 6 oz. 186
   potato, mashed, plain, 6 oz. 105
   rice pilaf, 3 oz. 112
   sliced tomatoes, 3 slices 13
pies, "Mother Butler," ⅙ pie:
   apple 430
   apple, with *Equal* 370
   cheesecake pie 470
     blueberry topping, 3 oz. 106
     cherry topping, 3 oz. 115
   cherry 540
   chocolate pecan 790
   coconut cream 480
   Dutch apple 440
   French silk 650
   German chocolate 580
   key lime 600

* Add bread; choice of soup, salad, or fruit; and choice of vegetable

Denny's, pies *(cont.)*
   lemon meringue 460
   pecan 600
other desserts:
   banana split sundae, 19 oz. 894
   chocolate cake, 4 oz. 370
   hot fudge cake sundae, 8 oz. 687
   sundae, double scoop, 6 oz., without topping 375
   sundae, single scoop, 3 oz., without topping 188
   tapioca, 4 oz. 127
   toppings, 2 oz.:
      blueberry 71
      chocolate 317
      fudge 201
      strawberry 77
coffee, flavored, 8 oz.:
   French vanilla 76
   hazelnut 66
   Irish cream 73
   raspberry iced tea, 16 oz. 78

DOMINO'S PIZZA

calories

cheese pizza, 12″ medium pie:
   deep dish, 2 of 8 slices 467
   hand-tossed, 2 of 8 slices 349
   thin crust, ¼ pie 273
   "Add a Topping":
      anchovies 23
      bacon 82
      beef, precooked 56
      cheddar cheese 57
      extra cheese 49
      ham 18
      mushrooms, fresh or canned 4
      olives, green 12
      olives, ripe 14
      onion 4
      pepperoni 62
      peppers, banana or green 3
      pineapple tidbits 10

sausage, Italian 55
cheese pizza, 14" large pie:
   deep dish, 2 of 12 slices 464
   hand-tossed, 2 of 12 slices 319
   thin crust, 1/6 pie 255
   "Add a Topping":
      anchovies 23
      bacon 75
      beef, precooked 44
      cheddar cheese 48
      extra cheese 46
      ham 17
      mushrooms, fresh or canned 3
      olives, green 11
      olives, ripe 12
      onion 3
      pepperoni 55
      peppers, banana 3
      peppers, green 2
      pineapple tidbits 8
      sausage, Italian 44
cheese pizza, 6" deep dish, 1 pie:
   plain 591
   "Add a Topping":
      anchovies 45
      bacon 82
      beef, precooked 44
      cheddar cheese 86
      extra cheese 59
      ham 17
      mushrooms, fresh or canned 2
      olives, green 10
      olives, ripe 11
      onion 3
      pepperoni 50
      peppers, banana 3
      peppers, green 2
      pineapple tidbits 5
      sausage, Italian 44
Buffalo wings:
   barbecue, 1 piece 50
   hot, 1 piece 45

Domino's Pizza (cont.)
breadstick, 1 piece 78
cheesy bread, 1 piece 103
salad, small 22
salad, large 39
Marzetti salad dressings, 1.5 oz.:
    blue cheese 220
    Caesar, creamy 200
    French, honey 210
    Italian, house 220
    Italian, light 20
    ranch 260
    ranch, fat free 40
    Thousand Island 200

GODFATHER'S PIZZA, one slice

                               calories

cheese, original crust:
    mini, ¼ pie 131
    medium, ⅛ pie 231
    large, 1/10 pie 258
    jumbo, 1/10 pie 382
cheese, golden crust:
    medium, ⅛ pie 212
    large, 1/10 pie 242
combo, original crust:
    mini, ¼ pie 176
    medium, ⅛ pie 306
    large, 1/10 pie 338
    jumbo, 1/10 pie 503
combo, golden crust:
    medium, ⅛ pie 271
    large, 1/10 pie 305

HÄAGEN-DAZS ICE CREAM SHOP

                               calories

ice cream, ½ cup:
    butter pecan or macadamia nut 320
    Brownies a la Mode (Exträas) 280
    Cappuccino Commotion (Exträas) 310

Caramel Cone Explosion (Exträas) 310
chocolate, cookies and cream, coffee, rum raisin, or vanilla . 270
chocolate chip, coffee chip, pralines and cream, or vanilla
   fudge 290
chocolate chocolate, Belgian 330
chocolate chocolate chip or chocolate chocolate mint 300
chocolate peanut butter, deep 370
Cookie Dough Dynamo (Exträas) 300
macadamia brittle or Swiss chocolate almond 300
Midnight Cookies and Cream 300
strawberry 250
Strawberry Cheesecake Craze (Exträas) 280
vanilla Swiss almond 310
ice cream bar, uncoated, 1 bar:
   chocolate 200
   coffee or vanilla 190
sorbet, ½ cup:
   banana strawberry or orchard peach 140
   chocolate 130
   mango 120
   raspberry 120
   strawberry 130
   Zesty Lemon 120
sorbet, soft-serve, mango or raspberry, ½ cup 100
yogurt, soft-serve, ½ cup:
   chocolate, nonfat, or vanilla, nonfat 110
   chocolate mousse, nonfat .80
   coffee 140
   vanilla mousse, nonfat 70

HARDEE'S

                                             calories

breakfast items:
   Big Country Breakfast, bacon 820
   Big Country Breakfast, sausage 1,000
   biscuit:
      Apple Cinnamon 'N' Raisin 200
      bacon and egg 570
      bacon, egg, and cheese 610
      country ham 430
      ham 400

Hardee's, **breakfast items, biscuit** *(cont.)*

    ham, egg, and cheese 540
    jelly 440
    Rise 'N' Shine 390
    sausage 510
    sausage and egg 630
    Ultimate Omelet 570
  Biscuit 'N' Gravy 510
  Frisco Breakfast Sandwich, ham 500
  Hash Rounds, regular 230
  pancakes, 3 pieces 280
burgers and sandwiches:
  Big Roast Beef sandwich 460
  The Boss 570
  cheeseburger 310
  cheeseburger, mesquite bacon 370
  cheeseburger, quarter pound double 470
  chicken fillet sandwich 480
  Cravin' Bacon cheeseburger 690
  Fisherman's Fillet 560
  Frisco burger 720
  grilled chicken sandwich 350
  hamburger 270
  hamburger, the works 530
  Hot Ham 'N' Cheese 310
  Mushroom 'N' Swiss burger 490
  roast beef sandwich, regular 320
fried chicken:
  breast 370
  leg 170
  thigh 330
  wing 200
sides:
  baked beans, 5 oz. 170
  coleslaw, 4 oz. 240
  fries, large 430
  fries, medium 350
  fries, small 240
  gravy, 1.5 oz. 20
  mashed potato, 4 oz. 70
salads:
  garden 220

```
    grilled chicken. . . . . . . . . . . . . . . . . . . . . . . . . 150
    side . . . . . . . . . . . . . . . . . . . . . . . . . . . . . . .25
dressings:
    French, fat free . . . . . . . . . . . . . . . . . . . . . . . .70
    ranch . . . . . . . . . . . . . . . . . . . . . . . . . . . . . 290
    Thousand Island . . . . . . . . . . . . . . . . . . . . . . 250
desserts and shakes:
    Big Cookie . . . . . . . . . . . . . . . . . . . . . . . . . . 280
    cone, chocolate . . . . . . . . . . . . . . . . . . . . . . . 180
    cone, Cool Twist, vanilla/chocolate . . . . . . . . . . . 180
    cone, vanilla . . . . . . . . . . . . . . . . . . . . . . . . . 170
    peach cobbler, 6 oz. . . . . . . . . . . . . . . . . . . . . 310
    shake, chocolate . . . . . . . . . . . . . . . . . . . . . . 370
    shake, peach . . . . . . . . . . . . . . . . . . . . . . . . 350
    shake, strawberry . . . . . . . . . . . . . . . . . . . . . 420
    shake, vanilla . . . . . . . . . . . . . . . . . . . . . . . . 350
    sundae, hot fudge . . . . . . . . . . . . . . . . . . . . . 290
    sundae, strawberry . . . . . . . . . . . . . . . . . . . . 210
```

JACK-IN-THE-BOX

calories

```
breakfast:
    Breakfast Jack. . . . . . . . . . . . . . . . . . . . . . . . 300
    Country Crock Spread, .2 oz. . . . . . . . . . . . . . . .25
    croissant, sausage . . . . . . . . . . . . . . . . . . . . . 670
    croissant, supreme . . . . . . . . . . . . . . . . . . . . . 570
    hash browns . . . . . . . . . . . . . . . . . . . . . . . . . 160
    jelly, grape, .5 oz. . . . . . . . . . . . . . . . . . . . . . .40
    pancake platter . . . . . . . . . . . . . . . . . . . . . . . 400
    pancake syrup, 1½ oz. . . . . . . . . . . . . . . . . . . 120
    sandwich, sourdough . . . . . . . . . . . . . . . . . . . 380
    sandwich, ultimate . . . . . . . . . . . . . . . . . . . . . 620
    scrambled egg pocket . . . . . . . . . . . . . . . . . . . 430
sandwiches:
    cheeseburger, double . . . . . . . . . . . . . . . . . . . 450
    cheeseburger, regular . . . . . . . . . . . . . . . . . . . 320
    cheeseburger, ultimate . . . . . . . . . . . . . . . . . 1,030
    chicken . . . . . . . . . . . . . . . . . . . . . . . . . . . . 400
    chicken, Caesar . . . . . . . . . . . . . . . . . . . . . . . 520
    chicken, spicy crispy . . . . . . . . . . . . . . . . . . . 560
    chicken, supreme . . . . . . . . . . . . . . . . . . . . . . 620
```

Jack-in-the-Box, sandwiches *(cont.)*

chicken fajita pita 290
chicken fillet, grilled 430
hamburger, regular 280
hamburger, quarter-pounder 510
hamburger, sourdough, grilled 670
Jumbo Jack 560
Jumbo Jack with cheese 650
entrees:
chicken teriyaki bowl 580
taco 190
taco, monster 283
salads:
chicken, garden 200
side 70
finger foods:
chicken strips, 4 pieces 290
chicken strips, 6 pieces 450
egg rolls, 3 pieces 440
egg rolls, 5 pieces 750
jalapeños, stuffed, 7 pieces 420
jalapeños, stuffed, 10 pieces 600
potato wedges with bacon, cheddar 800
side dishes:
fries, jumbo 400
fries, seasoned, curly 360
fries, regular 350
fries, small 220
fries, super scoop 590
onion rings 380
sauces:
barbeque, 1 oz. 45
buttermilk, .9 oz. 130
soy, .3 oz. 5
sweet and sour, 1 oz. 40
tartar, 1 oz. 150
dressings, 2 oz.:
blue cheese 210
buttermilk, house 290
Italian, low-calorie 25
Thousand Island 250

condiments:

cheese, American, 1 slice	.45
cheese, Swiss-style, 1 slice	.40
croutons, .4 oz.	.50
hot sauce, 1 pkt.	5
ketchup, 1 pkt.	.10
mayonnaise, 1 pkt.	150
mustard, 1 pkt.	5
salsa, 1 oz.	.10

desserts:

apple turnover	350
carrot cake	370
cheesecake	310
cheesecake, chocolate chip cookie dough	360

shakes:

chocolate or cappuccino	630
strawberry	640
vanilla	610

KFC

calories

chicken, *Original Recipe:*

breast	400
drumstick or whole wing	140
thigh	250

chicken, *Extra Tasty Crispy:*

breast	470
drumstick	190
thigh	370
wing, whole	200

chicken, *Hot & Spicy:*

breast	530
drumstick	190
thigh	370
wing, whole	210

chicken, *Tender Roast:*

breast, with skin	251
breast, without skin	169
drumstick, with skin	.97
drumstick, without skin	.67
thigh, with skin	207

KFC, chicken, *Tender Roast* (cont.)
thigh, without skin 106
wing, with skin 121
chicken potpie 770
Crispy Strips, 3 pieces 261
Hot Wings, 6 pieces 471
Kentucky Nuggets, 6 pieces 284
sandwiches, chicken:
BBQ flavored 256
Original Recipe 497
sides and specials:
BBQ baked beans 190
biscuit, 2-oz. piece 180
coleslaw 180
corn bread, 2-oz. piece 228
corn on the cob 190
garden rice 120
green beans 45
macaroni and cheese, 4 oz. 180
mashed potatoes with gravy 120
Mean Greens 70
potato salad 230
potato wedges 280
red beans and rice 130

LITTLE CAESARS

	calories
Baby Pan!Pan!, 2 squares	616
Crazy Bread, 1 piece	106
Crazy Sauce, 6 oz.	.74
Pan!Pan!, 1 medium slice:	
cheese only	181
pepperoni	199
Pizza!Pizza!, 1 medium slice:	
cheese only	201
pepperoni	220
salads, individual:	
antipasto	176
Caesar	140
Greek	168
tossed	116

dressings, 1.5 oz.:
    blue cheese 160
    Caesar 255
    French 166
    Greek 268
    Italian 200
    Italian, fat free 15
    ranch 221
    Thousand Island 183
sandwiches, cold deli-style
    ham and cheese 728
    Italian 740
    veggie 647
sandwiches, hot oven-baked:
    Cheeser 822
    Meatsa 1,036
    pepperoni 899
    supreme 894
    veggie 669

LONG JOHN SILVER'S

        calories

fish, seafood, and chicken:
    chicken, batter-dipped, 1 piece 120
    chicken, *Flavorbaked,* 1 piece 110
    chicken, popcorn, 3.3 oz. 250
    clams, 3 oz. 300
    fish, batter-dipped, 1 piece 170
    fish, *Flavorbaked,* 1 piece 90
    fish, popcorn, 3.6 oz. 290
    shrimp, batter-dipped, 1 piece 35
    shrimp, popcorn, 3.3 oz. 280
sandwiches:
    chicken, *Flavorbaked* 290
    fish, batter-dipped, without sauce 320
    fish, *Flavorbaked* 320
    Ultimate Fish 430
sides, 1 serving:
    cheese sticks, 1.6 oz. 160
    coleslaw 140
    corn cobbette, plain, 1 piece 80

Long John Silver's, sides _(cont.)_

corn cobbette, with butter, 1 piece	140
French fries, 3 oz.	250
green beans	.30
hush puppy, 1 piece	.60
potato, baked	210
rice pilaf	140
side salad	.25

dressings:

French, fat free, 1½ oz.	.50
Italian, 1 oz.	130
ranch, 1 oz.	170
ranch, fat free, 1½ oz.	.50
Thousand Island, 1 oz.	110

sauces and condiments:

honey mustard, .4 oz.	.20
malt vinegar, .3 oz.	0
margarine, .2 oz.	.35
shrimp sauce, .4 oz.	.15
sour cream, 1 oz.	.60
sweet 'n' sour, .4 oz.	.20
tartar sauce, .4 oz.	.35

McDONALD'S

calories

breakfast biscuits:

plain	260
bacon, egg, and cheese	440
sausage	430
sausage and egg	510

breakfast dishes:

burrito	320
eggs, scrambled, 2	160
hash browns	130
hot cakes, plain	310
hot cakes, with syrup and margarine	580
sausage	170

breakfast muffins:

English	140
Egg McMuffin	290
Sausage McMuffin	360

    Sausage McMuffin, with egg 440
Danish and muffin:
    apple bran muffin 300
    apple Danish 360
    cheese Danish 410
    cinnamon roll 400
sandwiches:
    Arch Deluxe 550
    Arch Deluxe, with bacon 590
    Big Mac 560
    cheeseburger 320
    Crispy Chicken Deluxe 500
    Fish Filet Deluxe 560
    Grilled Chicken Deluxe 440
    hamburger 260
    Quarter Pounder 420
    Quarter Pounder, with cheese 530
Chicken McNuggets:
    4 pieces 190
    6 pieces 290
    9 pieces 430
Chicken McNuggets sauces, 1 pkt.:
    barbeque 45
    honey 45
    honey mustard 50
    hot mustard 60
    light mayonnaise 40
    sweet and sour 50
french fries:
    small 210
    large 450
    Super Size 540
salads:
    garden 35
    grilled chicken salad deluxe 120
salad croutons, 1 pkg. 50
salad dressings, 1 pkg.:
    Caesar 160
    ranch 230
    red French, reduced calorie 160
    vinaigrette, lite 50

McDonald's (cont.)
desserts and shakes:

baked apple pie	260
chocolate chip cookie	170
ice cream cone, vanilla, reduced fat	150
McDonaldland Cookies, 1 pkg.	180
shake, chocolate, strawberry, or vanilla, small	360
sundae, hot caramel	360
sundae, hot fudge	340
sundae, strawberry	290
sundae nuts, ¼ oz.	.40

PIZZA HUT

	calories
Bigfoot, 1 slice:	
cheese	186
pepperoni	205
pepperoni, mushroom, and sausage	214
breadsticks, 5 pieces	750
hand-tossed, 1 slice of medium pie:	
beef	260
cheese	235
ham	213
Meat Lovers	314
pepperoni	238
Pepperoni Lovers	306
pork topping	268
sausage, Italian	267
supreme	284
supreme, super	296
Veggie Lovers	216
pan pizza, 1 slice of medium pie:	
beef	286
cheese	261
ham	239
Meat Lovers	340
pepperoni	265
Pepperoni Lovers	332
pork topping	294
sausage, Italian	293
supreme	311

QUINCY'S

calories

breakfast items:
    apples, escalloped, 3.5 oz. 120
    bacon, 1/4 oz. 35
    corned beef hash, 4.5 oz. 210
    eggs, scrambled, 2 oz. .95
    ham, 1.5 oz. 90
    oatmeal, 1 oz. 175
    pancakes, 1.5 oz. 95
    sausage gravy, 4 oz. 70
    sausage links, 2 oz. 225
    sausage patties, 2 oz. 230
    steak fingers, 3.5 oz. 360
    syrup, 1 oz. 75
beef entrees:
    fillet with bacon, 8 oz.* 340
    sirloin tips with mushroom gravy, 6 oz. 196
    sirloin tips with pepper and onions, 5 oz. 203
    steak, chopped, 8 oz.* 499
    steak, country, with gravy, 9 oz. 530
    steak, cowboy, 14 oz.* 580

* *Weight before cooking*

Quincy's, beef entrees *(cont.)*

steak, New York strip, 10 oz. 450
steak, porterhouse, 17 oz.* 683
steak, ribeye, 10 oz.* 452
steak, sirloin, junior, 5.5 oz.* 194
steak, sirloin, large, 10 oz.* 368
steak, sirloin, regular, 8 oz.* 285
steak, strip, smothered, 10 oz.* 622
steak, T-bone, 13 oz.* 521

other entree items:

chicken, grilled, 5 oz. 120
chicken fillet, homestyle, 3 oz. 217
chicken, roasted, with herbs, 14 oz. 875
chicken, roasted BBQ, 14 oz. 941
salmon, grilled, 7 oz. 228
shrimp, breaded, 7 oz. 546
steak and shrimp, 9 oz. 677

sandwiches, 1 piece:

burger, ⅓ lb. 565
burger, bacon cheese 663
chicken, grilled 324
chicken, spicy BBQ 368
steak, Philly cheese 588
steak, smothered 429

side dishes, 4 oz., except as noted:

apples, with cinnamon 172
beans, BBQ 114
beans, green 61
broccoli spears 34
broccoli spears, with cheese sauce, 5 oz. 92
corn 96
potato, baked, plain, 6 oz. 115
potatoes, fries, steak 358
potatoes, mashed 54
rice pilaf 119

bread, 2 oz.:

banana nut 165
biscuit 270
corn bread 140
roll, yeast 160

* *Weight before cooking*

soups, 6 oz.:
    broccoli, cream of 170
    chili 235
    clam chowder 180
    vegetable beef 90
salad dressings, 1 oz.:
    blue cheese 155
    French 125
    French, light 85
    honey mustard 100
    Italian 135
    Italian, light 20
    Italian, light, creamy 65
    Parmesan peppercorn 150
    ranch 110
    Thousand Island, light 65
desserts:
    brownie pudding cake, 4 oz. 310
    cobbler, apple, 6 oz. 255
    cobbler, cherry, 6 oz. 410
    cobbler, peach, 6 oz. 305
    cookie, chocolate chip or sugar, ½ oz. 60
    pudding, banana, 5 oz. 240
    yogurt, frozen, 4 oz. 135
    yogurt toppings, caramel or fudge, 1 oz. 105

RED LOBSTER

                                             calories

appetizers and soups:
    broccoli-cheese soup 160
    calamari 350
    chicken fingers 390
    clam chowder, 6 oz. 130
    crab add-on 60
    crab-shrimp cakes 480
    lobster quesadilla 760
    mozzarella sticks 730
    mushrooms, fresh fried 790
    mushrooms, stuffed 420
    mushrooms, lobster stuffed 400
    seafood gumbo, 6 oz. 120

Red Lobster, appetizers and soups (cont.)

shrimp cocktail, 6 shrimp only	.50
shrimp in shell, 6 oz.	110
zucchini, Parmesan	620

dinner entrees, 8 oz.:

Admiral's Feast	1,060
catfish, Santa Fe	340
chicken breast, grilled	230
chicken breast teriyaki, grilled	240
chicken Fresco	1,320
chicken, smothered	530
clam strips	720
cod/haddock, Atlantic, baked	220
crab Alfredo	1,170
crab legs, snow	110
fish and shrimp combo	730
Fisherman's platter, broiled	600
lobster, live Maine, steamed, 1¼ lb.	160
lobster, live Maine, stuffed, 2 lb.	430
lobster, shrimp, and scallop scampi	870
lobster tail, rock, broiled, 1 tail	190
mahi mahi, lemon pepper, grilled	240
Neptune's feast	1,210
Seafarer's platter, broiled	450
shrimp, fried, 12 large	500
shrimp carbonara	1,290
shrimp combo	380
shrimp feast	470
shrimp popcorn	580
shrimp Milano	1,190
shrimp and chicken	340
steak, New York strip	560
steak and fried shrimp	780
steak and lobster tail	570

lunch entrees, 5 oz.:

catfish, Santa Fe	180
chicken fingers	390
chicken Fresco	660
clam strips	360
crab Alfredo	590
fish nuggets	320
flounder, baked	190

flounder, fried 230
lobster, shrimp, and scallop scampi 430
Sailor's platter 250
seafood broil 310
shrimp carbonara 650
shrimp, fried 270
shrimp Milano 590
shrimp, popcorn 380
shrimp scampi 110
lunch sandwiches:
catfish, blackened 340
cheeseburger, grilled 580
chicken, grilled 290
chicken, Cajun, grilled 370
fish, broiled 300
fish, classic 520
fish:
catfish, 8 oz. (dinner) 220
catfish, 5 oz. (lunch) 130
cod, Atlantic, 8 oz. 200
cod, Atlantic, 5 oz. 110
flounder, 8 oz. 220
flounder, 5 oz. 130
grouper, 8 oz. 220
grouper, 5 oz. 130
haddock, 8 oz. 210
haddock, 5 oz. 120
halibut, 8 oz. 260
halibut, 5 oz. 150
mahi mahi, 8 oz. 220
mahi mahi, 5 oz. 130
perch, 8 oz. 220
perch, 5 oz. 130
perch, yellow lake, 8 oz. 220
perch, yellow lake, 5 oz. 130
pollock, 8 oz. 220
pollock, 5 oz. 120
red rockfish, 8 oz. 230
red rockfish, 5 oz. 130
red snapper, 8 oz. 240
red snapper, 5 oz. 140
salmon, Atlantic, 8 oz. 340

Red Lobster, fish *(cont.)*

salmon, Atlantic, 5 oz.	200
salmon, king, 8 oz.	420
salmon, king, 5 oz.	250
salmon, sockeye, 8 oz.	410
salmon, sockeye, 5 oz.	240
sole, 8 oz.	220
sole, 5 oz.	130
swordfish, 8 oz.	290
swordfish, 5 oz.	170
trout, lake, 8 oz.	340
trout, lake, 5 oz.	200
walleye, 8 oz.	210
walleye, 5 oz.	120

seasonings for fish:

blackened fish, dinner	.70
blackened fish, lunch	.50
broiled fish, dinner	.45
broiled fish, lunch	.35
grilled fish, dinner	.35
grilled fish, lunch	.25
lemon pepper, dinner	.35
lemon pepper, lunch	.30
Santa Fe style, dinner	.60
Santa Fe style, lunch	.40

children's menu:

chicken fingers, fried	680
chicken tenders, grilled	580
hamburger	920
shrimp, fried	650
shrimp, popcorn	650
shrimp, popcorn with cheese sticks	750
spaghetti with cheese sticks	830

salads, no dressing:

chicken, grilled	320
shrimp Caesar	240

side dishes:

applesauce, 4 oz.	.90
bread, garlic cheese, 1 piece	140
broccoli, 3 oz.	.25
coleslaw, 4 oz.	190
potato, baked, flesh only, 8 oz.	130

potato, french fried, 4 oz. 350
potato, twice-baked 430
rice pilaf, 4 oz. 180
salad, Caesar, with dressing 240
salad, garden, without dressing 50
vegetables, roasted, 6 oz. 120
vegetables, roasted, 4 oz. 80
dressings/condiments:
blue cheese dressing 170
butter, melted, 1 fl. oz. 200
buttermilk ranch dressing 110
Caesar dressing, 1 oz. 170
cocktail sauce, 1 oz. 30
Dijon honey mustard 140
marinara sauce 50
ranch dressing, fat free .50
sassy sauce, 1 oz. 80
tartar sauce, 1 oz. 160
vinaigrette dressing, red wine, light 50
desserts:
carrot cake, 6.5 oz. 730
cheesecake, 5 oz. 530
Fudge Overboard 620
ice cream, 4.5 fl. oz. 140
pie, key lime, 5 oz. 450
raspberry cobbler, 3 oz. 530
Sensational 7 790

ROY ROGERS

calories

breakfast items:
bagel, plain 300
bagel, cinnamon raisin 300
Big Country Breakfast Platter, with bacon 740
Big Country Breakfast Platter, with ham 710
Big Country Breakfast Platter, with sausage 920
biscuit, plain 390
biscuit, bacon 420
biscuit, bacon and egg 470
biscuit, *Cinnamon 'N' Raisin* 370
biscuit, ham and cheese 450

Roy Rogers, breakfast items (cont.)

biscuit, ham and egg 460
biscuit, ham, egg, and cheese 500
biscuit, sausage 510
biscuit, sausage and egg 560
hash rounds 230
orange juice 140
pancakes, 3 pieces, plain 280
pancakes, 3 pieces, with 2 strips bacon 350
pancakes, 3 pieces, with 1 sausage 430
sourdough sandwich, ham, egg, and cheese 480
sandwiches:
bacon cheeseburger 490
bacon cheeseburger, sourdough 730
cheeseburger 300
cheeseburger, 1/4 lb. 470
chicken, grilled 340
chicken, grilled, sourdough 500
chicken fillet 500
Fisherman's Fillet, seasonal 490
hamburger 260
hamburger, 1/4 lb. 430
roast beef 260
chicken, fried:
breast 370
leg 170
thigh 330
wing 200
1/4 Roy's Roaster:
dark meat 490
dark meat, with skin off 190
white meat 500
white meat, with skin off 190
chicken nuggets, 6 pieces 290
chicken nuggets, 9 pieces 460
salads:
chicken, grilled 120
garden 190
side 140
potatoes:
baked 130
baked, with margarine 240

baked, with margarine and sour cream 300
fries, regular 350
fries, large 430
mashed, 5 oz. 92
gravy for mashed potatoes 20
sides:
   baked beans, 5 oz. 160
   coleslaw, 5 oz. 295
   corn bread 310
vanilla frozen yogurt cone 180

SIZZLER

calories

hot entrees:
   chicken breast, hibachi, with pineapple, 5 oz. 193
   chicken breast, lemon-herb, 5 oz. 140
   chicken breast, Santa Fe, 5 oz. 150
   chicken patty, Malibu 310
   hamburger on bun, with lettuce, tomato 626
   salmon, 8 oz. 247
   shrimp, broiled, 5 oz. 150
   shrimp, fried, 4 pieces 223
   shrimp, mini, 4 oz. 152
   shrimp scampi, 5 oz. 143
   steak, Dakota Ranch, 6 oz. 316
   steak, Dakota Ranch, 8 oz. 421
   steak, Dakota Ranch, 9.5 oz. 500
   swordfish, 8 oz. 315
side dishes:
   cheese toast 273
   french fries, 4 oz. 358
   potato, baked, flesh only, 4 oz. 105
   rice pilaf, 6 oz. 256
sauces, 1½ oz.:
   buttery dipping sauce 330
   cocktail sauce 40
   hibachi sauce 57
   Malibu sauce 283
   sour dressing 89
   tartar sauce 170

Sizzler (cont.)
hot bar:
   chicken wings, 1 oz. 73
   focaccia bread, 2 pieces 108
   marinara sauce, 1 oz. 13
   meatballs, 4 pieces 157
   nacho cheese sauce, 2 oz. 120
   pasta, fettuccine, 2 oz. .80
   pasta, spaghetti, 2 oz. .80
   potato skins, 2 oz. 160
   refried beans, ¼ cup 62
   saltines, 2 pieces 25
   taco filling, 2 oz. 103
   taco shell, 1 piece 50
hot bar, soup, 4 oz.:
   broccoli cheese 139
   chicken noodle 31
   clam chowder 118
   minestrone 36
   vegetable sirloin 60
salads, prepared, 2 oz.:
   carrot and raisin 130
   Chinese chicken 54
   jicama, spicy 16
   Mediterranean Minted Fruit 29
   Mexican Fiesta 54
   potato, old-fashioned .84
   potato, red herb 121
   pasta, seafood Louis .64
   seafood Louis 56
   teriyaki beef 49
   tuna pasta 133
salad bar:
   alfalfa sprouts, ¼ cup 2
   avocado, half 153
   bean sprouts, ¼ cup 8
   beets, ¼ cup 13
   bell peppers, 2 oz. 8
   broccoli, ½ cup 12
   cabbage, red, ¼ cup 5
   cantaloupe, ½ cup 28
   carrots, ¼ cup 12

cucumber, 2 oz. 7
grapes, ½ cup 29
honeydew melon, ½ cup .30
jicama, 2 oz. 13
kiwifruit, 2 oz. 35
lettuce, iceberg, 1 cup 7
lettuce, Romaine, 1 cup 9
mushrooms, ¼ cup 4
onions, red, 2 tbsp. 8
pineapple, ½ cup 38
spinach, ½ cup 6
strawberries, ½ cup 22
tomatoes, cherry, ¼ cup .12
watermelon, ½ cup 26
zucchini, ¼ cup 5
dressings, 1 oz.:
blue cheese 111
guacamole 42
honey mustard 160
Italian, lite 14
Parmesan, Italian 100
ranch 120
ranch, lite 90
rice vinegar, Japanese .10
salsa 7
sour dressing 60
Thousand Island 143
salad toppings:
bacon bits, real, 1 tbsp. 27
cottage cheese, 2 oz. 51
eggs, 1 oz. 44
garbanzo beans, ¼ cup 63
kidney beans, ¼ cup 52
olives, 1 oz. 62
peaches, ¼ cup 34
peas, ¼ cup 31
turkey ham, 1 oz. 62
dessert bar:
ice cream, chocolate or vanilla, 4 oz. 136
chocolate syrup, 1 oz. .90
strawberry topping, 1 oz. 70
whipped topping, 1 tbsp. 12

SUBWAY

---

calories

sandwiches:

bologna, jumbo 446
bologna, junior 270
ham, jumbo 259
ham, junior 208
roast beef, jumbo 348
roast beef, junior 232
Subway Seafood & Crab, jumbo 472
Subway Seafood & Crab, jumbo, with lite mayo 348
Subway Seafood & Crab, junior 279
Subway Seafood & Crab, junior, with lite mayo 238
tuna, jumbo 632
tuna, jumbo, with lite mayo 406
tuna, junior 332
tuna, junior, with lite mayo 257
turkey breast, jumbo 290
turkey breast, junior 218

cold submarines, 6":

Classic Italian B.M.T. 434
ham 273
mixed cold cuts 347
roast beef 299
Subway Club 300
Subway Seafood & Crab 415
Subway Seafood & Crab, with lite mayo 333
tuna 522
tuna, with lite mayo 372
turkey breast 276
turkey breast and ham 275
Veggie Delite 223

hot submarines, 6":

chicken breast, roasted 321
meatball 411
steak and cheese 363
Subway Melt 361

salads:

bread bowl 290
chicken breast fillet, roasted 143
Subway Club 123

TACO BELL

calories

Taco Bell, breakfast items *(cont.)*

burrito, grande 420
quesadilla, cheese 390
quesadilla with bacon 460
quesadilla with sausage 440

burritos:
bacon cheeseburger 560
bean 380
big beef *Burrito Supreme* 520
Burrito Supreme 440
chicken 400
chicken, light 310
chicken *Burrito Supreme* 550
chicken *Burrito Supreme,* light 430
chicken club 540
chili cheese 330
7 layer 540

quesadillas:
cheese 370
chicken 420

fajitas:
chicken or steak 460
chicken *Supreme* 500
steak *Supreme* 510
veggie 420
veggie *Supreme* 460

tacos/tostada:
BLT soft taco 340
Double Decker Taco 340
Double Decker Taco Supreme 390
kid's soft taco, chicken 240
kid's soft taco, chicken, light 180
kid's soft taco roll-up 290
soft taco 210
soft taco, chicken 250
soft taco, chicken, light 180
soft taco, steak 200
soft *Taco Supreme* 260
taco 170
Taco Supreme 220
tostada 200

specialty items:

beef *MexiMelt*	300
cinnamon twists	140
Mexican pizza	570
Mexican rice	190
nachos	310
nachos *BellGrande*	750
nachos supreme	430
pintos 'n cheese	190
taco salad	840
taco salad, without shell	420

sides and condiments:

cheese, cheddar	.30
cheese, cheddar, nonfat	.10
cheese, pepper jack	.25
green sauce	5
guacamole	.35
nacho cheese sauce	120
picante sauce	0
pico de gallo	5
ranch dressing	136
red sauce	.10
salsa	.25
sour cream	.40
sour cream, nonfat	.20
taco sauce, hot or mild	0

TACO JOHN'S

calories

burritos:

bean	387
beef	449
combination	418
meat and potato	503
ranch	447
smothered, platter	1,031
super	465
chimichanga platter	979
enchilada platter, double	967

fajitas, chicken:

burrito	370

Taco John's, **fajitas, chicken** *(cont.)*
    salad, without dressing 557
    soft shell 200
Mexi Rolls with nacho cheese 863
nachos, super 919
sampler platter 1,406
Sierra chicken fillet sandwich 534
tacos:
    crispy 182
    kid's meal, with crispy taco 579
    kid's meal, with soft shell taco 617
    soft shell 230
    Taco Bravo 346
    taco burger 280
sides and condiments:
    beans, refried 357
    chili 350
    Mexican rice 567
    nachos 333
    nacho cheese 300
    Potato Oles 363
    Potato Oles, large 484
    Potato Oles, with nacho cheese 483
    salad dressing, house 114
    sour cream 60
desserts:
    choco taco 320
    churro 147
    flauta, apple 84
    flauta, cherry 143
    flauta, cream cheese 181
    Italian ice 80

TCBY

calories

all flavors, soft serve yogurt, ½ cup:
    regular 130
    nonfat 110
    nonfat, no sugar 80
all flavors, sorbet, ½ cup 100

premium nonfat yogurt, ½ cup:

apple pie à la mode	120
banana split	110
cappuccino	120
chocolate, brown/white	120
chocolate sundae, chewy	120
peach cobbler	110
raspberry cheesecake	120
strawberry shortcake	120
vanilla caramel custard	120

Yog-A-Bar, 1 bar:

orange or raspberry swirl	80
vanilla, chocolate dipped	120
vanilla, with toasted almonds	190
vanilla, with *Heath* toffee	190

WENDY'S

calories

sandwiches:

bacon cheeseburger, Jr.	380
Big Bacon Classic	570
cheeseburger, Jr. or Kid's Meal	320
cheeseburger deluxe, Jr.	360
chicken, grilled	310
chicken, breaded	440
chicken, spicy	410
chicken club	470
hamburger, single, plain	360
hamburger, single, with everything	420
hamburger, Jr. or Kid's Meal	270

sandwich components:

American cheese	70
American cheese, Jr.	45
bacon, 1 slice	20
bun, kaiser	190
bun, sandwich	160
burger patty, ¼ lb.	200
burger patty, 2 oz.	100
chicken patty, grilled	110
chicken patty, breaded	230
chicken patty, spicy	210

Wendy's, sandwich components *(cont.)*

honey mustard, reduced calorie, 1 tsp.	.25
ketchup, 1 tsp.	.10
lettuce, 1 leaf	0
mayonnaise, 1½ tsp.	.30
mustard, ½ tsp.	0
onion, 4 rings	0
pickles, 4 slices	0
tomato, 1 slice	5
chicken nuggets, 5 pieces	210

nuggets sauces, 1 oz.:

barbecue or sweet and sour	.50
honey mustard	130
spicy Buffalo wing	.25

chili:

small, 8 oz.	210
large, 12 oz.	340
cheddar cheese, shredded, 2 tbsp.	.70
saltine crackers, 2 pieces	.25

baked potatoes:

plain	310
bacon and cheese	540
broccoli and cheese	470
cheese	570
chili and cheese	620
sour cream and chive	380
sour cream or whipped margarine, 1 pkt.	.60

fries:

small, 3.2 oz.	260
medium, 4.6 oz.	380
Biggie, 5.6 oz.	460

salads-to-go, fresh, without dressing:

deluxe garden	110
grilled chicken	200
grilled chicken Caesar	260
side	.60
side, Caesar	110
taco	590
soft breadstick, 1 piece	130

salad dressing, 2 tbsp., except as noted:

blue cheese	170
French	120

French, fat free 30
French, sweet red 130
Italian, reduced fat and calorie 40
Italian Caesar 150
ranch, *Hidden Valley* 90
ranch, *Hidden Valley,* reduced fat and calorie 60
salad oil, 1 tbsp. 130
Thousand Island 130
wine vinegar, 1 tbsp. 0
Garden Spot salad bar:
applesauce, 2 tbsp. 30
bacon bits, 2 tbsp. 45
banana and strawberry glaze, ¼ cup 30
broccoli or cauliflower, ¼ cup 0
cantaloupe, 1 slice 15
carrots, ¼ cup 5
cheese, shredded, imitation, 2 tbsp. 50
chicken salad, 2 tbsp. 70
chow mein noodles, ¼ cup 35
coleslaw, 2 tbsp. 45
cottage cheese, 2 tbsp. 30
croutons, 2 tbsp. 30
cucumbers, 2 slices 0
eggs, hard-cooked, 2 tbsp. 40
green peas, 2 tbsp. 15
green pepper, 2 pieces 0
honeydew, 1 slice 20
lettuce, 1 cup 10
mushrooms, ½ cup 0
orange, 2 slices 15
Parmesan blend, grated, 2 tbsp. 70
pasta salad, 2 tbsp. 25
peaches, 1 slice 15
pepperoni, 6 slices 30
pineapple chunks, 4 pieces 20
potato salad, 2 tbsp. 80
pudding, chocolate or vanilla, ¼ cup 70
red onion, 3 rings 0
seafood salad, ¼ cup 70
sesame breadstick, 1 piece 15
strawberry, 1 piece 10
sunflower seeds and raisins, 2 tbsp. 80

Wendy's, Garden Spot salad bar *(cont.)*
    tomato wedge, 1 piece 5
    turkey ham, diced, 2 tbsp. 50
    watermelon, 1 wedge 20
desserts:
    chocolate chip cookie, 1 piece 270
    Frosty, small 340
    Frosty, medium 460
    Frosty, large 570

"HEALTHY WEIGHTS" FOR MEN AND WOMEN*

Height (without shoes)	Weight in pounds (without clothing)	
	19 to 34 years	35 years and over
5'0"	97–128	108–138
5'1"	101–132	111–143
5'2"	104–137	115–148
5'3"	107–141	119–152
5'4"	111–146	122–157
5'5"	114–150	126–162
5'6"	118–155	130–167
5'7"	121–160	134–172
5'8"	125–164	138–178
5'9"	129–169	142–183
5'10"	132–174	146–188
5'11"	136–179	151–194
6'0"	140–184	155–200
6'1"	144–189	159–205
6'2"	148–195	164–210
6'3"	152–200	168–216
6'4"	156–205	173–222

Source: Report of the Dietary Guidelines Advisory Committee on the Dietary Guidelines for Americans, 1990.

* The lower weights generally apply to women, the higher to men.

HOW MANY CALORIES TO MAINTAIN YOUR DESIRABLE WEIGHT?

Desirable weight	18–35 years	35–55 years	55–75 years
Women Daily Maintenance Calories*			
99	1,700	1,500	1,300
110	1,850	1,650	1,400
121	2,000	1,750	1,550
128	2,100	1,900	1,600
132	2,150	1,950	1,650
143	2,300	2,050	1,800
154	2,400	2,150	1,850
165	2,550	2,300	1,950
Men Daily Maintenance Calories*			
110	2,200	1,950	1,650
121	2,400	2,150	1,850
132	2,550	2,300	1,950
143	2,700	2,400	2,050
154	2,900	2,600	2,200
165	3,100	2,800	2,400
176	3,250	2,950	2,500
187	3,300	3,100	2,600

* Based on moderate activity. If your life is very active, add calories; if you lead a sedentary life, subtract calories. Prepared by the Food and Nutrition Board of the National Academy of Sciences, National Research Council.

Index